ECGs MADE EASY

Barbara Aehlert, RN, BSPA
Southwest EMS Education, Inc.
Phoenix, AZ/Pursley, TX

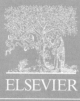
MOSBY JEMS

ELSEVIER

Fourth Edition

3251 Riverport Lane
Maryland Heights, Missouri 63043

ECGs MADE EASY, FOURTH EDITION   ISBN: 978-0-323-06924-3

Notice

Knowledge and best practice in this field are constantly changing. As new research and experience broaden our knowledge, changes in practice, treatment and drug therapy may become necessary or appropriate. Readers are advised to check the most current information provided (i) on procedures featured or (ii) by the manufacturer of each product to be administered, to verify the recommended dose or formula, the method and duration of administration, and contraindications. It is the responsibility of the practitioner, relying on their own experience and knowledge of the patient, to make diagnoses, to determine dosages and the best treatment for each individual patient, and to take all appropriate safety precautions. To the fullest extent of the law, neither the Publisher nor the Author assumes any liability for any injury and/or damage to persons or property arising out of or related to any use of the material contained in this book.

The Publisher

ISBN: 978-0-323-06924-3

Executive Editor: Linda Honeycutt Dickison
Associate Developmental Editor: Mary Jo Adams
Publishing Services Manager: Julie Eddy
Senior Project Manager: Andrea Campbell
Design Direction: Maggie Reid

Printed in China

Last digit is the print number: 9   8   7   6   5   4   3   2   1

Preface to the Fourth Edition

This book is designed for use by paramedic, nursing, and medical students; ECG monitor technicians; nurses; and other allied health personnel working in emergency departments, critical care units, post-anesthesia care units, operating rooms, and telemetry units wishing to master the skill of basic ECG recognition. This book may be used alone or as part of a formal course of instruction in basic dysrhythmia recognition.

The information presented in this book focuses on the essential information you need to know to interpret ECGs and understand their significance. Each ECG rhythm is described and accompanied by a sample rhythm strip. Possible patient signs and symptoms related to the rhythm and, where appropriate, current recommended treatment for the rhythm is discussed. Additional rhythm strips are provided for practice at the end of each chapter. All rhythm strips shown in this text were recorded in lead II unless otherwise noted.

In the fourth edition of this book, more practice ECG strips have been added. The Stop & Review exercises at the end of each chapter are self-assessment exercises that allow you to check your learning.

Every attempt has been made to provide information that is consistent with current literature, including current resuscitation guidelines. However, medicine is a dynamic field. Resuscitation guidelines change, new medications and technology are being developed, and medical research is ongoing. As a result, be sure to learn and follow local protocols as defined by your medical advisors.

Best regards,

Barbara Aehlert

Acknowledgments

I would like to thank Andrew Baird, CEP; James Bratcher; Holly Button, CEP; Gretchen Chalmers, CEP; Thomas Cole, CEP; Brent Haines, CEP; Paul Honeywell, CEP; Timothy Klatt, RN; Bill Loughran, RN; Andrea Lowrey, RN; Joe Martinez, CEP; Stephanos Orphanidis, CEP; Jason Payne, CEP; Steve Ruehs, CEP; Patty Seneski, RN; David Stockton, CEP; Jason Stodghill, CEP; Dionne Socie, CEP; Kristina Tellez, CEP; and Fran Wojculewicz, RN for providing many of the rhythm strips used in this text.

I would also like to thank the text reviewers for their comments and suggestions, which helped to improve the clarity of the information presented in this text.

About the Author

Barbara Aehlert is the President of Southwest EMS Education, Inc., in Phoenix, Arizona, and Pursley, Texas. She has been a registered nurse for more than 30 years, with clinical experience in medical/surgical and critical care nursing and more than 20 years experience in prehospital education. Barbara is an active CPR, First Aid, ACLS, and PALS instructor.

Publisher Acknowledgments

Tim Brisbin, RN, BSN, NREMT-P
Center for Prehospital Medicine
Charlotte, North Carolina

Chip Boehm, RN, EMT-P/FF, Level III I/C
Portland Fire Department
Portland, Maine

Joanne McCall, RN, MA, CEN, CFN, SANE-A
Senior Education Specialist, Emergency Services
Providence Park Hospital
Novi, Michigan

Larry Richmond, AS, EMT-P, CCEMT-P, EMS I/C
Mountain Plains Health Consortium
Rapid City, South Dakota

Everett Stephens, MD, FAAEM
Department of Emergency Medicine
University of Louisville
Louisville, Kentucky

Contents

Anatomy and Physiology

OBJECTIVES

After reading this chapter, you should be able to:

1. Describe the location of the heart.
2. Distinguish between the apex and base of the heart.
3. Identify and describe the chambers of the heart and the vessels that enter or leave each.
4. Explain stroke volume and ejection fraction.
5. Describe the structure and location of the pericardium, epicardium, myocardium, and endocardium.
6. Name and identify the location of the atrioventricular (AV) and semilunar (SL) valves.
7. Explain atrial kick.
8. Discuss the function of the chordae tendineae and papillary muscles.
9. Explain how heart sounds are created and their clinical significance.
10. Beginning with the right atrium, describe blood flow through the normal heart and lungs to the systemic circulation.
11. Identify the phases of the cardiac cycle.
12. Name the primary branches and areas of the heart supplied by the right and left coronary arteries.
13. Define the terms acute coronary syndrome, chronotropy, inotropy, and dromotropy.
14. Compare and contrast the effects of sympathetic and parasympathetic stimulation of the heart.
15. Name the primary neurotransmitter of the sympathetic and parasympathetic divisions of the autonomic nervous system.
16. Describe the effects of stimulation of alpha-receptors, beta-1-receptors, beta-2-receptors, and dopaminergic receptors.
17. Identify and define the components of cardiac output.

LOCATION OF THE HEART

[OBJECTIVES 1, 2]

The heart is a hollow muscular organ that lies in the space between the lungs (**mediastinum**) in the middle of the chest. It sits behind the sternum and just above the diaphragm (Figure 1-1). Approximately two thirds of the heart lies to the left of the midline of the sternum. The remaining third lies to the right of the sternum.

The **base** of the heart is its upper portion and is formed mainly by the left atrium, with a small amount of right atrium. It lies at approximately the level of the second rib, immediately in front of the esophagus and descending aorta. The heart's **apex**, or lower portion, is formed by the tip of the left ventricle. The apex lies just

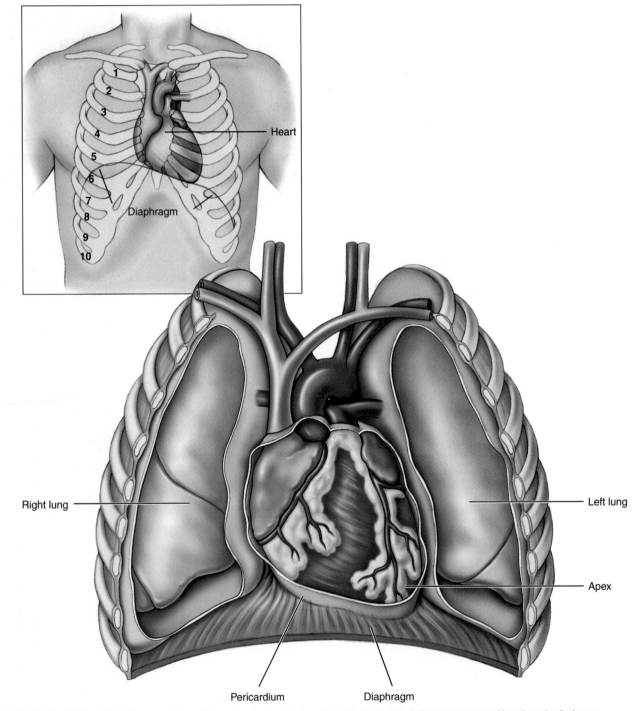

Figure 1-1   The heart lies in the space between the lungs (mediastinum) in the middle of the chest. It sits behind the sternum and just above the diaphragm.

above the diaphragm, between the fifth and sixth ribs, in the midclavicular line.

SIZE AND SHAPE OF THE HEART

The adult heart is approximately 5 inches (12 cm) long, 3½ inches (9 cm) wide, and 2½ inches (6 cm) thick. It typically weighs between 250 and 350 g (about 11 oz) and is about the size of its owner's fist (Figure 1-2). The weight of the heart is about 0.45% of a man's body weight and about 0.40% of a woman's. A person's heart size and weight are influenced by their age, body weight and build, frequency of physical exercise, and heart disease.

HEART CHAMBERS

Atria

[OBJECTIVE 3]
The heart has four chambers (Figure 1-3). The two upper chambers are the right and left **atria**. The atria have thin walls. Their purpose is to *receive* blood. The right atrium receives blood low in oxygen from:

- The superior vena cava, which carries blood from the head and upper extremities
- The inferior vena cava, which carries blood from the lower body
- The coronary sinus, which is the largest vein that drains the heart

The left atrium receives freshly oxygenated blood from the lungs via the right and left pulmonary veins. The wall of the right atrium is about 2 mm thick and the wall of the left atrium is about 3 mm thick. Blood is pumped from the atria

through an atrioventricular valve and into the ventricles. The valves of the heart are discussed later in this chapter.

ECG Pearl

Think of the atria as "holding tanks" or "reservoirs" for blood.

Ventricles

[OBJECTIVES 3, 4]
The heart's two lower chambers are the right and left **ventricles**. The walls of the ventricles are much thicker than those of the atria. Their purpose is to *pump* blood. The right ventricle pumps blood to the lungs. The left ventricle pumps blood out to the body. When the left ventricle contracts, it normally produces an impulse that can be felt at the apex of the heart (**apical impulse**). This occurs because as the left ventricle contracts, it rotates forward. In a normal heart, this causes the apex of the left ventricle to hit the chest wall. You may be able to see the apical impulse in thin individuals. The apical impulse is also called the **point of maximal impulse** (PMI) because it is the site where the left ventricular contraction is most strongly felt.

The outside surface of the heart has grooves called sulci. The coronary arteries and their major branches lie in these grooves. The coronary **sulcus** (groove) encircles the outside of the heart and separates the atria from the ventricles. It contains the coronary blood vessels and epicardial fat.

Two Functional Pumps

The right and left sides of the heart are separated by an internal wall of connective tissue called a **septum**. The *interatrial septum* separates the right and left atria. The *interventricular*

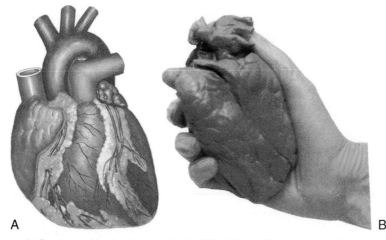

A   B

Figure 1-2   The adult heart weighs approximately 250 to 350 g and is about the size of its owner's fist.

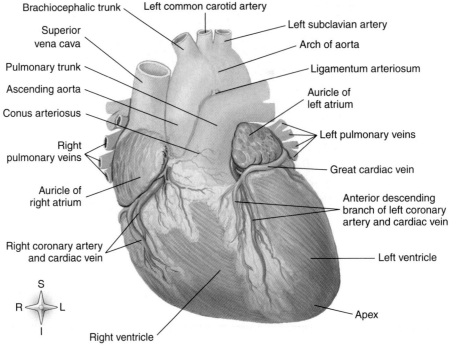

Brachiocephalic trunk
Left common carotid artery
Superior vena cava
Left subclavian artery
Pulmonary trunk
Arch of aorta
Ascending aorta
Ligamentum arteriosum
Conus arteriosus
Auricle of left atrium
Right pulmonary veins
Left pulmonary veins
Great cardiac vein
Auricle of right atrium
Anterior descending branch of left coronary artery and cardiac vein
Right coronary artery and cardiac vein
Left ventricle
Apex
Right ventricle

Figure 1-3   Anterior view of the heart and great vessels.

septum separates the right and left ventricles (Figure 1-4, *A*). The septa separate the heart into two functional pumps. The right atrium and right ventricle make up one pump. The left atrium and left ventricle make up the other (Figure 1-4, *B*).

The job of the right side of the heart is to pump unoxygenated blood to and through the lungs to the left side of the heart. This is called the *pulmonary circulation*. The right side of the heart is a low-pressure system. The left side of the heart is a high-pressure pump. The job of the left heart is to receive oxygenated blood and pump it out to the rest of the body. This is called the *systemic circulation*.

Blood is carried from the heart to the organs of the body through arteries, arterioles, and capillaries. Blood is returned to the right heart through venules and veins. The left ventricle is a high-pressure chamber. Its wall is much thicker than the right ventricle (the right ventricle is about 3–5 mm thick; the left ventricle is about 13–15 mm). This is because the left ventricle must overcome a lot of pressure and resistance from the arteries and contract forcefully in order to pump blood out to the body. Because the wall of the left ventricle is much thicker than the right, the interventricular septum normally bulges to the right.

Each ventricle holds about 150 mL of blood when it is full. They normally eject about half this volume (70–80 mL) with each contraction. **Stroke volume** is the amount of blood ejected from a ventricle with each heartbeat. The *percentage* of blood pumped out of a heart chamber with each contraction is called the **ejection fraction**. Ejection fraction is used as a measure of ventricular function. A normal ejection fraction is between 50% and 65%. A person is said to have impaired ventricular function when the ejection fraction is less than 40%.

Examples of patients who may have a poor ejection fraction include those with congestive heart failure, severe cardiomyopathy, or myocardial damage from a previous heart attack.

ECG Pearl

To better understand the pressure differences among the chambers of the heart, consider the following:
- The pressure within the right atrium is normally between 2 and 6 mm Hg. The pressure within the right ventricle is normally between 0 and 8 mm Hg when the chamber is at rest (diastole) and between 15 and 25 mm Hg during contraction (systole).
- The pressure within the left atrium is normally between 8 and 12 mm Hg. The pressure within the left ventricle is normally between 8 and 12 mm Hg when the chamber is at rest (diastole) and between 110 and 130 mm Hg during contraction (systole).

SURFACES OF THE HEART

The front (anterior) surface of the heart lies behind the sternum and costal cartilages. It is formed by portions of the right atrium and the left and right ventricles. However, because the heart is tilted slightly toward the left in the chest, the right ventricle is the area of the heart that lies most directly behind the sternum. The heart's left side (left lateral surface) is made up mostly of the left ventricle. The heart's bottom (inferior) surface is formed by both the right and left ventricles. The inferior surface of the heart is also called the diaphragmatic

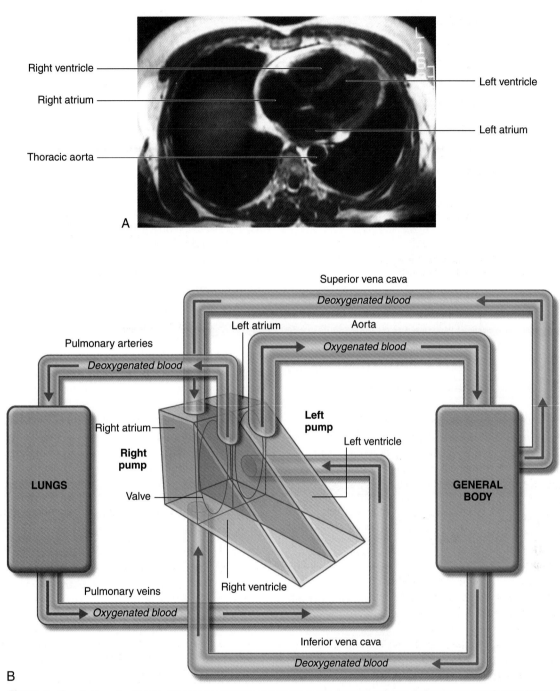

Figure 1-4 **A,** Magnetic resonance image of the midthorax, showing the heart's chambers and septa. **B,** The heart has two functional pumps.

surface. Figure 1-5 shows the surfaces of the heart. Note that the posterior surface of the heart is not shown.

LAYERS OF THE HEART

[OBJECTIVE 5]
The walls of the heart are made up of three tissue layers: the endocardium, myocardium, and epicardium (Table 1-1). The heart's innermost layer, the **endocardium**, is made up of a thin, smooth layer of epithelium and connective tissue and lines the heart's inner chambers, valves, chordae tendineae, and papillary muscles. It is continuous with the innermost layer of the arteries, veins, and capillaries of the body. This creates a continuous, closed circulatory system (Figure 1-6).

The **myocardium** (middle layer) is a thick, muscular layer that consists of cardiac muscle fibers (cells) responsible for the pumping action of the heart. The myocardium is subdivided into two areas. The innermost half of the myocardium is called the subendocardial area. The outermost half is called the subepicardial area. The muscle fibers of the

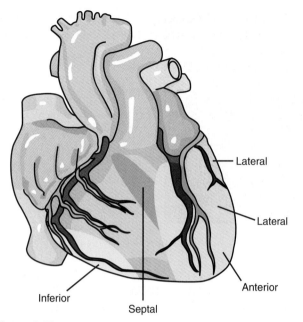

Figure 1-5   Surfaces of the heart. Posterior surface not shown.

TABLE **1-1**	Layers of the Heart Wall
EPICARDIUM	• External layer of the heart
	• Coronary arteries, blood capillaries, lymph capillaries, nerve fibers, nerves, and fat are found in this layer
MYOCARDIUM	• Middle and thickest layer of the heart
	• Responsible for heart's pumping action
ENDOCARDIUM	• Innermost layer of the heart
	• Lines heart's inner chambers, valves, chordae tendineae, and papillary muscles
	• Continuous with innermost layer of arteries, veins, and capillaries of body

myocardium are separated by connective tissues that have a rich supply of capillaries and nerve fibers.

We already mentioned that the thickness of the myocardium varies from one heart chamber to another. This variation in thickness is related to the amount of resistance that must be overcome to pump blood out of the different chambers. For example, the atria encounter little resistance when pumping blood to the ventricles. As a result, the atria have a thin myocardial layer. On the other hand, the ventricles must pump blood to either the lungs (the right ventricle) or the rest of the body (the left ventricle). So, the ventricles have a much thicker myocardial layer than the atria. The wall of the left ventricle is three times thicker than that of the right because the left ventricle propels blood to most vessels of the body. The right ventricle moves blood only through the blood vessels of the lungs and then into the left atrium.

The heart's outermost layer is called the **epicardium**. The epicardium is continuous with the inner lining of the pericardium at the heart's apex. The epicardium contains blood capillaries, lymph capillaries, nerve fibers, and fat. The main coronary arteries lie on the epicardial surface of the heart. They feed this area first before entering the myocardium and supplying the heart's inner layers with oxygenated blood. **Ischemia** is a decreased supply of oxygenated blood to a body part or organ. The heart's subendocardial area is at the greatest risk of ischemia because this area has a high demand for oxygen and is fed by the most distal branches of the coronary arteries.

The **pericardium** is a double-walled sac that encloses the heart and helps protect it from trauma and infection. The rough outer layer of the pericardial sac is called the *fibrous parietal pericardium*. It anchors the heart to some of the structures around it, such as the sternum and diaphragm, by means of ligaments. This helps prevent excessive movement of the heart in the chest with changes in body position. The

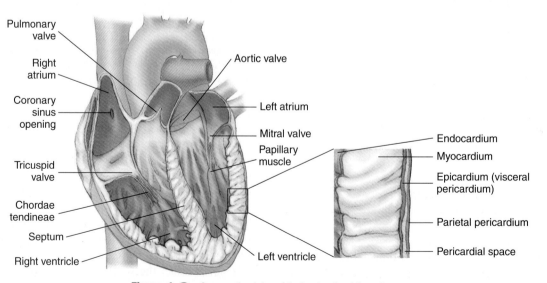

Figure 1-6   Cross-sectional view of the heart wall and tissue layers.

inner layer, the *serous pericardium*, consists of two layers: parietal and visceral. The parietal layer lines the inside of the fibrous pericardium. The visceral layer (also called the epicardium) adheres to the outside of the heart and forms the outer layer of the heart muscle.

Between the visceral and parietal layers is a space (the pericardial space) that normally contains about 20 mL of serous fluid. This fluid acts as a lubricant, preventing friction as the heart beats. If the pericardium becomes inflamed (pericarditis), more serous fluid is secreted. Pericarditis can be caused by a bacterial or viral infection, rheumatoid arthritis, destruction of the heart muscle in a heart attack, and other causes. Heart surgery or trauma to the heart, such as a stab wound, can cause a rapid buildup of blood in the pericardial space.

The buildup of excess blood or fluid in the pericardial space compresses the heart. This can affect the heart's ability to relax and fill with blood between heartbeats. If the heart cannot adequately fill with blood, the amount of blood the ventricles can pump out to the body (cardiac output) will be decreased. As a result, the amount of blood returning to the heart is also decreased. These changes can result in a life-threatening condition called *cardiac tamponade*. The amount of blood or fluid in the pericardial space needed to impair the heart's ability to fill depends on:

- The rate at which the buildup of blood or fluid occurs.
- The ability of the pericardium to stretch and accommodate the increased volume of fluid.

The rapid buildup of as little as 100 to 150 mL of fluid or blood can be enough to result in signs and symptoms of shock. On the other hand, 1000 mL of fluid may build up over a longer period without any significant effect on the heart's ability to fill. This is because the pericardium accommodates the increased fluid by stretching over time.

The symptoms of cardiac tamponade can be relieved by removing the excess fluid from the pericardial sac. **Pericardiocentesis** is a procedure in which a needle is inserted into the pericardial space and the excess fluid is sucked out (aspirated) through the needle. If scarring is the cause of the tamponade, surgery may be necessary to remove the affected area of the pericardium.

CARDIAC MUSCLE

Cardiac muscle is found only in the heart. Cardiac muscle fibers make up the walls of the heart. These fibers have striations, or stripes, similar to that of skeletal muscle. Each muscle fiber is made up of many muscle cells (Figure 1-7, *A*). Each muscle cell is enclosed in a membrane called a **sarcolemma**. Within each cell (as with all cells) are **mitochondria**, the energy-producing parts of a cell, and hundreds of long, tube-like structures called **myofibrils**. Myofibrils are made up of many **sarcomeres**, the basic protein units responsible for contraction. The process of contraction requires adenosine triphosphate (ATP) for energy. The mitochondria that are interspersed between the myofibrils are important sites of ATP production.

The sarcolemma has holes in it that lead into tubes called T (transverse) tubules. T-tubules are extensions of the cell membrane. Another system of tubules, the **sarcoplasmic reticulum** (SR), stores calcium. Muscle cells need calcium in order to contract. Calcium is moved from the sarcoplasm of the muscle cell into the sarcoplasmic reticulum by means of "pumps" in the sarcoplasmic reticulum.

There are certain places in the cell membrane where sodium (Na+), potassium (K+), and calcium (Ca++) can pass. These openings are called pores or channels. There are specific channels for sodium (sodium channels), potassium (potassium channels), and calcium (calcium channels). When the muscle is relaxed, the calcium channels are closed. As a result, calcium cannot pass through the membrane of the sarcoplasmic reticulum. This results in a high concentration of calcium in the sarcoplasmic reticulum and a low concentration in the sarcoplasm, where the muscle cells (sarcomeres) are found. If the muscle cells do not have calcium available to them, contraction is inhibited (the muscle stays relaxed).

T-tubules pass completely through the sarcolemma and go around the muscle cells. The job of the T-tubules is to conduct impulses from the cell's surface (sarcolemma) down into the cell to the sarcoplasmic reticulum. When an impulse travels along the membrane of the sarcoplasmic reticulum, the calcium channels open. Calcium rapidly leaves the sarcoplasmic reticulum and enters the sarcoplasm. The muscle cells are then stimulated to contract.

Much of the calcium that enters the cell's sarcoplasm comes from the interstitial fluid surrounding the cardiac muscle cells through the T-tubules. This is important because without the extra calcium from the T-tubules, the strength of a cardiac muscle contraction would be considerably reduced. Thus, the force of cardiac muscle contraction depends largely on the concentration of calcium ions in the extracellular fluid.

Each sarcomere is composed of thin filaments and thick filaments. The thin filaments are made up of actin and actin-binding proteins. Actin-binding proteins include tropomyosin and troponin-T, troponin-C, and troponin-I, among others. The thick filaments are made up of hundreds of myosin molecules. Contraction occurs when the muscle is stimulated. Projections on the thin actin filaments (Figure 1-7, *B*) interact with the thick myosin filaments and form crossbridges (Figure 1-7, *C*). The crossbridges use energy (ATP) to bend. This allows the actin filaments to slide over the myosin filaments toward the center of the sarcomere and overlap. This overlap causes shortening of the muscle cells, resulting in contraction. Actin-binding proteins hinder the formation of crossbridges with myosin. When crossbridge formation is hindered, the muscle is relaxed.

Cardiac muscle fibers are long branching cells that fit together tightly at junctions called *intercalated disks*. The

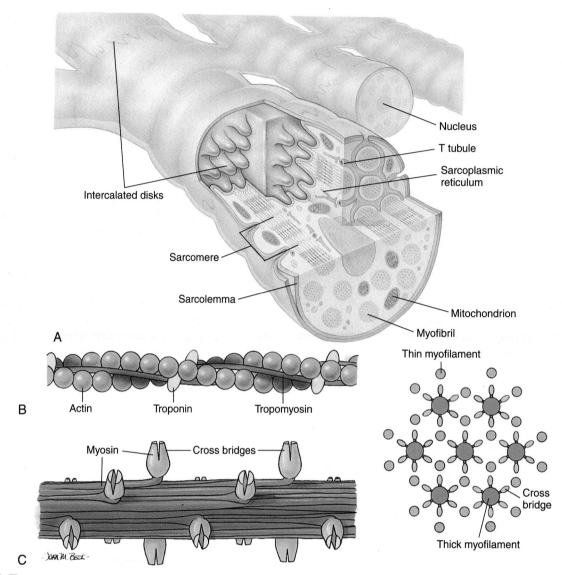

Intercalated disks

Sarcomere

Sarcolemma

Nucleus
T tubule
Sarcoplasmic reticulum
Mitochondrion
Myofibril

A

Thin myofilament

B   Actin   Troponin   Tropomyosin

Myosin   Cross bridges

Cross bridge

Thick myofilament

C

Figure 1-7   **A,** Cardiac muscle fiber. Unlike other types of muscle fibers, the cardiac muscle fiber is typically branched and forms junctions, called intercalated disks, with adjacent cardiac muscle fibers. **B,** Thin myofilament. **C,** Thick myofilament.

arrangement of these tight-fitting junctions gives an appearance of a **syncytium**, that is, resembling a network of cells with no separation between the individual cells. The intercalated disks fit together in such a way that they form gap junctions. Gap junctions allow cells to communicate with each other. They function as electrical connections and permit the exchange of nutrients, metabolites, ions, and small molecules. As a result, an electrical impulse can be quickly conducted throughout the wall of a heart chamber. This characteristic allows the walls of both atria (likewise, the walls of both ventricles) to contract almost at the same time.

When myocardial cells die, such as in a myocardial infarction (MI), substances in intracardiac cells pass through broken cell membranes and leak into the bloodstream. These substances (called *inflammatory markers, cardiac biomarkers,*

or *serum cardiac markers*) include creatine kinase (CK), creatine kinase myocardial band (CK-MB), myoglobin, troponin I (TnI), and troponin T (TnT). The presence of these substances in the blood can subsequently be measured by means of blood tests to verify the presence of an infarction.

The heart consists of two syncytiums: atrial and ventricular. The *atrial syncytium* consists of the walls of the right and left atria. The *ventricular syncytium* consists of the walls of the right and left ventricles. Normally, impulses can be conducted only from the atrial syncytium into the ventricular syncytium by means of the atrioventricular (AV) junction. The AV junction is a part of the heart's electrical system. This allows the atria to contract a short time before ventricular contraction. The heart's conduction system is discussed in more detail in Chapter 2.

HEART VALVES

[OBJECTIVES 6, 7, 8]

The heart has a skeleton. The skeleton is made up of four rings of thick connective tissue. This tissue surrounds the bases of the pulmonary trunk, aorta, and the heart valves. The heart's skeleton helps form the partitions (septa) that separate the atria from the ventricles. It also provides secure attachments for the valves and chambers of the heart (Figure 1-8).

There are four valves in the heart: two sets of atrioventricular (AV) valves and two sets of semilunar (SL) valves (Table 1-2). Their purpose is to make sure blood flows in one direction through the heart's chambers and prevent the backflow of blood.

Atrioventricular Valves

Atrioventricular (AV) valves separate the atria from the ventricles. The two AV valves consist of the following:
- Tough, fibrous rings (annuli fibrosi)
- Flaps (leaflets or cusps) of endocardium
- Chordae tendineae
- Papillary muscles

The tricuspid valve is the AV valve that lies between the right atrium and right ventricle. It consists of three separate cusps or flaps. It is larger in diameter and thinner than the mitral valve (Figure 1-9). The mitral (or bicuspid) valve has only two cusps. It lies between the left atrium and left ventricle (Figure 1-10). The AV valves open when a forward pressure gradient forces blood in a forward direction. They close when a backward pressure gradient pushes blood backward. The AV valves require almost no backflow to cause closure.[1]

ECG Pearl

The mitral valve is so named because it is thought to resemble a mitre (bishop's hat) when open.

The flow of blood from the superior and inferior venae cavae into the atria is normally continuous. About 70% of this blood flows directly through the atria and into the ventricles before the atria contract. As the atria fill with blood, the pressure within the atrial chamber rises. This pressure forces the tricuspid and mitral valves open and the ventricles begin to fill, gradually increasing the pressure within the ventricles. When the atria contract, an additional 10%

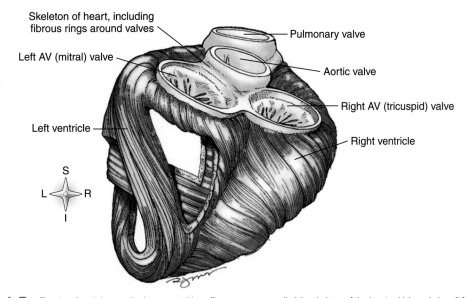

Figure 1-8 The rim of each heart valve is supported by a fibrous structure, called the skeleton of the heart, which encircles all four valves.

| TABLE 1-2 | Heart Valves | | |

Valve Type	Name	Right Heart vs. Left Heart	Location
Atrioventricular (AV)	Tricuspid	Right	Separates right atrium and right ventricle
	Mitral (bicuspid)	Left	Separates left atrium and left ventricle
Semilunar (SL)	Pulmonic	Right	Between right ventricle and pulmonary artery
	Aortic	Left	Between left ventricle and aorta

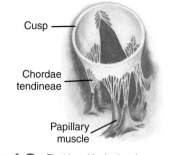

Cusp

Chordae
tendineae

Papillary
muscle

Figure 1-9   The tricuspid valve has three cusps or flaps.

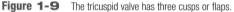

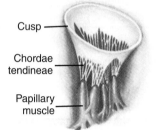

Cusp

Chordae
tendineae

Papillary
muscle

Figure 1-10   The mitral valve has two cusps or flaps.

to 30% of the returning blood is added to filling of the ventricles. This additional contribution of blood resulting from atrial contraction is called **atrial kick**. On the right side of the heart, blood low in oxygen empties into the right ventricle. On the left side of the heart, freshly oxygenated blood empties into the left ventricle. When the ventricles then contract (systole), the pressure within the ventricles rises sharply. The tricuspid and mitral valves completely close when the pressure within the ventricles exceeds that of the atria.

Chordae tendineae are thin strands of connective tissue. On one end, they are attached to the underside of the AV

valves. On the other end, they are attached to small mounds of myocardium called **papillary muscles**. Papillary muscles project inward from the lower portion of the ventricular walls. When the ventricles contract and relax, so do the papillary muscles. The papillary muscles adjust their tension on the chordae tendineae, preventing them from bulging too far into the atria. For example, when the right ventricle contracts, the papillary muscles of the right ventricle pull on the chordae tendineae. The chordae tendineae stretch, preventing the flaps of the tricuspid valve from bulging too far into the right atrium. Thus, the chordae tendineae and papillary muscles serve as anchors. Because the chordae tendineae are thin and stringlike, they are sometimes called "heart strings."

Semilunar Valves

The pulmonic and aortic valves are **semilunar (SL) valves**. The semilunar valves prevent backflow of blood from the aorta and pulmonary arteries into the ventricles (Figure 1-11). The SL valves have three cusps shaped like half-moons. The openings of the SL valves are smaller than the openings of the AV valves. The flaps of the SL valves are smaller and thicker than the AV valves. Unlike the AV valves, the semilunar valves are not attached to chordae tendineae.

When the ventricles contract, the SL valves open, allowing blood to flow out of the ventricles. When the right ventricle contracts, blood low in oxygen flows through the pulmonic valve into the right and left pulmonary arteries. When the left ventricle contracts, freshly oxygenated blood flows through the aortic valve into the aorta and out to the body. The SL valves close as ventricular contraction ends and the pressure in the pulmonary artery and aorta exceeds that of the ventricles. The location of the heart's AV and SL valves for auscultation is shown in Figure 1-12.

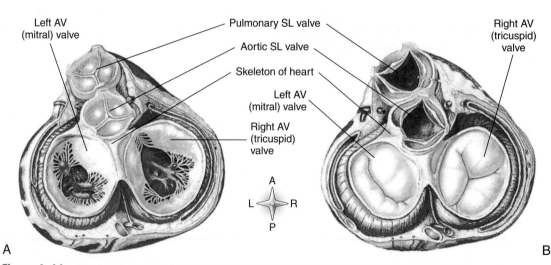

Left AV
(mitral) valve

Pulmonary SL valve

Aortic SL valve

Skeleton of heart

Left AV
(mitral) valve

Right AV
(tricuspid)
valve

Right AV
(tricuspid)
valve

A
L — R
P

A   B

Figure 1-11   AV and semilunar valves. **A,** AV valves are open, semilunar valves are closed. **B,** AV valves are closed, semilunar valves are open.

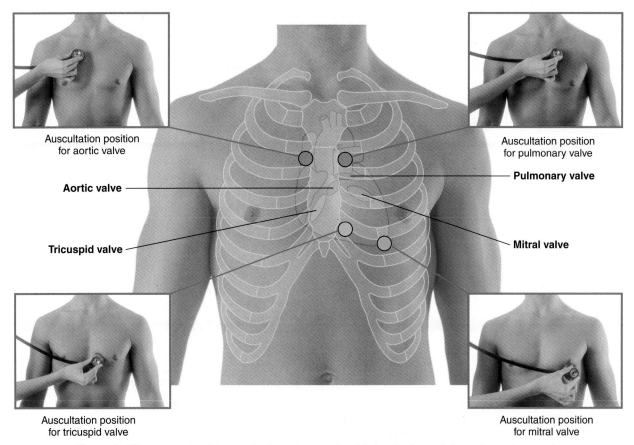

Figure 1-12 Anterior view of the chest showing the heart, location of the heart's valves, and where to listen to heart sounds.

ECG Pearl

The pulmonary trunk begins at the pulmonic valve and divides into the right and left pulmonary arteries. The sinus of Valsalva is a bulge at the base of the aorta formed by the thick leaflets of the aortic valve.

The heart's valves open and close in a specific sequence. This ensures a smooth flow of blood through the heart's chambers. Blood flow through the heart can be hampered if a valve does not function properly. Valvular heart disease is the term used to describe a malfunctioning heart valve. Types of valvular heart disease include:

- *Valvular stenosis.* If a valve narrows, stiffens, or thickens, the valve is said to be stenosed. The heart must work harder to pump blood through a stenosed valve.
- *Valvular prolapse.* If a valve flap inverts, it is said to prolapse. Prolapse can occur if one valve flap is larger than the other is. It can also occur if the chordae tendineae stretch markedly or rupture.
- *Valvular regurgitation.* Blood can flow backward, or regurgitate, if one or more of the heart's valves doesn't close properly. Valvular regurgitation is also known as valvular incompetence or valvular insufficiency.

Papillary muscles receive their blood supply from the coronary arteries. If a papillary muscle ruptures due to an inadequate blood supply (as in a myocardial infarction), the attached valve cusps will not completely close and may result in a murmur. If a papillary muscle in the left ventricle ruptures, the leaflets of the mitral valve may invert (prolapse). This may result in blood leaking from the left ventricle into the left atrium (regurgitation) during ventricular contraction. Blood flow to the body (cardiac output) could be decreased as a result.

HEART SOUNDS

[OBJECTIVE 9]
Heart sounds occur because of vibrations in the tissues of the heart caused by the closing of the heart's valves. Vibrations are created as blood flow is suddenly increased or slowed with the contraction and relaxation of the heart chambers and with the opening and closing of the valves.

Normal heart sounds are called S1 and S2. The first heart sound ("lubb") occurs during ventricular contraction when the tricuspid and mitral (AV) valves are closing. The second heart sound ("dupp") occurs during ventricular relaxation when the pulmonic and aortic (SL) valves are closing. A third heart sound is produced by ventricular filling. In persons younger than 40 years of age, the left ventricle normally permits rapid filling. The more rapid the ventricular filling, the greater the likelihood of hearing a third heart sound. A third heart sound (S3) heard in persons older than 40 years of age is considered abnormal. An abnormal third heart sound is frequently associated with heart failure. An S1-S2-S3 sequence is called a ventricular gallop or gallop rhythm. It sounds like Ken (S1) -tuck (S2) -y (S3).

ECG Pearl
S1 = sound one; S2 = sound two; S3 = sound three.

BLOOD FLOW THROUGH THE HEART

[OBJECTIVE 10]

The right atrium receives blood low in oxygen and high in carbon dioxide from the superior and inferior venae cavae and the coronary sinus (Figure 1-13). The coronary sinus is the largest vein that drains the heart. Blood flows from the right atrium through the tricuspid valve into the right ventricle. When the right ventricle contracts, the tricuspid valve closes. The right ventricle expels the blood through the pulmonic valve into the pulmonary trunk. The pulmonary trunk divides into a right and left pulmonary artery, each of which carries blood to one lung (pulmonary circuit).

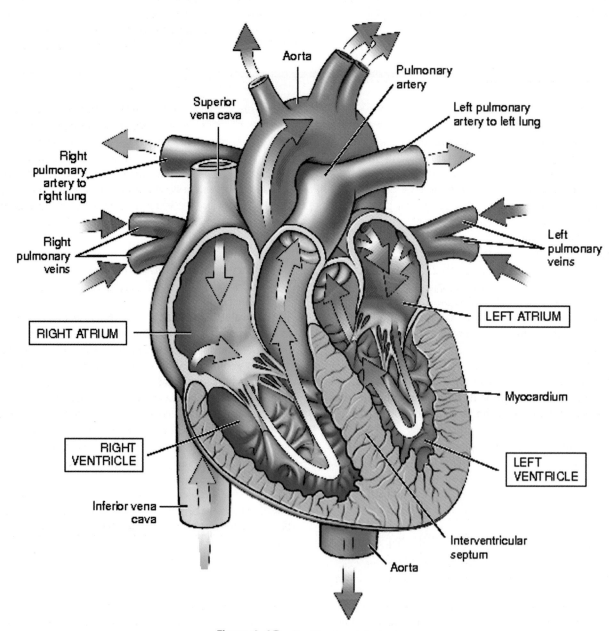

Figure 1-13   Blood flow through the heart.

Blood flows through the pulmonary arteries to the lungs. Blood low in oxygen passes through the pulmonary capillaries. There it comes in direct contact with the alveolar-capillary membrane, where oxygen and carbon dioxide are exchanged. Blood then flows into the pulmonary veins. The left atrium receives oxygenated blood from the lungs by the four pulmonary veins (two from the right lung and two from the left lung). Blood flows from the left atrium through the mitral (bicuspid) valve into the left ventricle. When the left ventricle contracts, the mitral valve closes. Blood leaves the left ventricle through the aortic valve to the aorta. Blood is distributed throughout the body (systemic circuit) through the aorta and its branches.

Blood from the tissues of the head, neck, and upper extremities is emptied into the superior vena cava. Blood from the lower body is returned to the inferior vena cava. The superior and inferior vena cavae carry blood into the right atrium.

CARDIAC CYCLE

[OBJECTIVE 11]

The cardiac cycle refers to a repetitive pumping process that includes all of the events associated with blood flow through the heart. The cycle has two phases for each heart chamber: systole and diastole. **Systole** is the period during which the chamber is contracting and blood is being ejected. Systole includes contraction of both atrial and ventricular muscle. **Diastole** is the period of relaxation during which the chambers are allowed to fill. Both the atria and ventricles have a diastolic phase. The myocardium receives its fresh supply of oxygenated blood from the coronary arteries during ventricular diastole. The cardiac cycle depends on the ability of the cardiac muscle to contract and on the condition of the heart's conduction system. The efficiency of the heart as a pump may be affected by abnormalities of the cardiac muscle, the valves, or the conduction system.

During the cardiac cycle, the pressure within each chamber of the heart rises in systole and falls in diastole. The heart's valves ensure that blood flows in the proper direction. Blood flows from one heart chamber to another from higher to lower pressure. These pressure relationships depend on the careful timing of contractions. The heart's conduction system provides the necessary timing of events between atrial and ventricular systole.

ECG Pearl

In a resting adult, each cardiac cycle lasts approximately 0.8 second. Atrial systole requires about 0.1 second. Ventricular systole requires about 0.3 second. Atrial diastole lasts about 0.7 second. Ventricular diastole lasts about 0.5 second during each cardiac cycle. Some processes occur at the same time, such as ventricular systole and atrial diastole. At rest, the rate of blood flow through the cardiovascular system is about 5000 mL/min.

Atrial Systole and Diastole

During atrial diastole, blood from the superior and inferior vena cavae and the coronary sinus enters the right atrium. The right atrium fills and distends. This pushes the tricuspid valve open and the right ventricle fills. The same sequence occurs a split second earlier in the left heart. The left atrium receives blood from the four pulmonary veins (two from the right lung and two from the left lung). The flaps of the mitral valve open as the left atrium fills. This allows blood to flow into the left ventricle.

The ventricles are 70% filled before the atria contract. Contraction of the atria forces additional blood (about 10% to 30% of the ventricular capacity) into the ventricles. This is called the atrial kick. Thus the ventricles become completely filled with blood during atrial systole. During atrial systole, blood does not flow into the atria because the pressure within the atria exceeds venous pressure. The atria then enter a period of atrial diastole, which continues until the start of the next cardiac cycle.

Ventricular Systole and Diastole

Ventricular systole occurs as atrial diastole begins. As the ventricles contract, blood is propelled through the systemic and pulmonary circulation and toward the atria. The SL valves close and the heart then begins a period of ventricular diastole. During ventricular diastole, the ventricles begin to passively fill with blood and both the atria and ventricles are relaxed. The cardiac cycle begins again with atrial systole and the completion of ventricular filling (Figure 1-14).

CORONARY CIRCULATION

The coronary circulation consists of coronary arteries and veins. With normal activity, 65% to 75% of the fresh oxygen in the blood is taken out by the myocardium by means of the coronary arteries. This is the highest removal rate of any tissue during normal activity and one that cannot be significantly improved. Thus the heart can improve its oxygen uptake only by increasing coronary blood flow. With strenuous activity, coronary blood flow can increase significantly to make sure there is an adequate supply of oxygen to the myocardium.

ECG Pearl

At rest, coronary blood flow averages about 250 mL/min. This represents 4% to 5% of the total cardiac output.

Coronary Arteries

[OBJECTIVE 12]

As you can see, the work of the heart is important. In order to ensure that it has an adequate blood supply, the heart makes sure to provide itself with a fresh supply of oxygenated

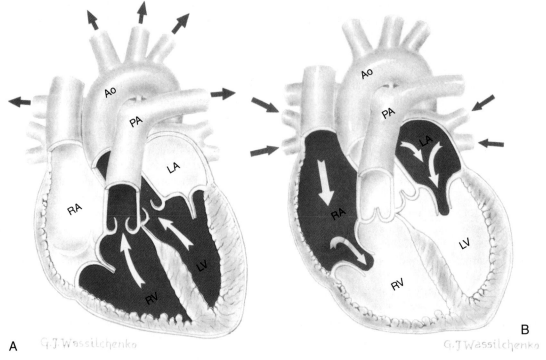

Figure 1-14 Blood flow during **(A)** systole and **(B)** diastole.

blood before supplying the rest of the body. This freshly oxygenated blood is supplied mainly by the branches of two vessels—the right and left coronary arteries. The right and left coronary arteries are the very first branches off the base of the aorta. The openings to these vessels lie just beyond the cusps of the aortic SL valve (Figure 1-15). When the heart contracts, blood flow to the tissues of the heart is significantly reduced because the heart's blood vessels are compressed. Thus, the coronary arteries fill when the ventricles are relaxed (diastole).

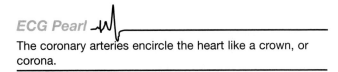

ECG Pearl

The coronary arteries encircle the heart like a crown, or corona.

The main coronary arteries lie on the outer (epicardial) surface of the heart. Coronary arteries that run on the surface of the heart are called epicardial coronary arteries. They branch into progressively smaller vessels, eventually becoming arterioles,

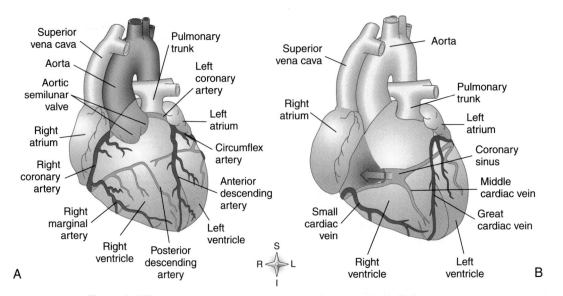

Figure 1-15 Anterior views of the coronary circulation. **A,** Coronary arteries. **B,** Coronary veins.

and then capillaries. Thus, the epicardium has a rich blood supply to draw from. Branches of the main coronary arteries penetrate into the heart's muscle mass and supply the subendocardium with blood. The diameter of these "feeder branches" (collateral circulation) is much narrower. The tissue supplied by these "feeder branches" gets enough blood and oxygen to survive, but they do not have much extra blood flow.

The three major coronary arteries include the left anterior descending (LAD) artery, circumflex (CX) artery, and the right coronary artery (RCA). A person is said to have coronary artery disease (CAD) if there is more than 50 percent diameter narrowing (stenosis) in one or more of these vessels.

ECG Pearl ⎍⩗⎍────────────

Coronary artery disease is classified as one-, two-, or three-vessel disease.

Since a heart attack (myocardial infarction) usually is caused by a blocked coronary artery, it is worthwhile to become familiar with the arteries that supply the heart. When myocardial ischemia or infarction is suspected, an understanding of coronary artery anatomy and the areas of the heart that they supply makes it possible to predict which coronary artery is blocked. The areas of the heart supplied by the three major coronary arteries are shown in Table 1-3.

Right Coronary Artery

The right coronary artery (RCA) originates from the right side of the aorta. It travels along the groove between the right atrium and right ventricle. A branch of the RCA supplies the:
- Right atrium
- Right ventricle
- Inferior surface of the left ventricle in about 85% of individuals
- Posterior surface of the left ventricle in 85%

- Sinoatrial (SA) node in about 60%
- Atrioventricular (AV) node in 85% to 90%

Left Coronary Artery

The left coronary artery (LCA) originates from the left side of the aorta. The first segment of the LCA is called the left main coronary artery. It is about the width of a soda straw and less than an inch long. The left main coronary artery supplies oxygenated blood to its two primary branches: the left anterior descending (LAD) (also called the *anterior interventricular*) artery and the circumflex artery (CX). These vessels are slightly smaller than the left main coronary artery.

The LAD can be seen on the outer (epicardial) surface on the front of the heart. It travels along the groove that lies between the right and left ventricles (anterior interventricular sulcus) toward the heart's apex. In more than 75% of patients, the LAD travels around the apex of the left ventricle and ends along the left ventricle's inferior surface. In the remaining patients, the LAD doesn't reach the inferior surface. Instead, it stops at or before the heart's apex. The major branches of the LAD are the septal and diagonal arteries. The septal branches of the LAD supply blood to the interventricular septum. The LAD supplies blood to:
- Anterior surface of left ventricle
- Part of lateral surface of left ventricle
- Most of the interventricular septum

The circumflex coronary artery circles around the left side of the heart. It is embedded in the epicardium on the back of the heart. The CX supplies blood to the:
- Left atrium
- Lateral surface of the left ventricle
- Inferior surface of the left ventricle in about 15% of individuals
- Posterior surface of the left ventricle in 15%
- SA node in about 40%
- AV node in 10% to 15%

TABLE 1-3 Coronary Arteries		
Coronary Artery and Its Branches	**Portion of Myocardium Supplied**	**Portion of Conduction System Supplied**
RIGHT Posterior descending Right marginal	• Right atrium • Right ventricle • Inferior surface of left ventricle (about 85%*) • Posterior surface of left ventricle (about 85%*)	• SA node (about 60%*) • AV node (85%–90%*) • Proximal portion of bundle of His • Part of posterior-inferior fascicle of left bundle branch
LEFT Anterior descending	• Anterior surface of left ventricle • Part of lateral surface of left ventricle • Most of the interventricular septum	• Most of right bundle branch • Anterior-superior fascicle of left bundle branch • Part of posterior-inferior fascicle of left bundle branch
Circumflex	• Left atrium • Part of lateral surface of left ventricle • Inferior surface of left ventricle (about 15%*) • Posterior surface of left ventricle (15%*)	• SA node (about 40%*) • AV node (10%–15%*)

*Prercentage of population

ECG Pearl

Blockage of the left main coronary artery has been referred to as the "widow maker" because of its association with sudden death.

Coronary Artery Dominance

In about 85% of people, the right coronary artery forms the posterior descending artery. In the remaining 15% of people, the circumflex artery forms the posterior descending artery. The coronary artery that forms the posterior descending artery is considered the "dominant" coronary artery. If a branch of the right coronary artery becomes the posterior descending artery, the coronary artery arrangement is described as a *right dominant system*. If the circumflex coronary artery branches and ends at the posterior descending artery, the coronary artery arrangement is described as a *left dominant system*. If damage to the posterior wall of the left ventricle is suspected, a cardiac catheterization usually is necessary to determine which coronary artery is involved.

Coronary Veins

The coronary (cardiac) veins travel alongside the arteries. Blood that has passed through the myocardial capillaries is drained by branches of the cardiac veins that join the coronary sinus. The coronary sinus is the largest vein that drains the heart. It lies in the groove (sulcus) that separates the atria from the ventricles. The coronary sinus receives blood from the great, middle, and small cardiac veins; a vein of the left atrium; and the posterior vein of the left ventricle. The coronary sinus drains into the right atrium. The anterior cardiac veins do not join the coronary sinus but empty directly into the right atrium.

ACUTE CORONARY SYNDROMES

[OBJECTIVE 13]

Acute coronary syndromes (ACSs) are conditions caused by a similar sequence of pathologic events—a temporary or permanent blockage of a coronary artery. This sequence of events results in conditions ranging from myocardial ischemia or injury to death (necrosis) of heart muscle. The usual cause of an ACS is the rupture of an atherosclerotic plaque. **Arteriosclerosis** is a chronic disease of the arterial system characterized by abnormal thickening and hardening of the vessel walls. **Atherosclerosis** is a form of arteriosclerosis in which the thickening and hardening of the vessel walls are caused by a buildup of fatlike deposits (plaque) in the inner lining of large- and middle-sized muscular arteries. As the fatty deposits build up, the opening of the artery slowly narrows and blood flow to the muscle decreases.

Complete blockage of a coronary artery may cause a heart attack (myocardial infarction). However, because plaque usually increases in size over months and years, other vascular pathways may enlarge as portions of a coronary artery become blocked. These vascular pathways (collateral circulation) serve as an alternative route for blood flow around the blocked artery to the heart muscle. Thus, the presence of collateral arteries may prevent infarction despite complete blockage of the primary artery.

ECG Pearl

Any artery in the body can develop atherosclerosis. If the coronary arteries are involved (coronary artery disease) and blood flow to the heart is decreased, angina pectoris or more serious signs and symptoms may result. If the arteries in the leg are involved (peripheral vascular disease), leg pain (claudication) may result. If the arteries supplying the brain are involved (carotid artery disease), a stroke or transient ischemic attack (TIA) may result.

Angina pectoris is chest discomfort or other related symptoms of sudden onset that may occur because the increased oxygen demand of the heart temporarily exceeds the blood supply. Angina is not a disease. It is a symptom of myocardial ischemia. Angina most often occurs in patients with coronary artery disease involving at least one coronary artery. However, it can be present in patients with normal coronary arteries. Angina also occurs in persons with uncontrolled high blood pressure or valvular

TABLE 1-4	Possible Causes of Myocardial Ischemia	
Inadequate Oxygen Supply	**Increased Myocardial Oxygen Demand**	
Anemia	Exercise	Cocaine, amphetamines
Hypoxemia	Smoking	Emotional stress
Coronary artery narrowing caused by a clot, vessel spasm, or rapid progression of atherosclerosis	Eating a heavy meal	Hypertension
	Fever	Exposure to cold weather
	Congestive heart failure	Aortic stenosis
	Rapid heart rate	Pheochromocytoma
	Obstructive cardiomyopathy	Thyrotoxicosis

heart disease. Possible causes of myocardial ischemia are shown in Table 1-4.

Angina means squeezing or tightening, not pain. The discomfort associated with angina occurs because of the stimulation of nerve endings by lactic acid and carbon dioxide that builds up in ischemic tissue. Common words used by patients experiencing angina to describe the sensation they are feeling are shown in Box 1-1. Some patients have difficulty describing their discomfort.

Chest discomfort associated with myocardial ischemia usually begins in the central or left chest and then radiates to the arm (especially the little finger [ulnar] side of the left arm), wrist, jaw, epigastrium, left shoulder, or between the shoulder blades (Figure 1-16). Ischemic chest discomfort is usually not sharp, worsened by deep inspiration, affected by moving muscles in the area where the discomfort is localized, or positional in nature.

Ischemia can occur because of increased myocardial oxygen demand (demand ischemia), reduced myocardial oxygen supply (supply ischemia), or both. If the cause of the ischemia is not reversed and blood flow restored to the affected area of the heart muscle, ischemia may lead to cellular injury and, ultimately, infarction. Ischemia can quickly resolve by reducing the heart's oxygen demand (by resting or slowing the heart rate with medications such as beta-blockers) or increasing blood flow by dilating the coronary arteries with drugs such as nitroglycerin (NTG). Early assessment, including obtaining a focused medical history, and emergency care are essential to prevent worsening ischemia.

Ischemia prolonged more than just a few minutes results in myocardial *injury*. Myocardial injury refers to myocardial tissue that has been cut off from or experienced a severe reduction in its blood and oxygen supply. Injured myocardial cells are still alive but will die (infarct) if the ischemia is not quickly corrected. If the blocked vessel can be quickly opened, restoring blood flow and oxygen to the injured area, no tissue death occurs. Methods to restore blood flow may include giving clot-busting drugs (fibrinolytics), coronary angioplasty, or a coronary artery bypass graft (CABG), among others. A **myocardial infarction** (MI) occurs when blood flow to the heart muscle stops or is suddenly decreased long enough to cause cell death.

Box **1-1**	Common Terms Patients Use To Describe Angina

"Heaviness"
"Pressing"
"Suffocating"
"Squeezing"
"Strangling"
"Constricting"
"Bursting"
"Burning"
"Griplike"
"A band across my chest"
"A weight in the center of my chest"
"A vise tightening around my chest"

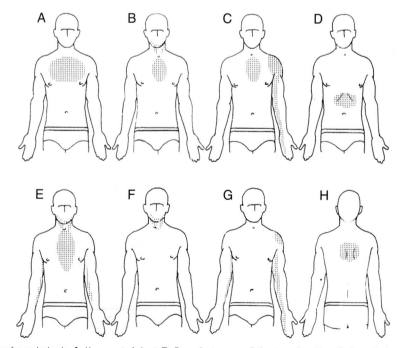

Figure 1-16   Common sites for anginal pain. **A,** Upper part of chest. **B,** Beneath sternum radiating to neck and jaw. **C,** Beneath sternum radiating down left arm. **D,** Epigastric. **E,** Epigastric radiating to neck, jaw, and arms. **F,** Neck and jaw. **G,** Left shoulder. **H,** Interscapular.

In the strictest sense, the term myocardial infarction relates to dead heart muscle tissue. In a practical sense, the term myocardial infarction is applied to the process that results in the death of myocardial tissue. Think of the "process" of MI as a continuum rather than the presence of dead heart tissue. If efforts are made to recognize the process of MI, patients may be identified earlier. If they are promptly treated, the loss of heart tissue may be avoided.[2]

HEART RATE

[OBJECTIVE 13]

The heart is affected by both the sympathetic and parasympathetic divisions of the autonomic nervous system (Figure 1-17). The sympathetic division prepares the body to function under stress ("fight-or-flight" response). The parasympathetic division conserves and restores body resources ("feed-and-breed" or "rest and digest" response). A review of the autonomic nervous system can be found in Table 1-5.

Chronotropy, **inotropy**, and **dromotropy** are terms used to describe effects on heart rate, myocardial contractility, and speed of conduction through the AV node. These terms are explained in Box 1-2.

Baroreceptors and Chemoreceptors

Baroreceptors are specialized nerve tissue (sensors). They are found in the internal carotid arteries and the aortic arch. These sensory receptors detect changes in blood pressure. When they are stimulated, they cause a reflex response in either the sympathetic or the parasympathetic divisions of the autonomic nervous system. For example, if the blood pressure decreases, the body will attempt to compensate by:

- Constricting peripheral blood vessels
- Increasing heart rate (chronotropy)
- Increasing the force of myocardial contraction (inotropy)

These compensatory responses occur because of a response by the sympathetic division. This is called a *sympathetic or adrenergic response*. If the blood pressure increases, the body will decrease sympathetic stimulation and increase the response by the parasympathetic division. This is called a *parasympathetic or cholinergic response*. The baroreceptors will be "reset" to a new "normal" after a few days of exposure to a specific pressure.

Chemoreceptors in the internal carotid arteries and aortic arch detect changes in the concentration of hydrogen ions (pH), oxygen, and carbon dioxide in the blood. The response to these changes by the autonomic nervous system can be sympathetic or parasympathetic.

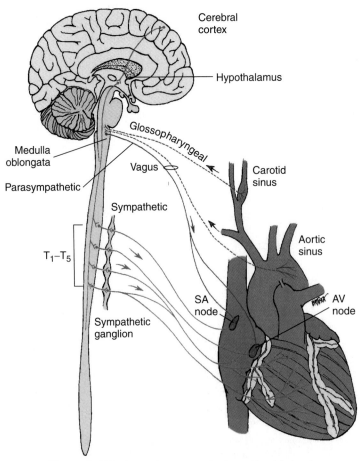

Figure 1-17   Autonomic nervous system innervation of the heart.

TABLE 1-5   A Review of the Autonomic Nervous System

	Sympathetic Division	Parasympathetic Division
General effect	Fight or flight	Feed and breed; rest and digest
Primary neurotransmitter	Norepinephrine	Acetylcholine
EFFECTS OF STIMULATION		
Abdominal blood vessels	Constriction (alpha-receptors)	No effect
Adrenal medulla	Increased secretion of epinephrine	No effect
Bronchioles	Dilation (beta-receptors)	Constriction
Blood vessels of skin	Constriction (alpha-receptors)	No effect
Blood vessels of skeletal muscle	Dilation (beta-receptors)	No effect
Cardiac muscle	Increased rate and strength of contraction (beta-receptors)	Decreased rate; decreased strength of atrial contraction, little effect on strength of ventricular contraction
Coronary blood vessels	Constriction (alpha-receptors) Dilation (beta-receptors)	Dilation

Box 1-2   Terminology

CHRONOTROPIC EFFECT
- Refers to a change in heart rate
- A positive chronotropic effect refers to an increase in heart rate
- A negative chronotropic effect refers to a decrease in heart rate

INOTROPIC EFFECT
- Refers to a change in myocardial contractility
- A positive inotropic effect results in an increase in myocardial contractility
- A negative inotropic effect results in a decrease in myocardial contractility

DROMOTROPIC EFFECT
- Refers to the speed of conduction through the AV junction
- A positive dromotropic effect results in an increase in AV conduction velocity
- A negative dromotropic effect results in a decrease in AV conduction velocity

Parasympathetic Stimulation

[OBJECTIVE 14, 15]
Parasympathetic (inhibitory) nerve fibers supply the sino-atrial node, atrial muscle, and the AV junction of the heart by the vagus nerves. Acetylcholine (Ach) is a chemical messenger (neurotransmitter) released when parasympathetic nerves are stimulated. Acetylcholine binds to parasympathetic receptors. The two main types of cholinergic receptors are nicotinic and muscarinic receptors. Nicotinic receptors are located in skeletal muscle. Muscarinic receptors are located in smooth muscle. Parasympathetic stimulation has the following actions:
- Slows the rate of discharge of the SA node
- Slows conduction through the AV node
- Decreases the strength of atrial contraction
- Can cause a small decrease in the force of ventricular contraction

Sympathetic Stimulation

[OBJECTIVES 14, 15, 16]
Sympathetic (accelerator) nerves supply specific areas of the heart's electrical system, atrial muscle, and the ventricular myocardium. When sympathetic nerves are stimulated, norepinephrine is released. Norepinephrine is a neurotransmitter. Remember: the job of the sympathetic division is to prepare the body for emergency or stressful situations. So, the release of norepinephrine results in the following predictable actions:
- Increased heart rate, force of contraction, conduction velocity, blood pressure, and cardiac output
- Dilation of smooth muscles of bronchi to improve oxygenation
- Shunting of blood from skin and blood vessels of internal organs to skeletal muscle
- Mobilization of stored energy to ensure an adequate supply of glucose for the brain and fatty acids for muscle activity
- Dilation of pupils
- Increased sweating

Sympathetic (adrenergic) receptors are located in different organs and have different physiologic actions when stimulated. There are five main types of sympathetic receptors: $alpha_1$, $alpha_2$, $beta_1$, $beta_2$, and dopamine (also called dopaminergic). A summary of sympathetic receptors is shown in Table 1-6.
- $Alpha_1$ receptors are found in the eyes, blood vessels, bladder, and male reproductive organs. Stimulation of $alpha_1$ receptor sites results in constriction.
- $Alpha_2$ receptor sites are found in parts of the digestive system and on presynaptic nerve terminals in the peripheral nervous system. Stimulation results in decreased secretions, peristalsis, and suppression of norepinephrine release.

TABLE 1-6	Sympathetic (Adrenergic) Receptors	
Receptor Type	**Location**	**Effects of Stimulation**
Alpha$_1$	Eye	Radial muscle contraction of iris causes increased pupil size
	Arterioles of skin, viscera, mucous membranes	Constriction, ↑ peripheral vascular resistance
	Veins	Constriction
	Bladder sphincters	Constriction
	Male reproductive organs	Ejaculation
Alpha$_2$	Digestive system	Decreased secretions, peristalsis
	Presynaptic nerve terminals in peripheral nervous system	Inhibits norepinephrine release
Beta$_1$	Heart	• ↑ heart rate • ↑ force of contraction • ↑ speed of conduction through AV node • ↑ oxygen consumption
	Kidneys	Renin release
Beta$_2$	Arterioles of heart, lungs, skeletal muscle	Dilation, ↑ organ perfusion
	Bronchi	Dilation
	Uterus	Relaxation
	Liver	Glycogenolysis (breakdown of glycogen to glucose)
Dopamine	Renal, mesenteric, and visceral blood vessels	Dilation

- Beta receptor sites are divided into beta$_1$ and beta$_2$. Beta$_1$ receptors are found in the heart and kidneys. Stimulation of beta$_1$ receptor sites in the heart results in increased heart rate, contractility, and, ultimately, irritability of cardiac cells. Stimulation of beta$_1$ receptor sites in the kidneys results in the release of renin into the blood. Renin promotes the production of angiotensin, a powerful vasoconstrictor. Beta$_2$ receptor sites are found in the arterioles of the heart, lungs, and skeletal muscle. Stimulation results in dilation. Stimulation of beta$_2$ receptor sites in the smooth muscle of the bronchi results in dilation.
- Dopamine receptors are found in the renal, mesenteric, and visceral blood vessels. Stimulation results in dilation.

ECG Pearl ⎯⌇⎯

Remember: Beta$_1$ receptors affect the heart (you have one heart); beta$_2$ receptors affect the lungs (you have two lungs).

THE HEART AS A PUMP

Venous Return

The heart functions as a pump to propel blood through the systemic and pulmonary circulations. As the heart chambers fill with blood, the heart muscle is stretched. The most important factor determining the amount of blood pumped out by the heart is the amount of blood flowing into the right heart from the systemic circulation (**venous return**).

Blood Pressure

The mechanical activity of the heart is reflected by the pulse and blood pressure. **Blood pressure** is the force exerted by the circulating blood volume on the walls of the arteries. **Peripheral vascular resistance** is the resistance to the flow of blood determined by blood vessel diameter and the tone of the vascular musculature. **Tone** is a term that may be used when referring to the normal state of balanced tension in body tissues.

Blood pressure is equal to cardiac output × peripheral vascular resistance. Cardiac output is discussed below. Blood pressure is affected by any condition that increases peripheral resistance or cardiac output. Thus an increase in either cardiac output or peripheral resistance typically results in an increase in blood pressure. Conversely, a decrease in either will result in a decrease in blood pressure.

Cardiac Output

[OBJECTIVE 17]

Cardiac output is the amount of blood pumped into the aorta each minute by the heart. It is defined as the **stroke volume** (amount of blood ejected from a ventricle with each heartbeat) multiplied by the heart rate. In the average adult, normal cardiac output is between 4 and 8 L/min. The cardiac output at rest is approximately 5 L/min (stroke volume of 70 mL multiplied by a heart rate of 70 beats/min).

Because the cardiovascular system is a closed system, the volume of blood leaving one part of the system must equal that entering another part. For example, if the left ventricle normally pumps 5 L/min, the volume flowing through the arteries, capillaries, and veins must equal 5 L/min. Thus, the cardiac output of the right ventricle (pulmonary blood flow) is normally equal to that of the left ventricle on a minute-to-minute basis.

Stroke Volume

Cardiac output may be increased by an increase in heart rate *or* stroke volume. Stroke volume is determined by the following:

- The degree of ventricular filling when the heart is relaxed (preload)
- The pressure against which the ventricle must pump (afterload)
- The myocardium's contractile state (contracting or relaxing)

Preload (end-diastolic volume) is the force exerted on the walls of the ventricles at the end of diastole. The volume of blood returning to the heart influences preload. More blood returning to the right atrium increases preload. Less blood returning decreases preload. Increased venous return increases preload. According to Starling's law of the heart, the greater the stretch of the cardiac muscle (within limits), the greater the resulting contraction (Figure 1-18). Heart muscle fibers stretch in response to the increased volume (preload) before contracting. Stretching of the muscle fibers allows the heart to eject the additional volume with increased force, thereby increasing stroke volume. So in the normal heart, the greater the preload, the greater the force of ventricular contraction and the greater the stroke volume, resulting in increased cardiac output. This is important so that the heart can adjust its pumping capacity in response to changes in venous return. For example, during

exercise, the heart muscle fibers stretch in response to increased volume (preload) before contracting. If, however, the ventricle is stretched beyond its physiologic limit, cardiac output may fall because of volume overload and overstretching of the muscle fibers. **Heart failure** is a condition in which the heart is unable to pump enough blood to meet the metabolic needs of the body. It may result from any condition that impairs preload, afterload, cardiac contractility, or heart rate.

Afterload is the pressure or resistance against which the ventricles must pump to eject blood. Afterload is influenced by the following:

- Arterial blood pressure
- The ability of the arteries to become stretched (arterial distensibility)
- Arterial resistance

The lower the resistance (lower afterload), the more easily blood can be ejected. Increased afterload (increased resistance) increases the heart's workload. Conditions that contribute to increased afterload include increased thickness of the blood (viscosity) and high blood pressure.

Cardiac output may be increased by an increase in heart rate *or* stroke volume. Increases in heart rate shorten all phases of the cardiac cycle. The most important is that the time the heart spends relaxing is less. If the length of time for ventricular relaxation is shortened, there is less time for them to fill adequately with blood. If the ventricles do not have time to fill, the following occur:

- The amount of blood sent to the coronary arteries is reduced
- The amount of blood pumped out of the ventricles will decrease (cardiac output)
- Signs of myocardial ischemia may be seen

When a rapid heart rate occurs with some specific types of abnormal heart rhythms, **vagal maneuvers** may be performed. Vagal maneuvers are methods used to stimulate the vagus nerve. When vagal maneuvers are performed, baroreceptors in the carotid arteries are stimulated in an attempt to slow conduction through the AV node. This should result in slowing of the heart rate. Common vagal maneuvers include asking the patient to cough, try to blow through an occluded straw, or bear down as if having a bowel movement.

The concentrations of extracellular ions also affect heart rate. Excess potassium (hyperkalemia) causes the heart to become dilated and flaccid (limp), slows the heart rate, and can dramatically alter conduction. An increase in calcium (hypercalcemia) causes almost the exact opposite effect to those of potassium, causing the heart to go into spastic contraction. Decreased calcium levels (hypocalcemia) cause the heart to become flaccid, similar to the effects of increased potassium levels.

Other factors that influence heart rate include hormone levels (e.g., epinephrine, norepinephrine), medications, stress, anxiety, fear, and body temperature. Heart rate increases when body temperature increases and decreases when body temperature decreases.

An increase in the force of the heart's contractions (and, subsequently, stroke volume) may occur because of many

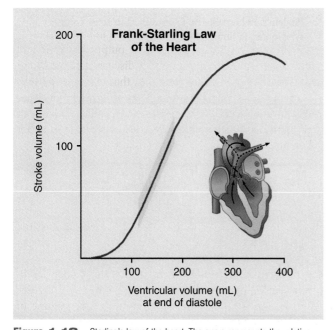

Figure 1-18 Starling's law of the heart. The curve represents the relationship between stroke volume and the ventricular volume at the end of diastole. The range of values observed in a typical heart is shaded. Note that if the ventricle has an abnormally large volume at the end of diastole (far right portion of the curve), the stroke volume cannot compensate.

conditions including norepinephrine and epinephrine release from the adrenal medulla, insulin and glucagon release from the pancreas, and medications, such as calcium, digitalis, dopamine, and dobutamine. A decrease in the force of contraction may result from many conditions including severe hypoxia, decreased pH, elevated carbon dioxide levels (hypercapnia), and medications, such as calcium channel blockers and beta-blockers.

Cardiac output varies depending on hormone balance, an individual's activity level and body size, and the body's metabolic needs. Factors that increase cardiac output include increased body metabolism, exercise, and the age and size of the body. Factors that may decrease cardiac output include **shock**, **hypovolemia**, and heart failure. Signs and symptoms of decreased cardiac output appear in Box 1-3. Heart failure may result from any condition that impairs preload, afterload, cardiac contractility, or heart rate. As the heart begins to fail, the body's compensatory mechanisms attempt to improve cardiac output by manipulating one or more of these factors.

Now that we have discussed heart rate, cardiac output, and stroke volume, let us review an important point. Remember that cardiac output may be increased by an increase in heart rate *or* stroke volume. Consider the following examples:

1. A patient has a stroke volume of 80 mL/beat. His heart rate is 70 beats/min. Is his cardiac output normal, decreased, or increased? Substitute numbers into the formula you already learned: CO = SV × HR. 5600 mL/min = 80 mL/beat × 70 beats/min. Cardiac output is normally between 4 and 8 L/min. This patient's cardiac output is within normal limits.

REFERENCES

1. Guyton AC, Hall JE: Heart muscle: The heart as a pump. In Textbook of medical physiology, ed 9, Philadelphia, 1996, WB Saunders.

| Box **1-3** | Signs and Symptoms of Decreased Cardiac Output |

- Cold, clammy skin
- Color changes in the skin and mucous membranes
- Dyspnea
- Orthopnea
- Crackles (rales)
- Changes in mental status
- Changes in blood pressure
- Dysrhythmias
- Fatigue
- Restlessness

2. Now, let us see what an increase in heart rate will do. If the patient's heart rate increases to 180 beats/min and his stroke volume remains at 80 mL/beat, what happens to his cardiac output? Using our formula again (CO = SV × HR) and substituting numbers, we end up with 14,400 mL/min = 80 mL/beat × 180 beats/min. This patient's cardiac output is increased.

3. What happens to cardiac output if the patient's heart rate is 70 beats/min but his stroke volume drops to 50 mL/beat? Using our formula one more time (CO = SV × HR) and substituting numbers, we end up with 3500 mL/min = 50 mL/beat × 70 beats/min. This patient's cardiac output is decreased. If the patient's heart rate increased to 90 beats/min to try to compensate for his failing pump, what would happen to his cardiac output? (4500 mL/min = 50 mL/beat × 90 beats/min). According to our example, the patient's cardiac output would increase—at least temporarily.

2. Phalen T, Aehlert B: The 12-lead ECG in acute coronary syndromes, St Louis, 2006, Elsevier.

STOP & REVIEW

Multiple Choice

In the space provided, identify the letter of the choice that best completes each statement or answers each question.

_____ 1. Movement of blood from the right ventricle to the lungs is called the
  a. systemic circulation.
  b. pulmonary circulation.

_____ 2. The _____ supplies the right atrium and ventricle with blood.
  a. right coronary artery
  b. left main coronary artery
  c. circumflex artery
  d. left anterior descending artery

_____ 3. The primary chemical mediator of the sympathetic division of the autonomic nervous system is
  a. dopamine.
  b. muscarine.
  c. acetylcholine.
  d. norepinephrine.

_____ 4. The circumflex artery is a branch of the
  a. left coronary artery.
  b. right coronary artery.
  c. left anterior descending artery.
  d. anterior interventricular artery.

_____ 5. The tricuspid valve
  a. is a semilunar valve.
  b. is located between the left ventricle and aorta.
  c. is located between the right atrium and right ventricle.
  d. is located between the right ventricle and pulmonary artery.

_____ 6. The anterior surface of the heart is made up mostly of the
  a. left atrium.
  b. right atrium.
  c. left ventricle.
  d. right ventricle.

_____ 7. The period during which a heart chamber is contracting and blood is being ejected is called
  a. systole.
  b. diastole.
  c. ischemia.
  d. infarction.

_____ 8. Which of the following is primarily responsible for parasympathetic stimulation of the heart?
  a. The vagus nerves
  b. The coronary sinus
  c. The carotid arteries
  d. The muscarinic nerves

Completion

In the blanks provided, write the words that best complete each sentence.

9. The _____ are the heart chambers that receive blood.

10. The inferior surface of the heart is also called the _____ surface.

11. The _____ are the heart chambers that pump blood.

12. The thick, muscular middle layer of the heart wall that contains the atrial and ventricular muscle fibers necessary for contraction is the _____.

Matching

Match the key terms in the left column with the definitions in the right column by placing the letter of each correct answer in the space provided.

_____ **13.** Right coronary artery

_____ **14.** Half-moon

_____ **15.** Chronotropic

_____ **16.** Endocardium

_____ **17.** Venous return

_____ **18.** Interatrial

_____ **19.** Tamponade

_____ **20.** Baroreceptors

_____ **21.** Pulmonic

_____ **22.** Atria

_____ **23.** Ejection fraction

_____ **24.** Myocardial ischemia

_____ **25.** Chemoreceptors

_____ **26.** Contracts

_____ **27.** Gap junctions

_____ **28.** Mediastinum

_____ **29.** Calcium

_____ **30.** Atrioventricular

_____ **31.** Ventricles

_____ **32.** Great vessels

a. Innermost layer of the heart

b. The percentage of blood pumped out of a heart chamber with each contraction.

c. Space between the lungs that contains the heart, great vessels, trachea, and esophagus, among other structures

d. Sensors in the internal carotid arteries and aortic arch that detect changes in the concentration of hydrogen ions (pH), oxygen, and carbon dioxide in the blood

e. A buildup of excess blood or fluid in the pericardial space can cause cardiac _____.

f. This type of heart valve separates an atrium and ventricle.

g. When actin and myosin filaments slide together, the cardiac muscle cell _____.

h. The amount of blood flowing into the right atrium each minute from the systemic circulation

i. A negative _____ effect refers to a decrease in heart rate.

j. One of the semilunar valves

k. Lower heart chambers

l. Coronary artery that supplies the SA node and AV node in most of the population

m. This typically results when the heart's demand for oxygen exceeds its supply from the coronary circulation

n. The _____ septum separates the right and left atria.

o. _____ in myocardial cells function as electrical connections and allow the cells to conduct electrical impulses very rapidly.

p. Specialized nerve tissue located in the internal carotid arteries and the aortic arch that detect changes in blood pressure

q. This electrolyte is very important in cardiac muscle contraction.

r. Pulmonary arteries and veins, aorta, superior and inferior vena cavae

s. A semilunar valve is shaped like a _____.

t. Upper chambers of the heart

Short Answer

33. Briefly describe parasympathetic innervation of the heart.

34. The right atrium receives blood low in oxygen from three vessels. Name them.
1.

2.

3.

35. List three types of sympathetic (adrenergic) receptor sites.
1.

2.

3.

36. Name the two main branches of the left coronary artery.
1.

2.

37. What factors affect afterload?

38. Define "atrial kick."

39. What effects can be expected from sympathetic stimulation of the heart?

40. Describe the function of the right atrium of the heart.

41. List six of the signs and symptoms of decreased cardiac output.

42. What effects can be expected from parasympathetic stimulation of the heart?

43. What factors affect stroke volume?

44. Your patient is a 62-year-old woman complaining of a "racing heart." Your examination of the patient reveals a pulse rate of 192 beats/min. Briefly explain why recognition of a rapid heart rate is important when providing patient care.

45. Label the following coronary arteries:
  · Circumflex
  · Posterior descending
  · Anterior descending
  · Marginal
  · Right coronary artery
  · Left main coronary artery

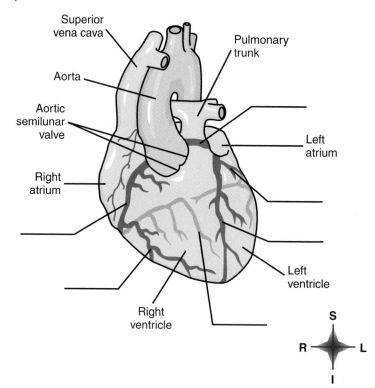

STOP & REVIEW ANSWERS

Multiple Choice

1. b

2. a

3. d

4. a

5. c

6. d

7. a

8. a

Completion

9. The *atria* are the heart chambers that receive blood.

10. The inferior surface of the heart is also called the *diaphragmatic* surface.

11. The *ventricles* are the heart chambers that pump blood.

12. The thick, muscular middle layer of the heart wall that contains the atrial and ventricular muscle fibers necessary for contraction is the *myocardium*.

Matching

13. l

14. s

15. i

16. a

17. h

18. n

19. e

20. p

21. j

22. t

23. b

24. m

25. d

26. g

27. o

28. c

29. q

30. f

31. k

32. r

Short Answer

33. Parasympathetic (inhibitory) nerve fibers supply the sinoatrial node, atrial muscle, and the AV junction of the heart by the vagus nerves.

34. The right atrium receives blood low in oxygen from:

1. The superior vena cava

2. The inferior vena cava

3. The coronary sinus

35. There are five main types of sympathetic (adrenergic) receptors: alpha$_1$, alpha$_2$, beta$_1$, beta$_2$, and dopamine (also called dopaminergic).

36. The left main coronary artery supplies oxygenated blood to its two primary branches: the left anterior descending (LAD) (also called the anterior interventricular) artery and the circumflex artery (CX).

37. Afterload is the pressure or resistance against which the ventricles must pump to eject blood. Afterload is influenced by the following:
Arterial blood pressure
The ability of the arteries to become stretched (arterial distensibility)
Arterial resistance

38. At the end of ventricular diastole, both atria simultaneously contract to eject 10% to 30% more blood into the ventricles.

39. Sympathetic stimulation of the heart results in increased heart rate, force of contraction, conduction velocity, blood pressure, and cardiac output.

40. The right atrium receives deoxygenated blood from the superior vena cava (which carries blood from the head and upper extremities), the inferior vena cava (which carries blood from the lower body), and the coronary sinus (which receives blood from the intracardiac circulation). Blood passes through the tricuspid valve to the right ventricle.

41.
- Cold, clammy skin
- Color changes in the skin and mucous membranes
- Dyspnea
- Orthopnea
- Crackles (rales)
- Changes in mental status
- Changes in blood pressure
- Dysrhythmias
- Fatigue
- Restlessness

42. Parasympathetic stimulation has the following actions:
- Slows the rate of discharge of the SA node
- Slows conduction through the AV node
- Decreases the strength of atrial contraction
- Can cause a small decrease in the force of ventricular contraction

43. Stroke volume is determined by the following:
- The degree of ventricular filling when the heart is relaxed (preload)
- The pressure against which the ventricle must pump (afterload)
- The myocardium's contractile state (contracting or relaxing)

44. Increases in heart rate shorten all phases of the cardiac cycle. The most important is that the time the heart spends relaxing is less. If the length of time for ventricular relaxation is shortened, there is less time for them to fill adequately with blood. If the ventricles do not have time to fill, the following occur:
- The amount of blood sent to the coronary arteries is reduced
- The amount of blood pumped out of the ventricles will decrease (cardiac output)
- Signs of myocardial ischemia may be seen

45.

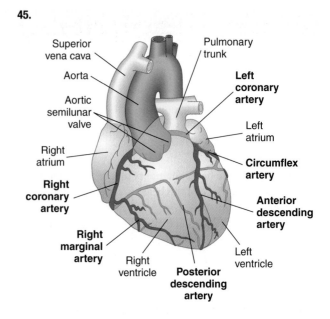

Basic Electrophysiology

OBJECTIVES

After reading this chapter, you should be able to:

1. Describe the two basic types of cardiac cells in the heart, where they are found, and their function.
2. Describe the primary characteristics of cardiac cells.
3. Define the events comprising the cardiac action potential and correlate them with the waveforms produced on the ECG.
4. Define the terms membrane potential, threshold potential, action potential, polarization, depolarization, and repolarization.
5. List the most important ions involved in cardiac action potential and their primary function in this process.
6. Define the absolute, relative refractory, and supernormal periods and their location in the cardiac cycle.
7. Describe the normal sequence of electrical conduction through the heart.
8. Describe the location, function, and (where appropriate), the intrinsic rate of the following structures: SA node, atrioventricular (AV) junction, bundle branches, and Purkinje fibers.
9. Differentiate the primary mechanisms responsible for producing cardiac dysrhythmias.
10. Describe reentry.
11. Explain the purpose of electrocardiographic monitoring.
12. Identify the limitations of the electrocardiogram (ECG).
13. Differentiate between frontal plane and horizontal plane leads.
14. Describe correct anatomic placement of the standard limb leads, augmented leads, and chest leads.
15. Relate the cardiac surfaces or areas represented by the electrocardiogram leads.
16. Identify the numeric values assigned to the small and large boxes on ECG paper.
17. Identify how heart rates, durations, and amplitudes may be determined from electrocardiographic recordings.
18. Define and describe the significance of each of the following as they relate to cardiac electrical activity: P wave, QRS complex, T wave, U wave, PR-segment, TP-segment, ST-segment, PR interval, QRS duration, and QT interval.
19. Recognize the changes on the electrocardiogram that may reflect evidence of myocardial ischemia and injury.
20. Define the term artifact and explain methods that may be used to minimize its occurrence.
21. Describe a systematic approach to the analysis and interpretation of cardiac dysrhythmias.

CARDIAC CELLS

Types of Cardiac Cells

[OBJECTIVE 1]

In general, cardiac cells have either a mechanical (contractile) or an electrical (pacemaker) function. **Myocardial cells** (working or mechanical cells) contain contractile filaments. When these cells are electrically stimulated, the contractile filaments slide together and the myocardial cell contracts. These myocardial cells form the thin muscular layer of the atrial walls and the thicker muscular layer of the ventricular walls (the myocardium). These cells do not normally generate electrical impulses on their own. They rely on pacemaker cells for this purpose.

Pacemaker cells are specialized cells of the heart's electrical system. Pacemaker cells also may be referred to as conducting cells or automatic cells. They are responsible for spontaneously generating and conducting electrical impulses.

Properties of Cardiac Cells

[OBJECTIVE 2]

When a nerve is stimulated, a chemical (neurotransmitter) is released. The chemical crosses the space between the end of the nerve and the muscle membrane (neuromuscular junction). The chemical binds to receptor sites on the muscle membrane and stimulates the receptors. An electrical impulse develops and travels along the muscle membrane, resulting in contraction. Thus a skeletal muscle normally contracts only after it is stimulated by a nerve.

The heart is unique because it has pacemaker cells that can generate an electrical impulse without being stimulated by a nerve. The ability of cardiac pacemaker cells to create an electrical impulse without being stimulated from another source is called **automaticity**. The heart's normal pacemaker (the sinoatrial node) usually prevents other areas of the heart from assuming this function because its cells depolarize more rapidly than other pacemaker cells. Normal concentrations of sodium (Na+), potassium (K+), and calcium (Ca++) are important in maintaining automaticity. Increased blood concentrations of these electrolytes decrease automaticity. Decreased concentrations of K+ and Ca++ in the blood increase automaticity.

Cardiac muscle is electrically irritable because of an ionic imbalance across the membranes of cells. **Excitability** (irritability) refers to the ability of cardiac muscle cells to respond to an outside stimulus. The stimulus may be from a chemical, mechanical, or electrical source. **Conductivity** refers to the ability of a cardiac cell to receive an electrical impulse and conduct it to an adjoining cardiac cell. All cardiac cells possess this characteristic. The intercalated disks present in the membranes of cardiac cells are responsible for the property of conductivity. They allow an impulse in any part of the myocardium to spread throughout the heart. The speed with which the impulse is conducted can be altered by factors such as sympathetic and parasympathetic stimulation and medications. **Contractility** refers to the ability of myocardial cells to shorten in response to an impulse. This results in contraction. The heart normally contracts in response to an impulse that begins in the sinoatrial (SA) node. The strength of the heart's contraction can be improved with certain medications, such as digitalis, dopamine, and epinephrine.

CARDIAC ACTION POTENTIAL

[OBJECTIVES 3, 4, 5]

Before the following discussion of the cardiac action potential, think about how a battery releases energy. A battery has two terminals; one terminal is positive and the other is negative. Charged particles exert forces on each other, and opposite charges attract. Electrons (negatively charged particles) are produced by a chemical reaction inside the battery. If a wire is connected between the two terminals, the circuit is completed and the stored energy is released. This allows electrons to flow quickly from the negative terminal along the wire to the positive terminal. If no wire is connected between the terminals, the chemical reaction does not take place and no current flow occurs. **Current** is the flow of electrical charge from one point to another.

Separated electrical charges of opposite polarity (positive versus negative) have potential energy. The measurement of this potential energy is called **voltage**. Voltage is measured between two points. In the battery example, the current flow is caused by the voltage, or potential difference, between the two terminals. Voltage is measured in units of volts or millivolts.

In the normal heart, electrical activity occurs because of changes that occur in the body's cells. Human body fluids contain **electrolytes,** which are elements or compounds that break into charged particles (**ions**) when melted or dissolved in water or another solvent. The main electrolytes that affect the function of the heart are Na+, K+, Ca++, and chloride (Cl$^-$). Body fluids that contain electrolytes conduct an electric current in much the same way as the wire in the battery example. Electrolytes move about in body fluids and carry a charge, just as electrons moving along a wire conduct a current. The **action potential** is a five-phase cycle that reflects the difference in the concentration of these charged particles across the cell membrane at any given time.

Polarization

In the body, ions spend a lot of time moving back and forth across cell membranes. As a result, a slight difference in the concentrations of charged particles across the membranes of cells is normal. Thus potential energy (voltage) exists because of the imbalance of charged particles. This imbalance makes the cells excitable.

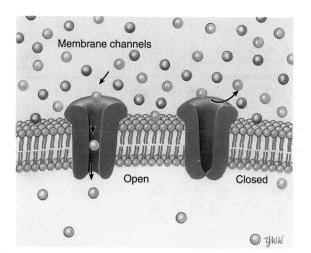

Figure 2-1   Cell membranes contain membrane channels. These channels are pores through which specific ions or other small, water-soluble molecules can cross the cell membrane from outside to inside.

Cell membranes contain pores or channels through which specific electrolytes and other small, water-soluble molecules can cross the cell membrane from outside to inside (Figure 2-1). When a cell is at rest, K+ leaks out of it. Large molecules such as proteins and phosphates remain inside the cell because they are too big to pass easily through the cell membrane. These large molecules carry a negative charge. This results in more negatively charged ions on the inside of the cell. When the inside of a cell is more negative than the outside, it is said to be in a **polarized state** (Figure 2-2). The voltage (difference in electrical charges) across the cell membrane is the **membrane potential**. Electrolytes are quickly moved from one side of the cell membrane to the other by means of pumps. These pumps require energy in the form of adenosine triphosphate (ATP) when

movement occurs against a concentration gradient. The energy expended by the cells to move electrolytes across the cell membrane creates a flow of current. This flow of current is expressed in volts. Voltage appears on an electrocardiogram (ECG) as spikes or waveforms. Thus an ECG is actually a sophisticated voltmeter.

Depolarization

For a pacemaker cell to "fire" (produce an impulse), a flow of electrolytes across the cell membrane must exist. When a cell is stimulated, the cell membrane changes and becomes **permeable** to Na+ and K+. Permeability refers to the ability of a membrane channel to allow passage of electrolytes once it is open. Na+ rushes into the cell through Na+ channels. This causes the inside of the cell to become more positive. A spike (waveform) is then recorded on the ECG. Threshold is the membrane potential at which the cell membrane becomes more positive. The stimulus that alters the electrical charges across the cell membrane may be electrical, mechanical, or chemical.

As described in the battery example, when opposite charges come together, energy is released. When the movement of electrolytes changes the electrical charge of the inside of the cell from negative to positive, an impulse is generated. The impulse causes channels to open in the next cell membrane and then the next. The movement of charged particles across a cell membrane causing the inside of the cell to become positive is called **depolarization** (Figure 2-3). Depolarization must take place before the heart can mechanically contract and pump blood. Depolarization occurs because of the movement of Na+ into the cell. Depolarization proceeds from the innermost layer of the heart (endocardium) to the outermost layer (epicardium).

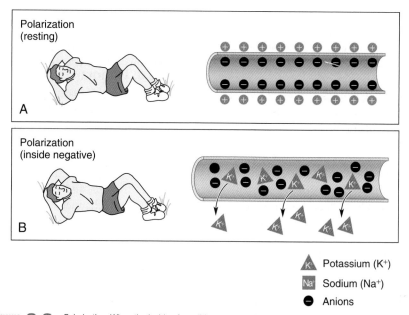

Figure 2-2   Polarization. When the inside of a cell is more negative than the outside it is said to be polarized.

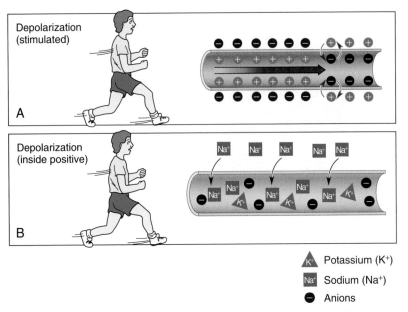

Depolarization
(stimulated)

A

Depolarization
(inside positive)

B

▲ Potassium (K⁺)

Na⁺ Sodium (Na⁺)

● Anions

Figure 2-3 Depolarization is the movement of ions across a cell membrane causing the inside of the cell to become more positive.

An impulse normally begins in the pacemaker cells found in the sinoatrial (SA) node of the heart. A chain reaction occurs from cell to cell in the heart's electrical conduction system until all the cells have been stimulated and depolarized. This chain reaction is a wave of depolarization. The chain reaction is made possible because of gap junctions that exist between the cells. Eventually the impulse is spread from the pacemaker cells to the working myocardial cells. The working myocardial cells contract when they are stimulated. When the atria are stimulated, a P wave is recorded on the ECG. Thus the P wave represents atrial depolarization. When the ventricles are stimulated, a QRS complex is recorded on the ECG. Thus the QRS complex represents ventricular depolarization.

ECG Pearl

Depolarization is *not* the same as contraction. Depolarization (an electrical event) is expected to result in contraction (a mechanical event). It is possible to see organized electrical activity on the cardiac monitor, yet evaluation of the patient reveals no palpable pulse. This clinical situation is called **pulseless electrical activity** (**PEA**).

Repolarization

After the cell depolarizes, it quickly begins to recover and restore its electrical charges to normal. The movement of charged particles across a cell membrane in which the inside of the cell is restored to its negative charge is called **repolarization**. The cell membrane stops the flow of Na+ into the cell and allows K+ to leave it. Negatively charged particles are left inside the cell. Thus the cell is returned to its resting state (Figure 2-4). This causes contractile proteins in the

working myocardial cells to separate (relax). The cell can be stimulated again if another electrical impulse arrives at the cell membrane. Repolarization proceeds from the epicardium to the endocardium. On the ECG, the ST-segment and T wave represent ventricular repolarization.

Phases of the Cardiac Action Potential

The action potential of a cardiac cell consists of five phases labeled 0 to 4. These phases reflect the rapid sequence of voltage changes that occur across the cell membrane during the electrical cardiac cycle. Phases 1, 2, and 3 have been referred to as *electrical systole*. Phase 4 has been referred to as *electrical diastole*. The configuration of the action potential varies depending on the location, size, and function of the cardiac cell. Figure 2-5 shows the action potential of a normal ventricular muscle cell.

Phase 0: Depolarization

The rapid entry of Na+ into the cell is largely responsible for phase 0 of the cardiac action potential. Phase 0 represents depolarization (Figure 2-6) and is called the rapid depolarization phase. Phase 0 also is called the *upstroke, spike,* or *overshoot*. Phase 0 begins when the cell receives an impulse. Na+ moves rapidly into the cell through the Na+ channels, K+ leaves the cell, and Ca++ moves slowly into the cell through Ca++ channels. The cell depolarizes and cardiac contraction begins. Phase 0 is represented on the ECG by the QRS complex.

The cells of the atria, ventricles, and the Purkinje fibers of the conduction system have many sodium channels. The SA and AV nodes of the heart have relatively few sodium channels. If the flow of sodium through the sodium channels is slowed or blocked, the heart rate slows, the cells

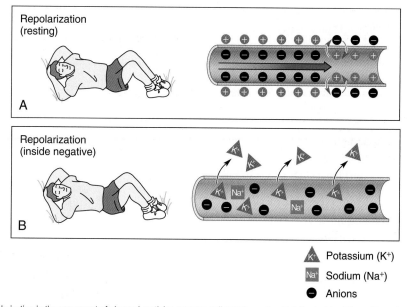

Potassium (K⁺)
Sodium (Na⁺)
Anions

Figure 2-4 Repolarization is the movement of charged particles across a cell membrane in which the inside of the cell is restored to its negative charge.

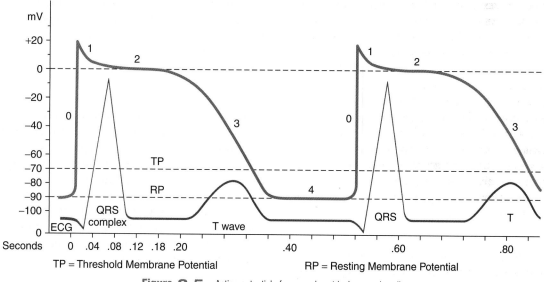

TP = Threshold Membrane Potential   RP = Resting Membrane Potential

Figure 2-5 Action potential of a normal ventricular muscle cell.

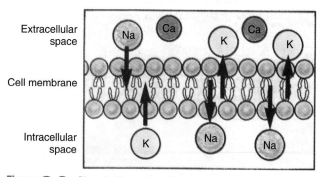

Figure 2-6 Phase 0 of the cardiac action potential represents depolarization. Na+ moves rapidly into the cell through Na+ channels. K+ leaves the cell and Ca++ moves slowly into the cell through Ca++ channels.

become less excitable, and the speed of conduction decreases. Phase 0 of the cardiac action potential immediately is followed by repolarization, which is divided into three phases.

Phase 1: Early Repolarization

During phase 1 of the cardiac action potential, the Na+ channels partially close, slowing the flow of Na+ into the cell. At the same time, Cl⁻ enters the cell and K+ leaves it through K+ channels. The result is a decrease in the number of positive electrical charges within the cell. This produces a small negative deflection in the action potential (see Figure 2-5).

Phase 2: Plateau Phase

Phase 2 is the plateau phase of the action potential (Figure 2-7). During this phase, Ca++ slowly enters the cell through Ca++ channels. The cells of the atria, ventricles, and the Purkinje fibers of the conduction system have many calcium channels. K+ continues to leave the cell slowly through K+ channels. The plateau phase allows cardiac muscle to sustain an increased period of contraction. The cells of the atria, ventricles, and Purkinje fibers spend less time in phase 2 if the flow of calcium through calcium channels is slowed or blocked. Medications such as calcium channel blockers slow the rate at which calcium passes through the cells (Box 2-1). Phase 2 is responsible for the ST-segment on the ECG. The ST-segment reflects the early part of repolarization of the right and left ventricles. Hypercalcemia and medications such as digitalis shorten the ST-segment.

Phase 3: Final Rapid Repolarization

Phase 3 begins with the downslope of the action potential. The cell rapidly completes repolarization as K+ quickly flows out of the cell. Na+ and Ca++ channels close, stopping the entry of Na+ and Ca++. The rapid movement of K+ out of the cell causes the inside to become progressively more electrically negative. The cell gradually becomes more sensitive to external stimuli until its original sensitivity is restored. Phase 3 of the action potential corresponds with the T wave (ventricular repolarization) on the ECG. Repolarization is complete by the end of phase 3. If potassium channels are blocked, the result is a longer action potential.

Phase 4: Resting Membrane Potential

Phase 4 is the resting membrane potential (return to resting state) (Figure 2-8). During phase 4, an excess of Na+ is inside the cell and an excess of K+ is outside the cell. The Na+/K+ pump is activated to move Na+ out of the cell and K+ back into the cell. The heart is polarized during this phase (i.e., ready for discharge). The cell will remain in this state until the cell membrane is reactivated by another stimulus.

The heart typically beats at a regular rate and rhythm. If this pattern is interrupted, an abnormal heart rhythm can

Box **2-1**	Examples of Calcium Channel Blockers

GENERIC NAME	TRADE NAME
diltiazem	Cardizem, Cardizem CD, Cardizem SR, Dilacor XR, Diltiazem XT, Tiazac
verapamil	Calan, Calan SR, Covera-HS, Isoptin, Isoptin SR, Verelan, Verelan PM
amlodipine	Norvasc
felodipine	Plendil
bepridil	Vascor
nisoldipine	Sular
nicardipine	Cardene, Cardene SR
nifedipine	Adalat, Adalat CC, Procardia, Procardia XL

result. Health care professionals use the terms **arrhythmia** and **dysrhythmia** interchangeably to refer to an abnormal heart rhythm. Medications used to correct irregular heartbeats and slow down hearts that beat too fast are called **antiarrhythmics**. Antiarrhythmic medications are classified by their effects on the cardiac action potential (Figure 2-9).

REFRACTORY PERIODS

[OBJECTIVE 6]

Refractoriness is a term used to describe the period of recovery that cells need after being discharged before they are able to respond to a stimulus. In the heart, the refractory period is longer than the contraction itself.

During the **absolute refractory period** (also known as the effective refractory period), the cell will not respond to further stimulation. This means that the myocardial working cells cannot contract and the cells of the electrical conduction system cannot conduct an electrical impulse—no matter how strong the stimulus. As a result, tetanic (sustained) contractions cannot be provoked in cardiac muscle. On the ECG, the absolute refractory period corresponds with the

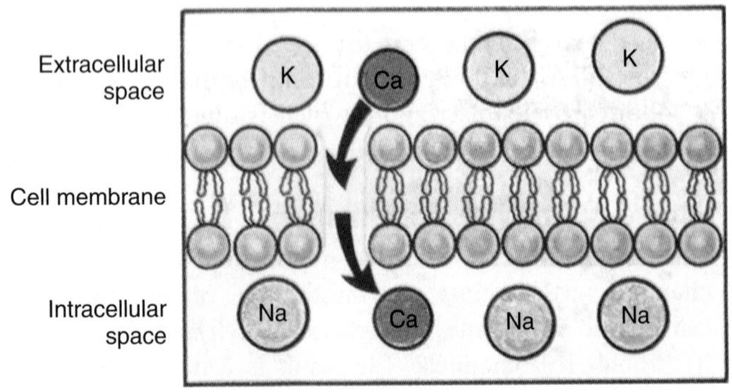

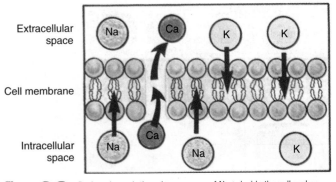

Figure 2-7 Phase 2 (plateau phase) of the cardiac action potential is caused by the slow inward movement of Ca++ and slow outward movement of K+ from the cell.

Figure 2-8 During phase 4, there is an excess of Na+ inside the cell and an excess of K+ outside the cell. The sodium-potassium pump is activated to move Na+ out of the cell and move K+ back into the cell.

Antiarrhythmic Drug Actions

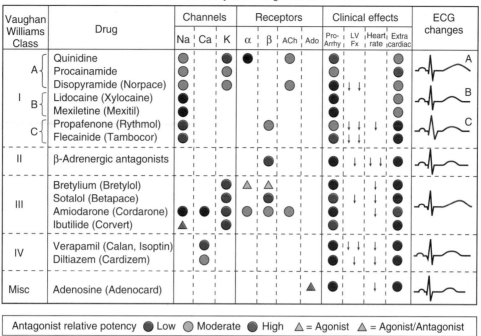

Vaughan Williams Class		Drug	Channels			Receptors				Clinical effects				ECG changes
			Na	Ca	K	α	β	ACh	Ado	Pro-Arrhy	LV Fx	Heart rate	Extra cardiac	
I	A	Quinidine	◐		●	●		◐		◐				●	A
		Procainamide	◐		◐					◐				●	
		Disopyramide (Norpace)	◐		◐			◐		●	↓ ↓	↓		●	B
	B	Lidocaine (Xylocaine)	●							●				●	
		Mexiletine (Mexitil)	●							●				●	C
	C	Propafenone (Rythmol)	●				◐			◐	↓ ↓	↓	↓	●	
		Flecainide (Tambocor)	●							◐	↓ ↓	↓		●	
II		β-Adrenergic antagonists					●			●	↓	↓ ↓ ↓		●	
III		Bretylium (Bretylol)			●	△	△			●				●	
		Sotalol (Betapace)			●		●			●	↓		↓	●	
		Amiodarone (Cordarone)	●	●	●	◐	◐	◐		◐		↓	↓	●	
		Ibutilide (Corvert)	△		●					◐				●	
IV		Verapamil (Calan, Isoptin)		◐						●	↓ ↓	↓	↓	●	
		Diltiazem (Cardizem)		◐						●	↓	↓	↓	●	
Misc		Adenosine (Adenocard)							△	●			↓	●	

Antagonist relative potency ● Low ◐ Moderate ● High △ = Agonist △ = Agonist/Antagonist

Figure 2-9 This figure is a modification of the Sicilian Gambit drug classification system and includes designation by the Vaughn-Williams system. The sodium channel blockers are subdivided into the A, B, and C subgroups based on their relative potency. The targets of antiarrhythmic drugs, listed across the columns, are the ion channels (sodium, calcium, and potassium) and the receptors (alpha-adrenergic, beta-adrenergic, cholinergic [ACH], and adenosinergic [ADO]). The next columns compare the drugs' clinical actions. These include proarrhythmic potential (Proarrhy) effects on left ventricular function (LV Fx), effects on heart rate (Heart Rate), and potential for extra cardiac side effects (Extra Cardiac). The ECG tracings indicate the changes (in color) that are caused by usual dosages of the drug (i.e., PR interval, QRS interval, and QT interval). The drugs are listed in rows with their brand names shown in parentheses. The symbols in the table indicate the drugs' relative potency as agonists or antagonists. The solid triangle indicates the biphasic effects of bretylium initially to release norepinephrine and act as an agonist and subsequently to block further release and act as an antagonist of adrenergic tone. The number of arrows and their direction indicate the magnitude and direction of effect of the drugs on heart rate and left ventricular function (i.e., inotropy).

onset of the QRS complex to the peak of the T wave. It includes phases 0, 1, 2, and part of phase 3 of the cardiac action potential (Figure 2-10).

During the **relative refractory period** (also known as the vulnerable period), some cardiac cells have repolarized to their threshold potential and can be stimulated to respond (depolarize) to a stronger than normal stimulus (see Figure 2-10). This period corresponds with the downslope of the T wave on the ECG.

After the relative refractory period is a **supernormal period**. A weaker than normal stimulus can cause cardiac cells to depolarize during this period. The supernormal period extends from the end of phase 3 to the beginning of phase 4 of the cardiac action potential. On the ECG, this corresponds with the end of the T wave. Dysrhythmias can develop during this period (Figure 2-11).

CONDUCTION SYSTEM

[OBJECTIVES 7, 8]
The specialized electrical (pacemaker) cells in the heart are arranged in a system of pathways called the **conduction system**. In the normal heart, the cells of the conduction

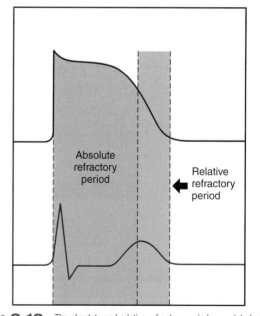

Figure 2-10 The absolute and relative refractory periods correlated with the action potential of a cardiac muscle cell and an ECG tracing.

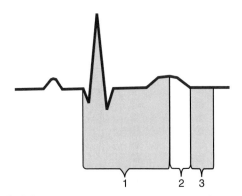

Figure 2-11   The absolute refractory period, (2) relative refractory period, and (3) the supernormal period.

system are interconnected. The conduction system makes sure that the chambers of the heart contract in a coordinated fashion. The pacemaker site with the fastest firing rate typically controls the heart.

Sinoatrial Node

The normal heartbeat is the result of an electrical impulse that begins in the SA node. In an adult, the SA node is about 10 to 20 mm long and 2 to 3 mm wide. Different types of cells are found in the SA node. Slightly less than half of the cells are thought to be pacemaker cells. The others are thought to be responsible for conducting the electrical impulse within the SA node and to its borders.

The heart's pacemaker cells have a built-in (intrinsic) rate that becomes slower and slower from the SA node down to the end of the His-Purkinje system. The intrinsic rate of the SA node is 60 to 100 beats/min. The SA node is normally the primary pacemaker of the heart because it has the fastest firing rate of all of the heart's normal pacemaker sites (Figure 2-12). Other areas of the heart can assume pacemaker responsibility if:

- The SA node fails to fire (generate an impulse)
- The SA node fires too slowly
- The SA node fails to activate the surrounding atrial myocardium

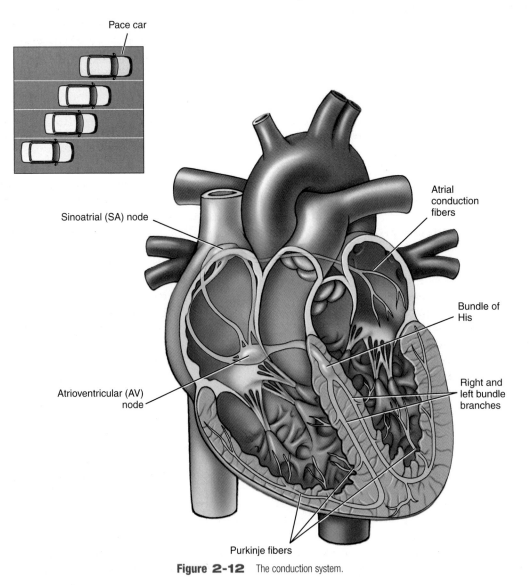

Figure 2-12   The conduction system.

The SA node is located in the upper posterior part of the right atrium where the superior vena cava and the right atrium meet. It lies less than 1 mm from the epicardial surface and is richly supplied by sympathetic and parasympathetic nerve fibers. Stimulation of sympathetic nerves will result in an increase in heart rate. The heart rate normally increases during exercise or stress. Stimulation of the vagus nerve will result in a decrease in heart rate. The heart rate normally slows during rest or sleep. The SA node receives its blood supply from the SA node artery that runs lengthwise through the center of the node. The SA node artery originates from the right coronary artery in about 60% of people and from the circumflex artery in the remaining 40%.

The fibers of the SA node directly connect with the fibers of the atria. As the impulse leaves the SA node, it is spread from cell to cell in wavelike form across the atrial muscle. As the impulse spreads, it stimulates the right atrium, the interatrial septum, and then the left atrium. This results in contraction of the right and left atria at almost the same time. It normally takes about 50 milliseconds for an impulse to travel from the SA node, through the atrial muscle, and down to the AV node. Because a fibrous skeleton separates the atrial myocardium from the ventricular myocardium, the electrical stimulus affects only the atria.

Conduction through the AV node begins before atrial depolarization is completed. The impulse is spread to the AV node by three internodal pathways. They have been identified as the anterior, middle, and posterior internodal pathways. These pathways consist of a mixture of working myocardial cells and specialized conducting fibers. The anterior internodal pathway (tract) is called Bachmann's bundle, the middle Wenckebach's bundle, and the posterior Thorel's pathway. Bachmann's bundle conducts impulses to the left atrium.

Atrioventricular Junction

The internodal pathways merge gradually with the cells of the AV node. Depolarization and repolarization are slow in the AV node, making this area vulnerable to blocks in conduction (AV blocks). The **AV junction** is the AV node and the nonbranching portion of the bundle of His (Figure 2-13). This area consists of specialized conduction tissue that provides the electrical links between the atria and ventricles. When the AV junction is bypassed by an abnormal pathway, the abnormal route is called an **accessory pathway**. An accessory pathway is an extra bundle of working myocardial tissue that forms a connection between the atria and ventricles outside the normal conduction system.

Atrioventricular Node

The **AV node** is a group of cells located in the floor of the right atrium immediately behind the tricuspid valve and near the opening of the coronary sinus. In an adult, the AV node is about 22 mm long, 10 mm wide, and 3 mm thick. The AV node is supplied by the right coronary artery in 85% to 90%

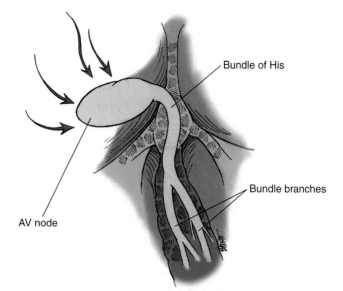

Figure 2-13   The AV junction consists of the AV node and the nonbranching portion of the bundle of His.

of the population. In the remainder, the circumflex artery provides the blood supply. The AV node is supplied by both sympathetic and parasympathetic nerve fibers.

As the impulse from the atria enters the AV node, there is a delay in conduction of the impulse to the ventricles. This delay occurs in part because the fibers in the AV junction are smaller than those of atrial muscle and have few gap junctions. If this delay did not occur, the atria and ventricles would contract at about the same time. The delay in conduction allows the atria to empty blood into the ventricles before the next ventricular contraction begins. This increases the amount of blood in the ventricles, increasing stroke volume.

The AV node has been divided into three functional regions according to their action potentials and responses to electrical and chemical stimulation (Figure 2-14):
- Atrionodal (AN) or upper junctional region (also called the transitional zone)
- Nodal (N) region, the midportion of the AV node
- Nodal-His (NH) or lower junctional region where the fibers of the AV node merge gradually with the bundle of His

The primary delay in the spread of the electrical impulse from the atria to the ventricles occurs in the AN and N areas of the AV node.

ECG Pearl

When atrial rates are very fast (as in atrial fibrillation), the AV node helps regulate the number of impulses reaching the ventricles to protect them from dangerously fast rates.

Bundle of His

The AV junction is the AV node (the upper portion of the AV junction) and the nonbranching portion of the **bundle of His** (the lower portion of the AV junction). The bundle of

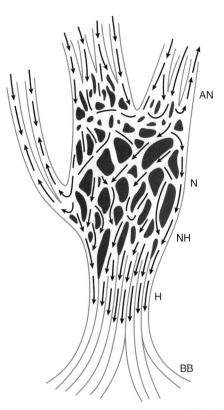

Figure 2-14 The AV junction. *AN,* atrionodal; *N,* nodal; *NH,* nodal-His; *H,* bundle of His; *BB,* bundle branches.

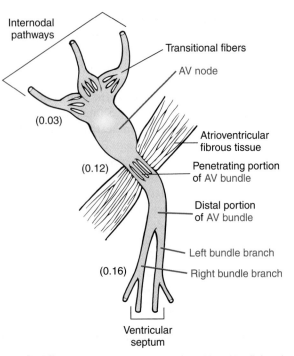

Figure 2-15 The AV node, bundle of His (AV bundle), and bundle branches. The numbers represent the time from the origin of an impulse in the SA node.

His is also called the common bundle or the atrioventricular bundle and is located in the upper portion of the interventricular septum. The AV junction has pacemaker cells capable of firing at a rate of 40 to 60 beats/min. The bundle of His conducts the electrical impulse to the right and left bundle branches (Figure 2-15).

The bundle of His receives a dual blood supply from branches of the left anterior and posterior descending coronary arteries. Because of this dual blood supply, the bundle of His is less vulnerable to ischemia. The term **His-Purkinje system** or His-Purkinje network refers to the bundle of His, bundle branches, and Purkinje fibers.

ECG Pearl

The speed of impulse conduction is fastest in the His-Purkinje system. It is slowest in the SA and AV nodes.

Right and Left Bundle Branches

The right bundle branch innervates the right ventricle. The left bundle branch spreads the electrical impulse to the interventricular septum and left ventricle, which is thicker and more muscular than the right ventricle. The left bundle branch divides into three divisions called **fascicles**. Fascicles are small bundles of nerve fibers. The three fascicles are called the anterior fascicle, posterior fascicle, and the septal fascicle. The anterior fascicle spreads the electrical impulse to the

anterior portions of the left ventricle. The posterior fascicle relays the impulse to the posterior portions of the left ventricle, and the septal fascicle relays the impulse to the midseptum.

Purkinje Fibers

The right and left bundle branches divide into smaller and smaller branches and then into a special network of fibers called the **Purkinje fibers**. These fibers spread from the interventricular septum into the papillary muscles. They continue downward to the apex of the heart, making up an elaborate web that penetrates about one third of the way into the ventricular muscle mass. The fibers then become continuous with the muscle cells of the right and left ventricles. The Purkinje fibers have pacemaker cells capable of firing at a rate of 20 to 40 beats/min (Table 2-1). The electrical impulse spreads rapidly through the right and left bundle branches and the Purkinje fibers to reach the ventricular muscle. The electrical impulse spreads from the endocardium to the myocardium, finally reaching the epicardial surface. The ventricular walls are stimulated to contract in a twisting motion that wrings blood out of the ventricular chambers and forces it into arteries.

TABLE **2-1** Normal Pacemaker Sites	
Pacemaker	**Beats/min**
SA node (primary pacemaker)	60-100
AV junction	40-60
Purkinje fibers	20-40

Figure 2-16 shows the sequence of activation through the conduction system. Remember that an electrical impulse precedes muscle contraction. As you can see in this figure, an impulse that begins in the SA node is not recorded on the ECG. However, the first upright waveform that you see (the P wave) shows the spread of that impulse throughout the atria (atrial depolarization). The AV node is stimulated at approximately the peak of the P wave. A summary of the conduction system is shown in Table 2-2. Figure 2-17 shows the time it takes for an impulse to reach different areas of the heart.

CAUSES OF DYSRHYTHMIAS

[OBJECTIVE 9]
Abnormal heart rhythms (dysrhythmias) are usually due to one of three basic mechanisms:
- Enhanced automaticity
- Triggered activity
- Reentry

Enhanced Automaticity

Enhanced automaticity is an abnormal condition in which one of the following occurs:

- Cardiac cells that are not normally associated with a pacemaker function begin to depolarize spontaneously *or*
- A pacemaker site other than the SA node increases its firing rate beyond that which is considered normal.

Possible reasons for enhanced automaticity are shown in Box 2-2. Examples of rhythms associated with enhanced automaticity include atrial flutter; atrial fibrillation; supraventricular tachycardia; premature atrial, junctional, or ventricular complexes; ventricular tachycardia or ventricular fibrillation; junctional tachycardia; accelerated idioventricular rhythm; and accelerated junctional rhythm.

Triggered Activity

Triggered activity results from abnormal electrical impulses that sometimes occur during repolarization, when cells are normally quiet. These abnormal electrical impulses are called afterdepolarizations. Triggered activity requires a stimulus to begin depolarization. It occurs when pacemaker cells from a site other than the SA node and myocardial working cells depolarize more than once after being stimulated by a single impulse.

Causes of triggered activity are shown in Box 2-3. Triggered activity can result in atrial or ventricular beats that

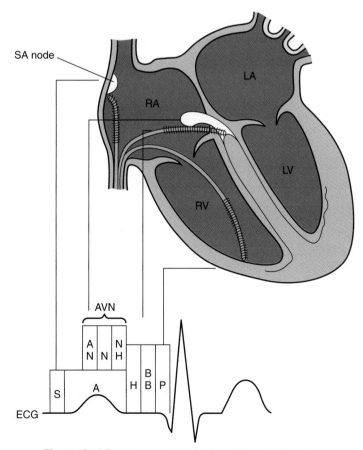

Figure 2-16 Sequence of activation through the conduction system.

TABLE **2-2**	Summary of the Conduction System			
Structure	**Location**	**Function**	**Intrinsic Pacemaker**	**Time Lapse from SA Node**
SA node	Right atrial wall just inferior to opening of superior vena cava	Primary pacemaker; initiates impulse that is normally conducted throughout the left and right atria	60-100 beats/min	0 sec
AV node	Floor of the right atrium immediately behind the tricuspid valve and near the opening of the coronary sinus	Receives impulse from SA node and delays relay of the impulse to the bundle of His, allowing time for the atria to empty their contents into the ventricles before the onset of ventricular contraction.		0.03 sec
Bundle of His	Superior portion of interventricular septum	Receives impulse from AV node and relays it to right and left bundle branches	40-60 beats/min	0.04 sec
Right and left bundle branches	Interventricular septum	Receives impulse from bundle of His and relays it to Purkinje fibers		0.17 sec
Purkinje fibers	Ventricular myocardium	Receives impulse from bundle branches and relays it to ventricular myocardium	20-40 beats/min	0.20-0.22 sec

occur alone, in pairs, in "runs" (three or more beats), or as a sustained ectopic rhythm. **Ectopic** refers to an impulse originating from a source other than the SA node. For example, an irritable site in the ventricles can produce episodic ventricular beats or a sustained, rapid rhythm such as ventricular tachycardia.

Reentry

[OBJECTIVE 10]
An impulse normally spreads through the heart only once after it is initiated by pacemaker cells. **Reentry** is the spread of an impulse through tissue already stimulated by that same impulse. An electrical impulse is delayed or blocked (or both) in one or more areas of the conduction system while

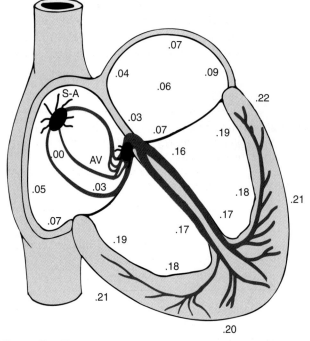

Figure 2-17 Transmission of the cardiac impulse through the heart showing the time of appearance (in fractions of a second) of the impulse in different parts of the heart.

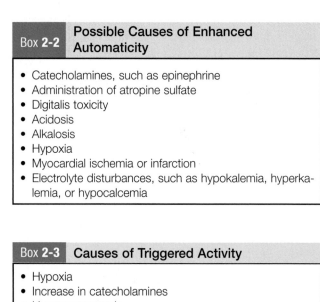

Box **2-2**	**Possible Causes of Enhanced Automaticity**

- Catecholamines, such as epinephrine
- Administration of atropine sulfate
- Digitalis toxicity
- Acidosis
- Alkalosis
- Hypoxia
- Myocardial ischemia or infarction
- Electrolyte disturbances, such as hypokalemia, hyperkalemia, or hypocalcemia

Box **2-3**	**Causes of Triggered Activity**

- Hypoxia
- Increase in catecholamines
- Hypomagnesemia
- Myocardial ischemia or injury
- Medications that prolong repolarization (such as quinidine)

the impulse is conducted normally through the rest of the conduction system. This results in the delayed electrical impulse entering cardiac cells that have just been depolarized by the normally conducted impulse. Reentry requires the following three conditions (Figure 2-18):

- A potential conduction circuit or circular conduction pathway
- A block within part of the circuit
- Delayed conduction with the remainder of the circuit

If the area the delayed impulse stimulates is relatively refractory, the impulse can cause depolarization of those cells, producing a single premature beat or repetitive electrical impulses. This can result in short periods of an abnormally fast heart rate. Common causes of reentry are shown in Box 2-4. Examples of rhythms associated with reentry are paroxysmal supraventricular tachycardia; ventricular tachycardia; and premature atrial, junctional, or ventricular complexes.

Escape Beats or Rhythms

Escape is the term used when the SA node slows down or fails to initiate depolarization, and a lower site spontaneously produces electrical impulses, assuming responsibility for pacing the heart. Escape beats or rhythms are protective mechanisms to maintain cardiac output. For example, the AV junction and ventricles are escape

Box **2-4**	Common Causes of Reentry

- Hyperkalemia
- Myocardial ischemia
- Some antiarrhythmic medications

pacemakers. If the SA node fails to fire, the escape pacemaker sites serve as a fail-safe mechanism to make sure another site steps in and assumes pacing responsibility. Examples of escape beats or rhythms include junctional escape beats, junctional rhythm, idioventricular rhythm (also known as a ventricular escape rhythm), and ventricular escape beats.

Conduction Disturbances

Conduction disturbances may occur because of trauma, drug toxicity, electrolyte disturbances, myocardial ischemia, or infarction. Conduction may be too rapid or too slow. Examples of rhythms associated with disturbances in conduction include AV blocks. AV blocks will be discussed in detail in Chapter 7.

THE ELECTROCARDIOGRAM

[OBJECTIVES 11, 12]

The electrocardiogram (ECG) records the electrical activity of a large mass of atrial and ventricular cells as specific waveforms and complexes. The electrical activity within the heart can be observed by means of electrodes connected by cables to an ECG machine. Think of the ECG as a voltmeter that records the electrical voltages (potentials) generated by depolarization of the heart's cells. The basic function of the ECG is to detect current flow as measured on the patient's skin.

ECG Pearl

The first ECG was introduced by Willem Einthoven, a Dutch physiologist, in the early 1900s. No matter how sophisticated the cardiac monitor, no matter how many additional features the monitor may include, the ECG is simply a display of the electrical activity recorded on the body's surface.

ECG monitoring may be used for the following purposes:

- Monitor a patient's heart rate
- Evaluate the effects of disease or injury on heart function
- Evaluate pacemaker function
- Evaluate the response to medications (such as antiarrhythmics)
- Obtain a baseline recording before, during, and after a medical procedure

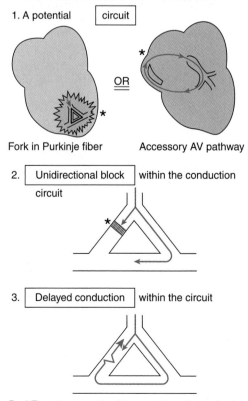

CONDITIONS REQUIRED FOR REENTRY

1. A potential circuit

OR

Fork in Purkinje fiber   Accessory AV pathway

2. Unidirectional block within the conduction circuit

3. Delayed conduction within the circuit

Figure 2-18   Reentry requires (1) a potential conduction circuit or circular conduction pathway, (2) a block within part of the circuit, and (3) delayed conduction with the remainder of the circuit.

The ECG *can* provide information about the following:
- The orientation of the heart in the chest
- Conduction disturbances
- Electrical effects of medications and electrolytes
- The mass of cardiac muscle
- The presence of ischemic damage

The ECG does *not* provide information about the mechanical (contractile) condition of the myocardium. To evaluate the effectiveness of the heart's mechanical activity, the patient's pulse and blood pressure are assessed.

ECG Pearl

A standard ECG does not directly record the activity of the heart's electrical system. These structures are too small to produce detectable voltage on the body surface. What you see on the ECG is the activation and recovery of the working cells of the heart.[5] It *is* possible to record signals from the heart's electrical system. However, this requires the use of specialized equipment, signal-averaging techniques, or the use of recording electrodes placed in the heart.

Electrodes

Electrode refers to the paper, plastic, or metal device that contains conductive media and is applied to the patient's skin. Electrodes are applied at specific locations on the patient's chest wall and extremities to view the heart's electrical activity from different angles and planes.

Three types of electrodes used for surface (skin) electrocardiography are the metal disk, metal suction cup, and the disposable disk. Disposable disk electrodes consist of an adhesive ring with a conductive substance in the center. The conductive media of the electrode conducts skin surface voltage changes through wires to a cardiac monitor. To minimize distortion (artifact), be sure the conductive jelly in the center of the electrode is not dry, and avoid placing the electrodes directly over bony areas (Skill 2-1).

One end of a monitoring cable is attached to the electrode and the other end to an ECG machine. The cable is a wire that attaches to the electrode and conducts current back to the cardiac monitor. Do not rely on the color-coding of ECG cables. Colors are not standard and often vary.

It is desirable to remove oil and dead cells from the patient's skin before applying electrodes. Skin oil and dead cells may be removed by a variety of techniques. For some time alcohol swabs were used for this purpose. The alcohol helped remove the oil, while a brisk rub with the swab eliminated some of the dead cells. However, while the alcohol works to remove the skin oil, it further dries out the skin. Therefore, most electrode manufacturers recommend NOT using alcohol. A brisk dry rub of the skin should be used instead. Many electrode manufacturers include an abrasive area on the disposable backing of the electrode for this purpose, but a gauze sponge works well, too. Specific skin prep tools are also commercially available. In some circumstances, small areas may need to be shaved or chest hair cut if the electrode(s) will not stick.

Leads

[OBJECTIVES 13, 14, 15]

A **lead** is a record (tracing) of electrical activity between two electrodes. Each lead records the *average* current flow at a specific time in a portion of the heart. Leads allow

---

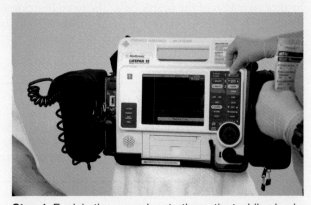

Step 1 Explain the procedure to the patient while checking your equipment. Make sure there are no loose pins in the end of the ECG cable and no frayed or broken cable or lead wires. Make sure the monitor has an adequate paper supply. Connect the ECG cable to the machine. Connect the lead wires to the ECG cable (if not already connected). Turn the power on to the monitor. Adjust the contrast on the screen if necessary.

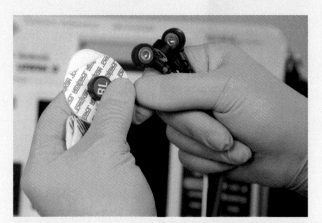

Step 2 Open a package of ECG electrodes. Make sure the electrode gel in the electrodes to be used is moist. Attach an electrode to each lead wire.

SKILL 2-1 ECG Monitoring—cont'd

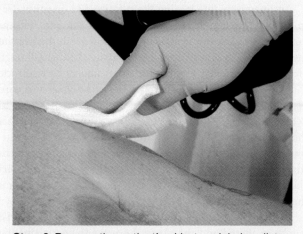

Step 3 Prepare the patient's skin to minimize distortion of the ECG tracing. Do this by briskly rubbing the skin with a dry gauze pad. Do not use alcohol, tincture of benzoin, or antiperspirant when prepping the skin. If electrodes will be applied to the patient's chest instead of limbs, shave small amounts of chest hair if needed before applying electrodes to ensure good contact.

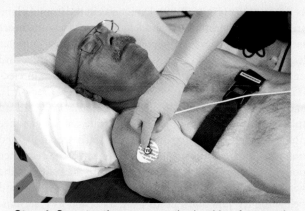

Step 4 One at a time, remove the backing from each electrode and apply them to the patient. Limb lead electrodes usually are placed on the wrists and ankles but may be positioned anywhere on the appropriate limb. To reduce muscle tension, make sure the patient's limbs are resting on a supportive surface. Do not apply electrodes over bony areas, broken skin, joints, skin creases, scar tissue, burns, or rashes. Connect the lead wires to the electrodes.

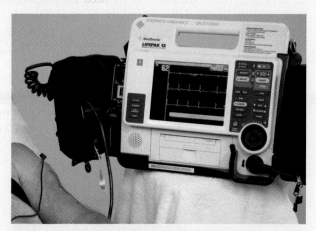

Step 5 Coach the patient to relax. Select the desired lead on the cardiac monitor. Adjust the ECG size if necessary. If the ECG size is set too low, the monitor will not detect QRS complexes and the heart rate display will be incorrect. Feel the patient's pulse and compare it with the heart rate indicator on the monitor. If not already preset, set the heart rate alarms on the monitor according to your agency's policy.

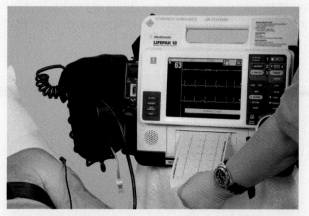

Step 6 Select the print or record button to obtain a copy of the patient's ECG. Interpret the ECG rhythm. Assess the patient to find out how he is tolerating the rate and rhythm. Attach the rhythm strip to the patient's hospital record or prehospital care report. Continue patient care.

viewing the heart's electrical activity in two different planes: frontal (coronal) and horizontal (transverse). A 12-lead ECG provides views of the heart in both the frontal and horizontal planes and views the surfaces of the left ventricle from 12 different angles. From this, ischemia, injury, and infarction affecting any area of the heart can be identified.

ECG Pearl

In this text, the word lead is used in two ways. Lead refers to both the actual tracing obtained and the position of the electrode. For example, the term "V_1 position" represents its proper location on the chest wall, while "lead V_1" refers to the tracing obtained from that position.[6]

Frontal Plane Leads

Frontal plane leads view the heart from the front of the body as if it were flat (Figure 2-19). Directions in the frontal plane are superior, inferior, right, and left. Six leads view the heart in the frontal plane: three bipolar leads and three unipolar leads. A **bipolar lead** is an ECG lead that has a positive and negative electrode. Each lead records the difference in electrical potential between two selected electrodes. Leads I, II, and III are called *standard limb leads* or *bipolar leads*. A lead that consists of a single positive electrode and a reference point is called a **unipolar lead**. These leads are also called *unipolar limb leads* or *augmented limb leads*. The reference point (with zero electrical potential) lies in the center of the heart's electrical field (left of the interventricular septum and below the AV junction). Leads aVR, aVL, and aVF are unipolar or augmented limb leads.

Standard Limb Leads

Leads I, II, and III make up the standard limb leads. If an electrode is placed on the right arm, left arm, and left leg, three leads are formed. Since each of these three leads has a distinct negative pole and a distinct positive pole; they are considered bipolar. The positive electrode is located at the left wrist in lead I, while leads II and III both have their positive electrode located at the left foot. The difference in electrical potential between the positive

pole and its corresponding negative pole is measured by each lead.

An imaginary line joining the positive and negative electrodes of a lead is called the **axis** of the lead. The axes of these three limb leads form an equilateral triangle with the heart at the center (Einthoven's triangle) (Figure 2-20). Although placement of the left leg electrode may appear to make the triangle out of balance, it is nevertheless an equilateral triangle because all electrodes are about equidistant from the electrical field of the heart.[2] Einthoven's triangle is a way of showing that the two arms and the left leg form apices of a triangle surrounding the heart. The two apices at the upper part of the triangle represent the points at which the two arms connect electrically with the fluids around the heart. The lower apex is the point at which the left leg connects with the fluids.[3]

Over the years, electrode placement for leads I, II, and III has been altered and moved to the patient's chest. This has been done to allow for patient movement and to minimize distortion on the ECG tracing. However, proper electrode positioning for these leads includes placement on the patient's extremities. Where the electrodes are placed on the extremity does not matter as long as bony areas are avoided.

Lead I records the difference in electrical potential between the left arm (+) and right arm (−) electrodes. The positive electrode is placed on the left arm and the negative electrode is placed on the right arm. The third electrode is a ground that minimizes electrical activity from other sources (Figure 2-21, *A*). Lead I views the lateral surface of the left ventricle.

Lead II records the difference in electrical potential between the left leg (+) and right arm (−) electrodes. The positive electrode is placed on the left leg and the negative electrode is placed on the right arm (Figure 2-21, *B*). Lead II views the

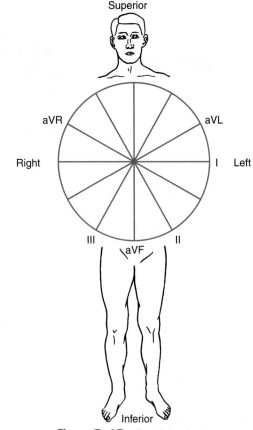

Figure 2-19 Frontal plane leads.

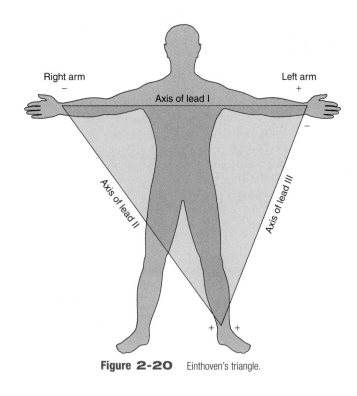

Figure 2-20 Einthoven's triangle.

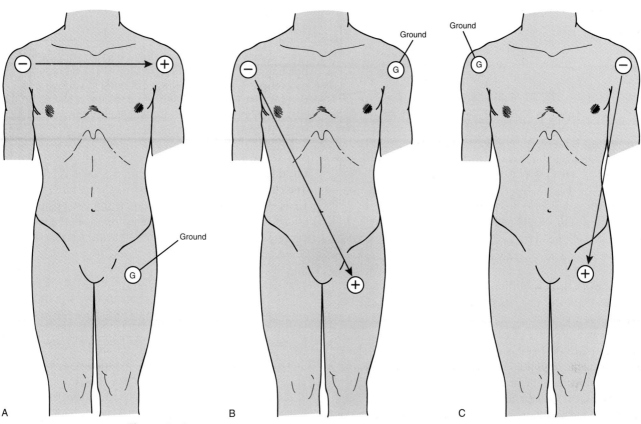

Figure 2-21 Electrode placement on the patient's limbs for **A,** Lead I. **B,** Lead II. and **C,** Lead III.

inferior surface of the left ventricle. This lead is commonly used for cardiac monitoring because positioning of the positive and negative electrodes in this lead most closely resembles the normal pathway of current flow in the heart.

Lead III records the difference in electrical potential between the left leg (+) and left arm (−) electrodes. In lead III the positive electrode is placed on the left leg and the negative electrode is placed on the left arm (Figure 2-21, C). Lead III views the inferior surface of the left ventricle. A summary of the standard limb leads can be found in Table 2-3.

ECG Pearl

Leads I, II, III, aVR, aVL, and aVF are obtained from electrodes placed on the patient's arms and legs. The deltoid area is suitable for electrodes attached to the arms and is easily accessed. Either the thigh or lower leg is suitable for the leg electrodes. Use the more convenient site, but keep the leads in a similar position. For example, keep the upper extremity electrodes on the deltoids—not one on the upper arm and one on the inner arm. Be sure that the patient's limbs are resting on a supportive surface. This decreases muscle tension in the patient's arms and legs and helps minimize distortion of the ECG tracing (artifact). Should circumstances require that the leads be placed on the torso, be certain to position them as close to the appropriate limb as possible.

TABLE 2-3	Standard Limb Leads		
Lead	Positive Electrode	Negative Electrode	Heart Surface Viewed
I	Left arm	Right arm	Lateral
II	Left leg	Right arm	Inferior
III	Left leg	Left arm	Inferior

Augmented Limb Leads

Leads aVR, aVL, and aVF are augmented limb leads. The electrical potential produced by the augmented leads is normally relatively small. The ECG machine augments (magnifies) the amplitude of the electrical potentials detected at each extremity by about 50% over those recorded at the bipolar leads. The "a" in aVR, aVL, and aVF refers to augmented. The "V" refers to voltage. The "R" refers to right arm, the "L" to left arm, and the "F" to left foot (leg). Therefore, the positive electrode in aVR is located on the right arm, aVL has a positive electrode at the left arm, and aVF has a positive electrode positioned on the left leg (Figure 2-22).

While leads aVR, aVL, and aVF have a distinct positive pole, they do not have a distinct negative pole. Since they have only one true pole, they are referred to as unipolar

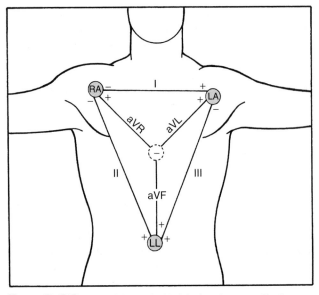

Figure 2-22   View of the standard limb leads and augmented leads.

 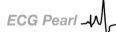

While it may not be immediately obvious, your patient's position can have an effect on the ECG. One reason for differences between tracings obtained in various positions is that while the electrode does not move when the patient changes position, the position of the heart does move relative to that electrode.[6]

Chest Leads

The chest leads are identified as V_1, V_2, V_3, V_4, V_5, and V_6. Each electrode placed in a "V" position is a positive electrode. The negative electrode is found at the electrical center of the heart. Thus the chest leads are also unipolar leads.

ECG Pearl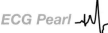

Because their location varies, do not use the nipples as landmarks for chest electrode placement. If your patient is a woman, place the electrodes for leads V_3-V_6 *under* the breast, rather than on the breast.

leads. In place of a single negative pole these leads have multiple negative poles, creating a negative field (central terminal), of which the heart is at the center. Theoretically, this makes the heart the negative electrode.[6] The augmented voltage leads are not the only unipolar leads in the standard 12-lead ECG. The chest leads, discussed in the next section, are also unipolar.

Lead aVR views the heart from the right shoulder (the positive electrode) and views the base of the heart (primarily the atria and the great vessels). This lead does not view any wall of the heart. Lead aVL combines views from the right arm and left leg (using the heart as a central terminal), with the "view" being from the left arm and oriented to the lateral wall of the left ventricle. Lead aVF combines views from the right arm and left arm toward the left leg, viewing the inferior surface of the left ventricle from the left leg. A summary of augmented leads can be found in Table 2-4.

Horizontal Plane Leads

Horizontal plane leads view the heart as if the body were sliced in half horizontally. Directions in the horizontal plane are anterior, posterior, right, and left. Six chest (precordial or "V") leads view the heart in the horizontal plane (Figure 2-23). This allows a view of the front and left side of the heart.

Lead V_1 is recorded with the positive electrode in the fourth intercostal space, just to the right of the sternum. Lead V_2 is recorded with the positive electrode in the fourth intercostal space, just to the left of the sternum. Lead V_3 is recorded with the positive electrode on a line midway between V_2 and V_4. Lead V_4 is recorded with the

TABLE 2-4	Augmented Leads	
Lead	**Positive Electrode**	**Heart Surface Viewed**
aVR	Right arm	None
aVL	Left arm	Lateral
aVF	Left leg	Inferior

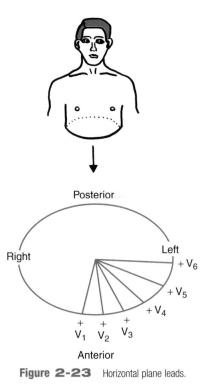

Figure 2-23   Horizontal plane leads.

positive electrode in the left midclavicular line in the fifth intercostal space. If a right ventricular myocardial infarction is suspected, lead V_4 may be moved to the same anatomic location but on the right side of the chest. The lead is then called V_4R and is viewed for ECG changes consistent with acute MI. Lead V_5 is recorded with the positive electrode in the left anterior axillary line at the same level as V_4. Lead V_6 is recorded with the positive electrode in the left midaxillary line at the same level as V_4. A summary of the chest leads can be found in Table 2-5. Skill 2-2 shows chest lead placement.

ECG Pearl

All of the electrode positions refer to the location of the gel. For example, the gel of the V_1 electrode, not the entire adhesive patch, is positioned in the fourth intercostal space, just to the right of the sternum.[6]

Right Chest Leads Other chest leads that are not part of a standard 12-lead ECG may be used to view specific surfaces of the heart. When a right ventricular myocardial infarction is suspected, right chest leads are used (Figure 2-24). Placement of right chest leads is identical to placement of the standard chest leads except it is done on the right side of the chest. If time does not permit obtaining all of the right chest leads, the lead of choice is V_4R. A summary of the right chest leads can be found in Table 2-6. Skill 2-3 shows placement of the right chest leads.

Posterior Chest Leads On a standard 12-lead ECG, no leads look directly at the posterior surface of the heart. Additional chest leads may be used for this purpose. These leads are placed further left and toward the back. All of the leads are placed on the same horizontal line as V_4 to V_6. Lead V_7 is placed at the posterior axillary line. Lead V_8 is placed at the angle of the scapula (posterior scapular line) and lead V_9 is placed over the left border of spine. Skill 2-4 shows placement of the posterior chest leads.

ECG Pearl

Fifteen- and 18-lead ECGs are being used with increasing frequency to help spot infarctions of the right ventricle and the posterior wall of the left ventricle. The 15-lead ECG uses all leads of a standard 12-lead plus leads V_4R, V_8, and V_9. An 18-lead ECG uses the 15-lead ECG plus leads V_5R, V_6R, and V_7.

Modified Chest Leads The modified chest leads (MCL) are bipolar chest leads that are variations of the unipolar chest leads. Each modified chest lead consists of a positive and negative electrode applied to a specific location on the chest. Accurate placement of the positive electrode is important. The modified chest leads are useful in detecting bundle branch blocks, differentiating right and left premature beats, and differentiating supraventricular tachycardia from ventricular tachycardia.

Lead MCL_1 is a variation of the chest lead V_1 and views the ventricular septum. The negative electrode is placed below the left clavicle toward the left shoulder, and the positive electrode is placed to the right of the sternum in the fourth intercostal space (Figure 2-25, A). In this lead the positive electrode is in a position to the right of the left ventricle. Because the primary wave of depolarization is directed toward the left ventricle, the QRS complex recorded in this lead will normally appear negative (Figure 2-25, B).

Lead MCL_6 is a variation of the chest lead V_6 and views the low lateral wall of the left ventricle. The negative electrode is placed below the left clavicle toward the left shoulder and the positive electrode is placed at the fifth intercostal space, left midaxillary line. An example of a typical ECG tracing recorded in this lead is shown in Figure 2-25, C.

ECG Pearl

Leads MCL_1 and V_1 are similar but not identical. In V_1, the negative electrode is calculated by the ECG machine at the center of the heart. In MCL_1, the negative electrode is located just below the left clavicle.[6]

What Each Lead "Sees"

Think of the positive electrode as an eye looking in at the heart. The part of the heart that each lead "sees" is determined by two factors. The first factor is the dominance of the left ventricle on the ECG and the second is the position of the positive electrode on the body. Because the ECG does not directly measure the heart's electrical activity, it does not "see" all of the current flowing through the heart. What the ECG sees from its vantage point on the body's surface is the net result of countless individual currents competing in a tug-of-war. For example, the QRS complex, which represents ventricular depolarization, is not a display of all the electrical

TABLE 2-5	Chest Leads	
Lead	Positive Electrode Position	Heart Surface Viewed
V_1	Right side of sternum, fourth intercostal space	Septum
V_2	Left side of sternum, fourth intercostal space	Septum
V_3	Midway between V_2 and V_4	Anterior
V_4	Left midclavicular line, fifth intercostal space	Anterior
V_5	Left anterior axillary line at same level as V_4	Lateral
V_6	Left midaxillary line at same level as V_4	Lateral

SKILL 2-2   **Chest Lead Placement**

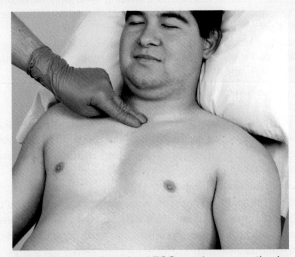

Step 1 An accurate 12-lead ECG requires correctly placing the electrodes. Begin positioning of the chest leads by placing your finger at the notch at the top of the sternum.

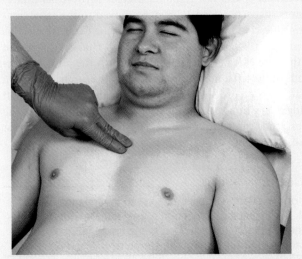

Step 2 Move your finger slowly downward until you feel a slight horizontal ridge or elevation. This is the angle of Louis (sternal angle), where the manubrium joins the body of the sternum.

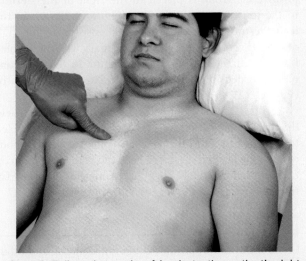

Step 3 Follow the angle of Louis to the patient's right until it articulates with the second rib.

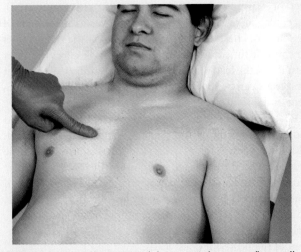

Step 4 Locate the second intercostal space (immediately below the second rib).

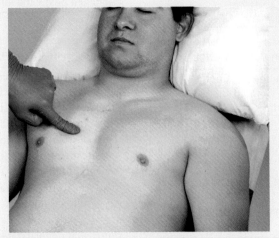

Step 5 From the second intercostal space, the third and fourth intercostal spaces can be found.

SKILL **2-2** Chest Lead Placement—cont'd

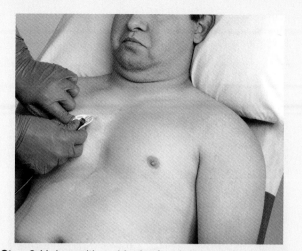

Step 6 V₁ is positioned in the fourth intercostal space just to the right of the sternum. Note: All the electrode positions refer to the location of the gel. For example, the gel of the V₁ electrode, not the entire adhesive patch, is positioned in the fourth intercostal space, just to the right of the sternum.

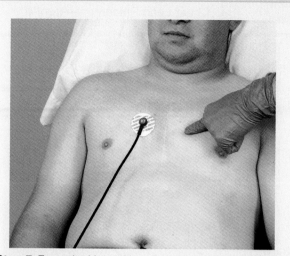

Step 7 From the V₁ position, find the corresponding intercostal space on the left side of the sternum.

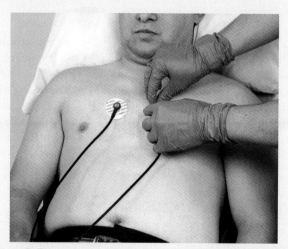

Step 8 Place the V₂ electrode in the fourth intercostal space just to the left of the sternum.

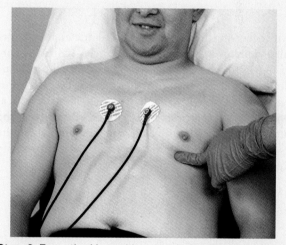

Step 9 From the V₂ position, locate the fifth intercostal space and follow it to the midclavicular line.

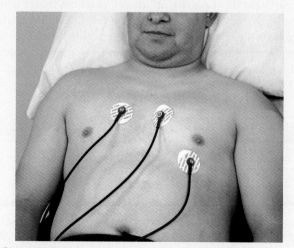

Step 10 Position the V₄ electrode in the fifth intercostal space in the midclavicular line.

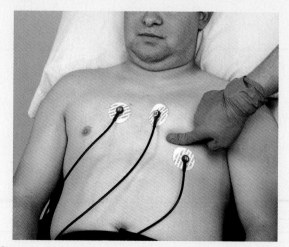

Step 11 V₃ is positioned halfway between V₂ and V₄.

(Continued)

SKILL 2-2 **Chest Lead Placement—cont'd**

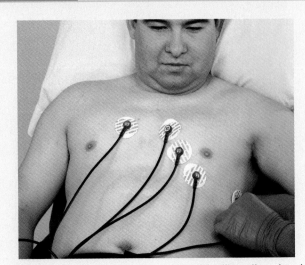

Step 12 V$_6$ is positioned in the midaxillary line, level with V$_4$.

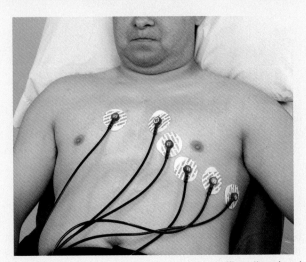

Step 13 V$_5$ is positioned in the anterior axillary line, level with V$_4$.

activity occurring in the right and left ventricles. It is the net result of a tug-of-war produced by the many individual currents in both the right and left ventricles. Since the left ventricle is much larger than the right, the left overpowers it. What is seen in the QRS complex is the additional electrical activity of the left ventricle (i.e., the portion that exceeds the right ventricle). Therefore, in a normally conducted beat, the QRS complex primarily represents the electrical activity occurring in the left ventricle.

The second factor, position of the positive electrode on the body, determines which portion of the left ventricle is seen by each lead. You can commit the view of each lead to memory, or you can easily reason it by remembering where the positive electrode is located. The view of each lead is listed in Table 2-7, while Figure 2-26 demonstrates the portion of the left ventricle that each lead views. Please note that aVR is not included in Table 2-7 or Figure 2-26.

ELECTROCARDIOGRAM PAPER

[OBJECTIVES 16, 17]
Remember that the ECG is a graphical representation of the heart's electrical activity. When you place electrodes on the patient's body and connect them to an ECG, the machine records the voltage (potential difference) between the electrodes. The needle (or pen) of the ECG moves a specific distance depending on the voltage measured. This recording is made on ECG paper.

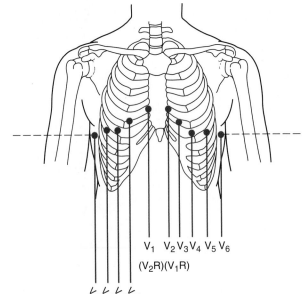

Figure 2-24 Anatomic placement of the left and right chest leads.

TABLE 2-6	Right Chest Leads and Their Placement
Lead	**Placement**
V$_1$R	Lead V$_2$
V$_2$R	Lead V$_1$
V$_3$R	Midway between V$_2$R and V$_4$R
V$_4$R	Right midclavicular line, fifth intercostal space
V$_5$R	Right anterior axillary line at same level as V$_4$R
V$_6$R	Right midaxillary line at same level as V$_4$R

SKILL 2-3   Right Chest Lead Placement

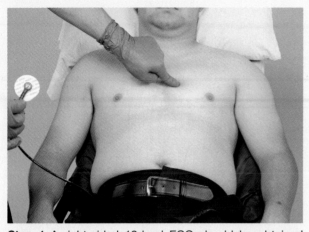

Step 1 A right-sided 12-lead ECG should be obtained when a right ventricular infarction is suspected. Placement of right chest leads is identical to placement of the standard chest leads except it is done on the right side of the chest. When obtaining right-sided and/or posterior leads, obtain a standard 12-lead first. Then move the cables for the standard chest leads to the electrodes for the additional leads. Any chest lead cable can be moved to obtain the right and/or posterior leads. Begin by placing the electrode for V_1R in the fourth intercostal space, just to the left of the sternum.

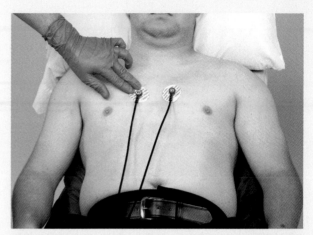

Step 2 From the V_1R position, find the corresponding intercostal space on the right side of the sternum. This is V_2R. Place the V_2R electrode in the fourth intercostal space, just to the right of the sternum.

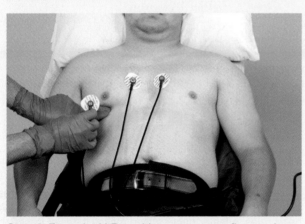

Step 3 From the V_2R position, move your fingers down, find the fifth intercostal space, and follow it to the midclavicular line. Place the V_4R electrode in the fifth intercostal space in the midclavicular line.

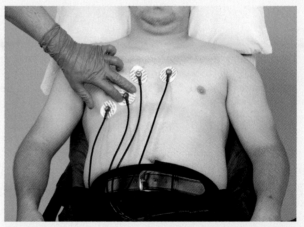

Step 4 Imagine a line between V_2R and V_4R. Position the V_3R electrode halfway between V_2R and V_4R on the imaginary line.

(Continued)

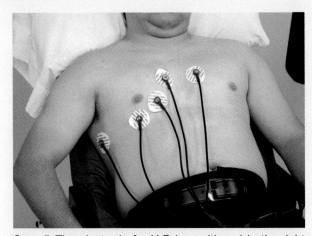

Step 5 The electrode for V₆R is positioned in the right midaxillary line, level with V₄R.

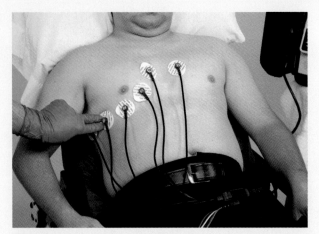

Step 6 Position V₅R in the right anterior axillary line, level with V₄R.

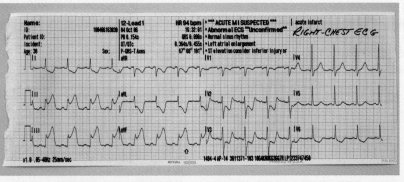

Step 7 Once these leads are printed, the correct lead must be handwritten onto the ECG to indicate the origin of the tracing. Clearly label the upper portion of the ECG tracing "right chest ECG." The computer-generated interpretation also must be disregarded in the event that the cables have been moved.

ECG paper is graph paper made up of small and large boxes measured in millimeters. The smallest boxes are 1 mm wide and 1 mm high (Figure 2-27, see p. 55). The horizontal axis of the paper corresponds with *time*. Time is used to measure the interval between or duration of specific cardiac events. Time is stated in seconds.

ECG paper normally records at a constant speed of 25 mm/sec. Thus each horizontal 1-mm box represents 0.04 second (25 mm/sec × 0.04 sec = 1 mm). Look closely at the boxes in Figure 2-27. You can see that the lines after every five small boxes on the paper are heavier. The heavier lines indicate one large box. Because each large box is the width of five small boxes, a large box represents 0.20 seconds. Five large boxes, each consisting of five small boxes, represent 1 second. Fifteen large boxes equal an interval of 3 seconds. Thirty large boxes represent 6 seconds.

The vertical axis of the ECG paper measures the *voltage* or *amplitude* of a waveform. Voltage is measured in millivolts (mV). Voltage may be a positive or negative value. Amplitude is measured in millimeters (mm). The ECG machine's sensitivity must be calibrated so that a 1-mV

ECG Pearl

The rate at which ECG paper goes through the printer is adjustable. A faster paper speed makes the rhythm appear slower and the QRS complex wider. Thus in cases of rapid heart rates, a faster paper speed makes it easier to see the waveforms and analyze the rhythm. A slower paper speed makes the rhythm appear faster and the QRS narrower.[6]

electrical signal will produce a deflection measuring exactly 10 mm tall (Figure 2-28). When properly calibrated, a small box is 1 mm high (0.1 mV), and a large box (equal to five small boxes) is 5 mm high (0.5 mV). Clinically, the height of a waveform is usually stated in millimeters, not millivolts.

Waveforms

[OBJECTIVE 18]

A **waveform** (deflection) is movement away from the baseline in a positive (upward) or negative (downward) direction (Box 2-5). Each waveform that you see on an

SKILL 2-4   Posterior Chest Lead Placement

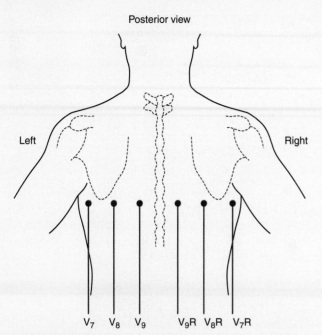

Posterior view

Left   Right

V₇   V₈   V₉   V₉R V₈R V₇R

Step 1 Posterior chest leads are used when a posterior infarction is suspected. First obtain and print a standard 12-lead ECG. Then locate the landmarks for the posterior leads: posterior axillary line, midscapular line, and left border of the spine. Leads V₇, V₈, and V₉ are on the same horizontal line as leads V₄, V₅, and V₆ on the front of the chest.

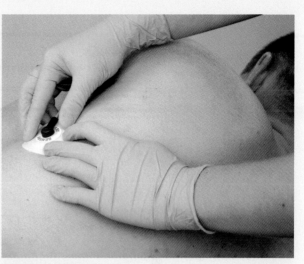

Step 2 Position the patient on his or her side. Find the posterior axillary line. Now locate the fifth intercostal space and place the V₇ electrode. Attach the V₄ lead wire to the V₇ electrode.

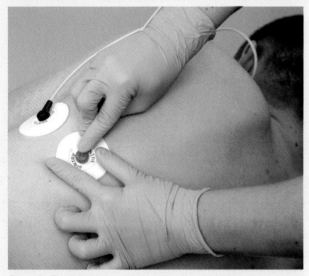

Step 3 Find the left midscapular line and fifth intercostal space. Place the V₈ electrode here. Attach the V₅ lead wire to the V₈ electrode.

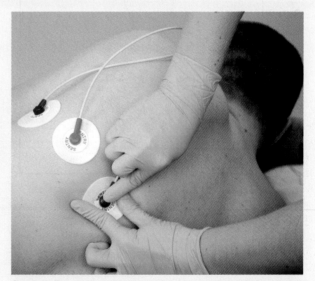

Step 4 Place the electrode for V₉ just left of the spinal column at the fifth intercostal space. Attach the V₆ lead wire to the V₉ electrode.

(Continued)

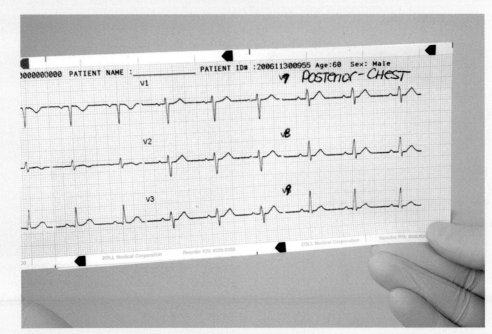

Step 5 Obtain and print the 12-lead ECG. Clearly label the upper portion of the ECG tracing "posterior chest ECG." Remember to relabel lead V_4 on the printout V_7, relabel V_5 to V_8, and V_6 to V_9.

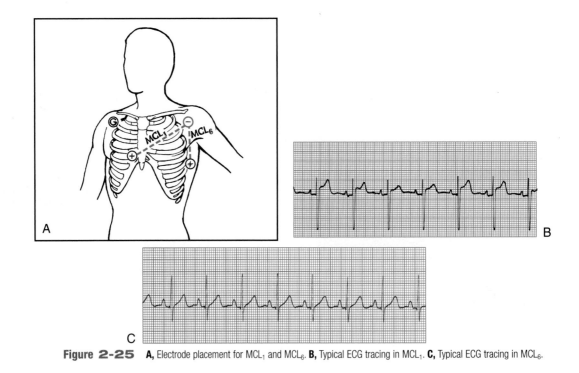

Figure 2-25   A, Electrode placement for MCL_1 and MCL_6. **B,** Typical ECG tracing in MCL_1. **C,** Typical ECG tracing in MCL_6.

ECG is related to a specific electrical event in the heart. Waveforms are named alphabetically, beginning with P, QRS, T, and U. When electrical activity is not detected, a straight line is recorded. This line is called the **baseline** or **isoelectric line**. If the wave of depolarization (electrical impulse) moves toward the positive electrode, the waveform recorded on ECG graph paper will be upright (positive deflection). If the wave of depolarization

TABLE 2-7	What Each Lead "Sees"
Leads	**Heart Surface Viewed**
II, III, aVF	Inferior
V_1, V_2	Septal
V_3, V_4	Anterior
I, aVL, V_5, V_6	Lateral

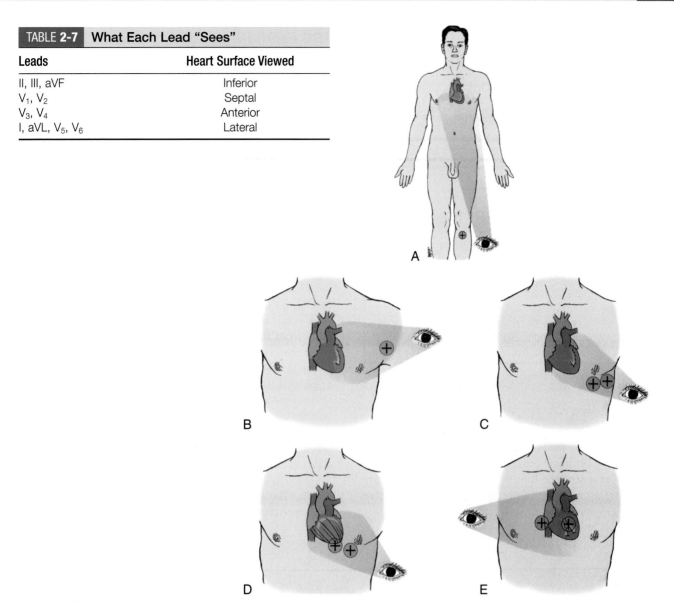

Figure 2-26 **A,** Leads II, III, and aVF each have their positive electrode positioned on the left leg. From the perspective of the left leg, each of them "sees" the inferior wall of the left ventricle. **B,** From their vantage point on the left arm, leads I and aVL "look" in at the lateral wall of the left ventricle. **C,** Leads V_5 and V_6 also "view" the lateral wall because they are positioned on the axillary area of the left chest. **D,** Leads V_3 and V_4 are positioned in the area of the anterior chest. From this perspective, these leads "see" the anterior wall of the left ventricle. **E,** The septal wall is "seen" by leads V_1 and V_2, which are positioned next to the sternum.

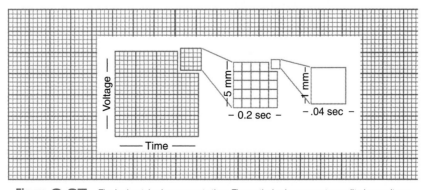

Figure 2-27 The horizontal axis represents time. The vertical axis represents amplitude or voltage.

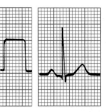

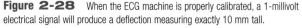

Figure 2-28   When the ECG machine is properly calibrated, a 1-millivolt electrical signal will produce a deflection measuring exactly 10 mm tall.

Box **2-5**	Terminology

Baseline (isoelectric line): A straight line recorded when electrical activity is not detected
Waveform: Movement away from the baseline in either a positive or negative direction
Segment: A line between waveforms; named by the waveform that precedes or follows it
Interval: A waveform and a segment
Complex: Several waveforms

moves away from the positive electrode, the waveform recorded will be inverted (downward or negative deflection). A **biphasic** (partly positive, partly negative) waveform or a straight line is recorded when the wave of depolarization moves perpendicularly to the positive electrode (Figure 2-29).

ECG Pearl

Possible Causes of Low Amplitude Waveforms
- Normal variant
- Obesity
- Emphysema
- Extensive myocardial infarction
- Pericardial effusion
- Pleural effusion
- Hypothyroidism
- Gain or lead selection on the cardiac monitor

P Wave

Remember that activation of the SA node occurs before the onset of the P wave. This event is not recorded on the ECG. However, the spread of that impulse throughout the atria (atrial depolarization) is observed. The first waveform in the cardiac cycle is the *P wave* (Box 2-6). The beginning of the P wave is recognized as the first abrupt or gradual movement away from the baseline; its end is the point at which the waveform returns to the baseline (Figure 2-30). The first half of the P wave is recorded when the electrical impulse that originated in the SA node stimulates the right atrium and reaches the AV node. The downslope of the P wave reflects stimulation of the left atrium. Thus the P wave represents atrial depolarization and the spread of the electrical impulse throughout the right and left atria. A P wave normally precedes each QRS complex.

The atria contract a fraction of a second after the P wave begins. The atria begin to repolarize at the same time as the ventricles depolarize. A waveform representing atrial

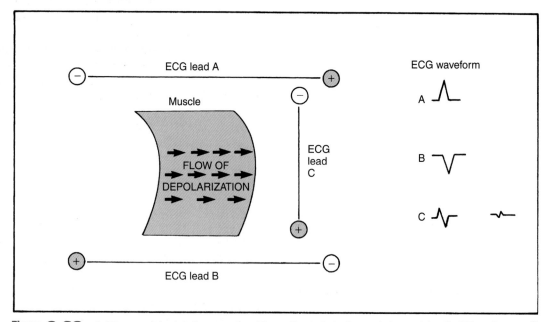

Figure 2-29   **A,** If the wave of depolarization moves toward the *positive* electrode, the waveform recorded on the ECG graph paper will be upright. **B,** If the wave of depolarization moves toward the *negative* electrode, the waveform produced will be inverted. **C,** A biphasic (partly positive, partly negative) waveform or a straight line is recorded when the wave of depolarization moves perpendicularly to the positive electrode.

Box 2-6 Normal Characteristics of the P Wave

- Smooth and rounded
- No more than 2.5 mm in height
- No more than 0.11 second in duration
- Positive in leads I, II, aVF, and V_2 through V_6

repolarization is usually not seen on the ECG because it is small and buried in the QRS complex.

Tall and pointed (peaked) or wide and notched P waves may be seen in conditions such as chronic obstructive pulmonary disease (COPD), congestive heart failure (CHF), or in valvular disease and may be indicative of atrial enlargement

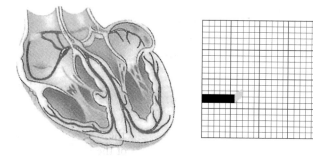

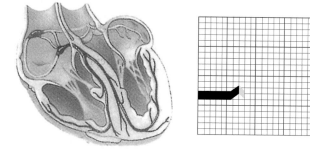

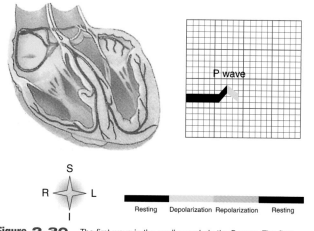

Figure 2-30 The first wave in the cardiac cycle is the P wave. The first half of the P wave reflects stimulation of the right atrium. The downslope of the P wave reflects stimulation of the left atrium.

(Figure 2-31). Enlargement of the right atrium produces an abnormally tall initial part of the P wave. The latter part of the P wave is prominent in left atrial enlargement.

P waves that begin at a site other than the SA node (ectopic P waves) may be positive or negative in lead II. If the ectopic pacemaker is in the atria, the P wave will be upright. If the ectopic pacemaker is in the AV junction, the P wave will be negative (inverted) in lead II.

QRS Complex
[OBJECTIVE 19]

A **complex** consists of several waveforms. The QRS complex consists of the Q wave, R wave, and S wave. It represents the spread of the electrical impulse through the ventricles (ventricular depolarization) (Figure 2-32). Ventricular depolarization normally triggers contraction of ventricular tissue. Thus, shortly after the QRS complex begins, the ventricles contract. The QRS complex is significantly larger than the P wave because depolarization of the ventricles involves a considerably greater muscle mass than depolarization of the atria. Atrial repolarization usually takes place during ventricular depolarization, but the QRS complex overshadows it on the ECG.

A QRS complex normally follows each P wave. One or even two of the three waveforms that make up the QRS complex may not always be present. The QRS complex begins as a downward deflection, the Q wave. A Q wave is **always** a negative waveform. The Q wave begins when the ECG leaves the isoelectric line in a downward direction and continues until it returns to the isoelectric line. The Q wave represents depolarization of the interventricular septum, which is activated from left to right. In lead II, the direction of the current flow is almost perpendicular to it, and more current is moving away from the positive electrode than is moving toward it. In lead MCL_1, depolarization of the interventricular septum will appear as a small, upright R wave. In this lead, this is the first deflection of a normal QRS complex.

It is important to differentiate normal (physiologic) Q waves from pathologic Q waves (Figure 2-33). With the exception of leads III and aVR, a normal Q wave in the limb leads is less than 0.04 second (one small box) in duration and less than one third the height of the R wave in that lead.

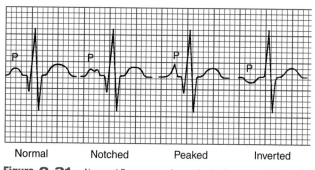

Normal Notched Peaked Inverted

Figure 2-31 Abnormal P waves may be notched, tall and pointed (peaked), or inverted (negative).

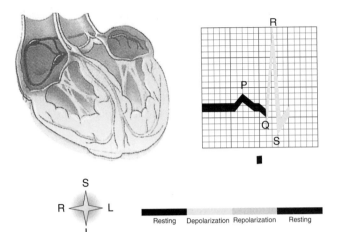

Figure 2-32   The QRS complex represents ventricular depolarization.

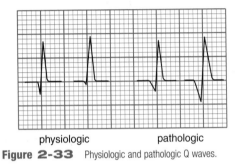

Figure 2-33   Physiologic and pathologic Q waves.

An abnormal (pathologic) Q wave is more than 0.04 second in duration or more than one third the height of the following R wave in that lead. Myocardial infarction is one possible cause of abnormal Q waves. In the early hours of infarction, an abnormal Q wave may not have developed to its full width or amplitude. Therefore, a single ECG tracing may not identify an abnormal Q wave. In a patient with a suspected MI, be sure to look at Q waves closely. Even if the initial ECG tracings do not show Q waves that are more than 0.04 second in duration or equal to or more than one third the amplitude of the QRS complex, pathology must be considered if the Q waves become wider or deeper in each subsequent tracing.

The QRS complex continues as a large, upright, triangular waveform known as the *R wave*. The R wave is the first positive (upright) waveform following the P wave. The S wave is the negative waveform following the R wave. An R wave is **always** positive and an S wave is **always** negative. The R and S waves represent simultaneous depolarization of the right and left ventricles. Because of its greater muscle mass, the QRS complex generally represents the electrical activity occurring in the left ventricle.

The QRS complex may appear predominantly positive, negative, or biphasic, depending on the lead. It is predominantly positive in leads that view the heart from the left (I, aVL, V_5, V_6) and in leads that look at the heart's inferior surface (II, III, aVF). In leads that view the heart from the

right side, the QRS complex is predominantly negative (aVR, V_1, V_2). The QRS is normally biphasic in leads V_3, V_4, and sometimes III.[4] A comparison of the waveforms recorded in the standard limb leads is shown in Figure 2-34.

QRS Measurement

The QRS duration is a measurement of the time required for ventricular depolarization. The width of a QRS complex is most accurately determined when it is viewed and measured in more than one lead. The measurement should be taken from the QRS complex with the longest duration and clearest onset and end. The beginning of the QRS complex is measured from the point where the first wave of the complex begins to deviate from the baseline. The point at which the last wave of the complex begins to level out or distinctly change direction at, above, or below the baseline marks the end of the QRS complex. The normal duration of the QRS complex is 0.10 second or less (Box 2-7). If an electrical impulse does not follow the normal ventricular conduction pathway, it will take longer to depolarize the myocardium. This delay in conduction through the ventricles produces a wider QRS complex.

ECG Pearl

Einthoven expressed the relationship between leads I, II, and III as the sum of any complex in leads I and III equals that of lead II. Thus, lead I + III = II. Stated another way, the voltage of a waveform in lead I plus the voltage of the same waveform in lead III equals the voltage of the same waveform in lead II. For example, when you look at leads I, II, and III, if the R wave in lead II does not appear to be the sum of the voltage of the R waves in leads I and III, the leads may have been incorrectly applied.

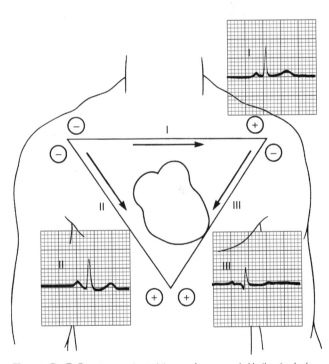

Figure 2-34   A comparison of the waveforms recorded in the standard limb leads.

Box 2-7 **Normal Characteristics of the QRS Complex**

- Normal duration of the QRS complex is 0.10 second or less
- With the exception of leads III and aVR, a normal Q wave in the limb leads is less than 0.04 seconds in duration and less than one third of the amplitude of the R wave in that lead

Abnormal QRS Complexes

- Duration of an abnormal QRS complex is greater than 0.10 second
- Duration of a QRS caused by an impulse originating in an ectopic pacemaker in the Purkinje network or ventricular myocardium is usually greater than 0.12 second and often 0.16 second or greater
- If the impulse originates in a bundle branch, the duration of the QRS may be only slightly greater than 0.10 second. For example, a QRS measuring 0.10 to 0.12 second is called an *incomplete* bundle branch block. A QRS measuring more than 0.12 second is called a *complete* bundle branch block. This is discussed in more detail in Chapter 9.
- Enlargement of the right ventricle produces an abnormally tall R wave; left ventricular enlargement produces an abnormally deep S wave.

QRS Variations

Although the term QRS complex is used, not every QRS complex contains a Q wave, R wave, and S wave. If the QRS complex consists entirely of a positive waveform, it is called an *R wave*. If the complex consists entirely of a negative waveform, it is called a *QS wave*. QS waves may be pathologic. If there are two positive deflections in the same complex, the second is called *R prime* and is written *R'*. If there are two negative deflections following an R wave, the second is called *S prime* and is written *S'*. Capital (upper case) letters are used to designate waveforms of relatively large amplitude, and small (lower case) letters are used to label relatively small waveforms (Figure 2-35).

T Wave

Ventricular repolarization is represented on the ECG by the T wave (Figure 2-36). The absolute refractory period is still present during the beginning of the T wave. At the peak of the T wave, the relative refractory period has begun. It is during the relative refractory period that a stronger than normal stimulus may produce ventricular dysrhythmias.

In the limb leads, lead II most commonly reveals the tallest T wave. The normal T wave is slightly asymmetric: the peak of the waveform is closer to its end than to the beginning, and the first half has a more gradual slope than the second half (Box 2-8). The beginning of the T wave is identified as the point where the slope of the ST-segment appears to

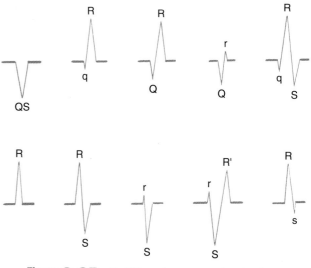

Figure 2-35 The QRS complex may appear in various forms.

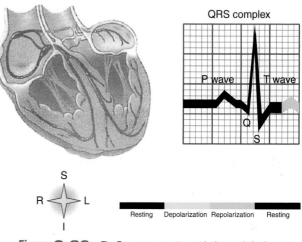

Figure 2-36 The T wave represents ventricular repolarization.

Box 2-8 | **Normal Characteristics of the T Wave**

- Slightly asymmetric
- Usually 5 mm or less in height in any limb lead or 10 mm or less in any chest lead
- Usually 0.5 mm or more in height in leads I and II

become abruptly or gradually steeper. The T wave ends when it returns to the baseline. It may be difficult to clearly determine the onset and end of the T wave. Examples of T waves are shown in Figure 2-37.

The direction of the T wave is normally the same as the QRS complex that precedes it. This is because depolarization begins at the endocardial surface and spreads to the epicardium. Repolarization begins at the epicardium and spreads to the endocardium.

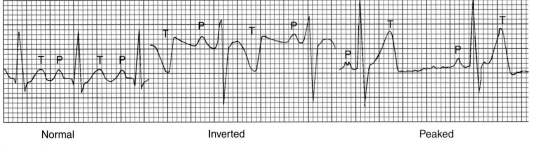

Normal Inverted Peaked

Figure 2-37 Examples of T waves.

Abnormal T Waves

- A T wave following an abnormal QRS complex is usually opposite in direction of the QRS. In other words, when the QRS complex points down, the T wave points up, and vice versa. This may be seen with ventricular beats or rhythms and in bundle branch block.
- Negative T waves suggest myocardial ischemia
- Tall, pointed (peaked) T waves are commonly seen in hyperkalemia
- Low-amplitude T waves may be seen in hypokalemia or hypomagnesemia
- Significant cerebral disease (such as subarachnoid hemorrhage) may be associated with deeply inverted T waves, often called cerebral T waves (Figure 2-38)
- Tall, broad T waves with internal pacemakers

U Wave

A U wave is a small waveform that, when seen, follows the T wave. The mechanism of the U wave is not definitely known. One theory suggests that it represents repolarization

ECG Pearl

T wave inversion, which may occur simultaneously with ST-segment elevation, suggests the presence of myocardial ischemia. The development of pathologic Q waves provides evidence that tissue death has occurred. A pathologic Q wave indicates the presence of dead myocardial tissue and subsequently, a loss of electrical activity.

of the Purkinje fibers. Normal U waves are small, round, and less than 1.5 mm in amplitude (Box 2-9). Possible causes of tall U waves include the following:

- Electrolyte imbalance (such as hypokalemia)
- Medications (such as quinidine, procainamide, disopyramide, amiodarone, digitalis, phenothiazines)
- Hyperthyroidism
- Central nervous system disease
- Long QT syndrome

U waves are most easily seen when the heart rate is slow and are difficult to identify when the rate exceeds 90 beats/min.

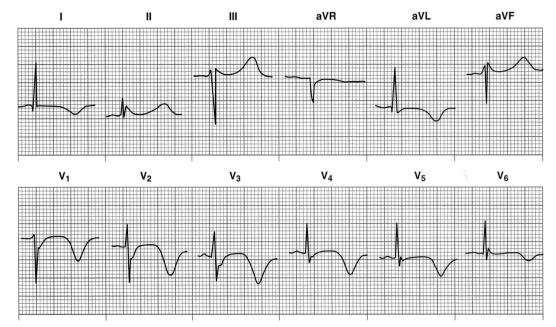

Figure 2-38 The ECG of a patient with acute subarachnoid hemorrhage shows giant T wave inversion. Subarachnoid hemorrhage may cause deeply inverted T waves, usually with markedly prolonged QT intervals, simulating the pattern seen in myocardial infarction.

Box **2-9**	Characteristics of the U Wave

- Rounded and symmetric
- Usually less than 1.5 mm in height and smaller than that of the preceding T wave
- In general, a U wave more than 1.5 mm in height in any lead is considered abnormal

When seen, they are normally tallest in leads V_2 and V_3 (Figure 2-39). U waves usually appear in the same direction as the T wave that precedes it. The amplitude of the normal U wave is usually proportional to the T wave in the same lead, ranging between 5% and 25% of the T wave's amplitude. Negative U waves are strongly suggestive of organic heart disease and may be seen in patients with ischemic heart disease.

Segments

[OBJECTIVES 18, 19]

A **segment** is a line between waveforms. It is named by the waveform that precedes or follows it.

PR-Segment

The PR-segment is the horizontal line between the end of the P wave and the beginning of the QRS complex (Figure 2-40). It is part of the PR interval and represents activation of the AV node, the bundle of His, the bundle branches, and the Purkinje fibers. The PR-segment appears isoelectric because the potentials generated by these structures are too small to produce detectable voltage on the body surface.[5] Atrial repolarization also occurs during this period.

The duration of the PR-segment depends on duration of the P wave and impulse conduction through the AV junction.[1] Most of the conduction delay during the PR-segment is a result of slow conduction within the AV node. The PR-segment may be depressed in patients with ventricular **hypertrophy** (an increase in the thickness of a heart chamber due to chronic pressure overload) or chronic pulmonary disease.

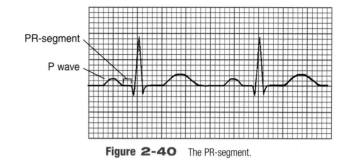

Figure 2-40 The PR-segment.

TP-Segment

The TP-segment is the portion of the ECG tracing between the end of the T wave and the beginning of the following P wave. When the heart rate is within normal limits, the TP-segment is usually isoelectric. With rapid heart rates, the TP-segment is often unrecognizable because the P wave encroaches on the preceding T wave.

ST-Segment

The portion of the ECG tracing between the QRS complex and the T wave is the ST-segment. The term *ST-segment* is used regardless of whether the final wave of the QRS complex is an R or an S wave. The ST-segment represents the early part of repolarization of the right and left ventricles (Figure 2-41). The normal ST-segment begins at the isoelectric line, extends from the end of the S wave, and curves gradually upward to the beginning of the T wave (Box 2-10). In the limb leads, the normal ST-segment is isoelectric (flat) but may normally be slightly elevated or depressed (usually by less than 1 mm).

The point where the QRS complex and the ST-segment meet is called the *junction* or *J-point* (Figure 2-42). Various conditions may cause displacement of the ST-segment from the isoelectric line in either a positive or negative direction. Myocardial ischemia, injury, and infarction are among the causes of ST-segment deviation. When looking for ST-segment

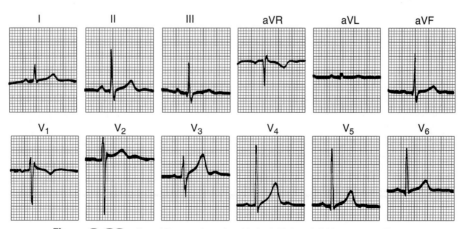

Figure 2-39 Normal U waves (best viewed in leads V_2 through V_4) in a 22-year-old man.

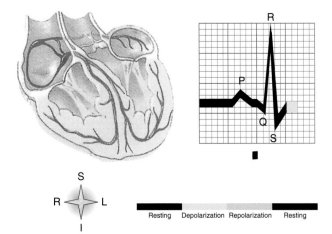

Figure 2-41   The ST-segment represents the early part of repolarization of the right and left ventricles.

Box **2-10**	**Normal Characteristics of the ST-segment**

- Begins with the end of the QRS complex and ends with the onset of the T wave
- In the limb leads, the normal ST-segment is isoelectric (flat) but may normally be slightly elevated or depressed (usually by less than 1 mm)
- In the chest leads, ST-segment deviation may vary from −0.5 to +2 mm

elevation or depression, we are particularly interested in the *early* portion of the ST-segment. First locate the J-point. Next use the TP-segment and the PR-segment to estimate the position of the isoelectric line. Then compare the level of the ST-segment to the isoelectric line (Figure 2-43). It may be difficult to clearly determine the J-point in patients with rapid heart rates or hyperkalemia. Although some deviation of the ST-segment from the isoelectric line can be a normal finding, the following findings are considered significant if they are seen in two or more leads facing the same anatomic area of the heart (also known as contiguous leads):

- ST-segment depression of more than 0.5 mm (suggests myocardial ischemia)
- ST-segment elevation of more than 1 mm (suggests myocardial injury)

There is some difference of opinion as to where ST-segment deviation should be measured. Some authorities simply measure deviation at the J-point while others look for displacement 0.04 second after the J-point. Still others measure ST-segment deviation 0.06 second after the J-point. Proper machine calibration is critical when analyzing ST-segments. The ST-segment criteria described here applies *only* when the monitor is adjusted to standard calibration.[6]

ST-segment elevation in the shape of a "smiley" face (upward concavity) is usually benign, particularly when it occurs in an otherwise healthy, asymptomatic patient (Figure 2-44). The appearance of coved ("frowny face") ST-segment elevation is called an *acute injury pattern*. Other

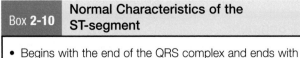

Figure 2-42   The point where the QRS complex and the ST-segment meet is called the "junction" or "J" point.

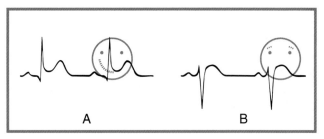

Figure 2-44   **A,** ST-segment elevation in the shape of a "smiley" face (upward concavity) is usually benign, particularly when it occurs in an otherwise healthy, asymptomatic patient. **B,** ST-segment elevation in the shape of a "frowny" face (downward concavity) is more often associated with an acute injury pattern.

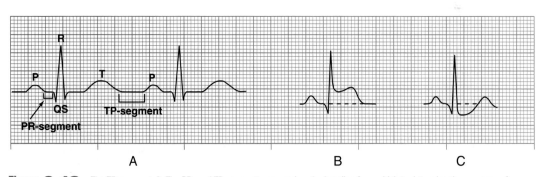

Figure 2-43   The TP-segment. **A,** The PR- and TP-segments are used as the baseline from which to determine the presence of ST-segment elevation or depression. **B,** ST-segment elevation. **C,** ST-segment depression.

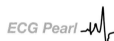

ST-segment elevation provides the strongest ECG evidence for the early recognition of myocardial infarction. In a patient experiencing an acute coronary syndrome, keep in mind that myocardial injury refers to myocardial tissue that has been cut off from or experienced a severe reduction in its blood and oxygen supply. The tissue is not yet dead and may be salvageable if the blocked vessel can be quickly opened, restoring blood flow and oxygen to the injured area.

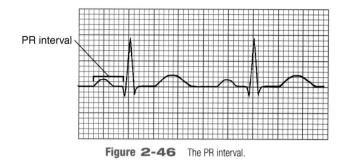

Figure 2-46 The PR interval.

causes of ST-segment elevation may represent a normal variant, pericarditis, or ventricular aneurysm, among other causes. Pericarditis causes ST-segment elevation in all or virtually all leads. ST-segments are discussed in more detail in Chapter 9.

Abnormal ST-Segments

- ST-segment depression of more than 0.5 mm is suggestive of myocardial ischemia
- ST-segment elevation of more than 1 mm in the limb leads or 2 mm in the chest leads is suggestive of myocardial injury
- A horizontal ST-segment (forming a sharp angle with the T wave) is suggestive of ischemia
- Digitalis causes a depression (scoop) of the ST-segment sometimes referred to as a "dig dip" (Figure 2-45)

Intervals

[OBJECTIVE 18]

PR Interval

An **interval** is a waveform and a segment. The P wave plus the PR-segment equals the PR interval (PRI) (Figure 2-46). The PR interval is measured from the point where the P wave leaves the baseline to the beginning of the QRS complex. The

term *PQ interval* is preferred by some because it is the period actually measured unless a Q wave is absent.

Remember that the P wave reflects depolarization of the right and left atria. The PR-segment represents the spread of the impulse through the AV node, bundle of His, right and left bundle branches, and the Purkinje fibers (Figure 2-47). The PRI does not include the duration of conduction from the SA node to the right atrium. The PRI changes with heart rate but normally measures 0.12 to 0.20 second in adults (Box 2-11). As the heart rate increases, the duration of the PR interval shortens. A conduction problem above the level of the bundle branches will largely affect the P wave and PR interval.

 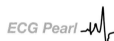

Measuring how quickly or slowly an electrical impulse spreads through the heart provides important information about the condition of the heart's conduction system and the muscle itself.

Abnormal PR Intervals

A long PRIs (greater than 0.20 sec) indicates the impulse was delayed as it passed through the atria or AV node. Prolonged PR intervals may be seen in patients taking beta-blockers or calcium channel blockers, first-degree AV block, hypothyroidism, and digitalis toxicity, among

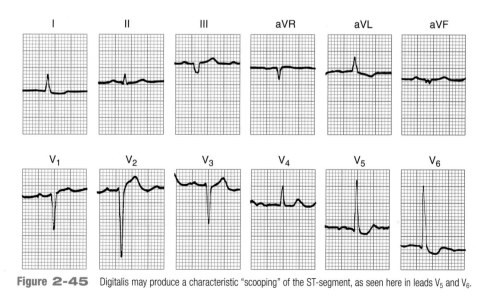

Figure 2-45 Digitalis may produce a characteristic "scooping" of the ST-segment, as seen here in leads V₅ and V₆.

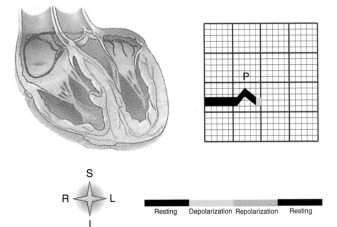

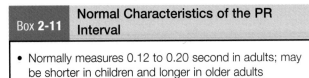

Resting   Depolarization Repolarization   Resting

Figure 2-47   The PR interval reflects depolarization of the right and left atria (P wave) and the spread of the impulse through the AV node, bundle of His, right and left bundle branches, and the Purkinje fibers (PR-segment).

Box 2-11	Normal Characteristics of the PR Interval

- Normally measures 0.12 to 0.20 second in adults; may be shorter in children and longer in older adults
- Normally shortens as heart rate increases

other conditions. The P wave associated with a prolonged PR interval may be normal or abnormal.

A PR interval of less than 0.12 second may be seen when the impulse originates in an ectopic pacemaker in the atria close to the AV node or in the AV junction. A shortened PR interval may also occur if the electrical impulse progresses from the atria to the ventricles through an abnormal conduction pathway that bypasses the AV node and depolarizes the ventricles earlier than usual.

QT Interval

[OBJECTIVE 18]

The QT interval represents total ventricular activity—the time from ventricular depolarization (activation) to repolarization (recovery). The QT interval is measured from the beginning of the QRS complex to the end of the T wave. In the absence of a Q wave, the QT interval is measured from the beginning of the R wave to the end of the T wave. The term *QT interval* is used regardless of whether the QRS complex begins with a Q or R wave.

To quickly determine the QT interval, measure the interval between two consecutive R waves (R-R interval) and divide the number by two. Measure the QT interval. If the measured QT interval is less than half the R-R interval, it is probably normal (Figure 2-48). A QT interval that is approximately half the R-R interval is considered borderline. A QT interval that is more than half the R-R interval is considered prolonged.

Many conditions, such as electrolyte disorders, and medications, such as amiodarone and sotalol, can prolong the QT interval. A prolonged QT interval indicates a lengthened relative refractory period (vulnerable period). This puts the ventricles at risk for life-threatening dysrhythmias, such as torsades de pointes (TdP). A prolonged QT interval may be congenital or acquired. Digitalis and hypercalcemia shorten the QT interval.

ECG Pearl

The duration of the QT interval varies according to age, gender, and heart rate. As the heart rate increases, the QT interval shortens (decreases). As the heart rate decreases, the QT interval lengthens (increases). Because of the variability of the QT interval with the heart rate, it can be measured more accurately if it is corrected (adjusted) for the patient's heart rate. The corrected QT interval is noted as QTc. Many clinicians do not consider the QT interval abnormally long unless the QT interval corrected for the heart rate exceeds 0.44 second.

R-R and P-P Intervals

The R-R (R wave-to-R wave) and P-P (P wave-to-P wave) intervals are used to determine the rate and regularity of a cardiac rhythm. To evaluate the regularity of the ventricular rhythm on a rhythm strip, the interval between two consecutive R waves is measured. The distance between succeeding R-R intervals is measured and compared. If the ventricular rhythm is regular, the R-R intervals will measure

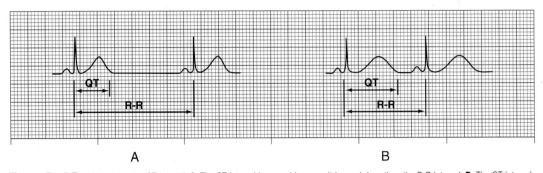

A   B

Figure 2-48   Measuring the QT interval. **A,** The QT interval is normal because it is much less than the R-R interval. **B,** The QT interval is prolonged because it is more than half the R-R interval.

the same. To evaluate the regularity of the atrial rhythm, the same procedure is used but the interval between two consecutive P waves is measured and compared to succeeding P-P intervals.

Figure 2-49 displays the ECG waveforms, and Figure 2-50 displays important ECG intervals discussed in this chapter.

Artifact

[OBJECTIVE 20]

Accurate ECG rhythm recognition requires a tracing in which the waveforms and intervals are free of distortion. Distortion of an ECG tracing by electrical activity that is noncardiac in origin is called **artifact**. Because artifact can mimic various cardiac dysrhythmias, including ventricular fibrillation, it is essential to evaluate the patient before initiating any medical intervention.

Artifact may be caused by loose electrodes, broken ECG cables or broken wires, muscle tremor, patient movement, external chest compressions, and 60-cycle interference. Proper preparation of the patient's skin and evaluation of the monitoring equipment (electrodes, wires) before use can minimize the problems associated with artifact.

Loose Electrodes

An irregular baseline may be identified by bizarre, irregular deflections of the baseline on the ECG paper. This may be the result of a broken lead wire, poor electrical contact, or a loose electrode (Figure 2-51). When hair is present in large quantities, it may interfere with electrode adhesion. When the gel is in contact with hair instead of skin, penetration will be hindered. A simple disposable razor may be used to remove hair before placing the electrodes, but many prefer to

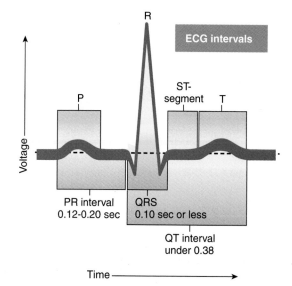

Figure 2-50 The ECG segments and intervals—PR interval, QRS duration, ST-segment, QT interval.

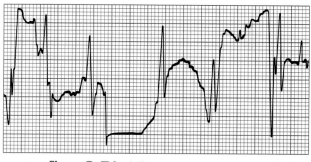

Figure 2-51 Artifact caused by a loose electrode.

use electric clippers instead. Whatever device is used, it is important to remove the hair in the area where the electrodes will be applied.

Patient Movement/Muscle Activity

A wandering baseline may occur because of normal respiratory movement (particularly when electrodes have been applied directly over the ribs) or because of poor electrode contact with the patient's skin. Seizures, shivering, tense muscles, or Parkinson's disease may cause muscle tremor artifact (Figure 2-52). Consider clipping the ECG cable to the patient's clothing to minimize excessive movement.

60-Cycle (AC) Interference

A phenomenon known as 60-cycle interference may be caused by improperly grounded electrical equipment or other electrical interference (Figure 2-53). If 60-cycle interference is observed, check for crossing of cable wires with other electrical wires (such as a bed control) or frayed and broken wires. Verify that all electrical equipment is properly grounded and that the cable electrode connections are clean.

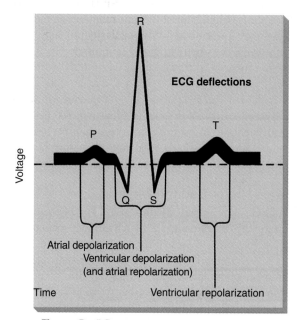

Figure 2-49 The ECG waveforms—P, QRS, and T.

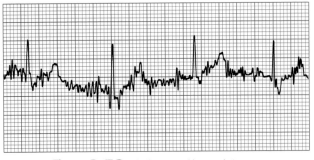

Figure 2-52 Artifact caused by muscle tremors.

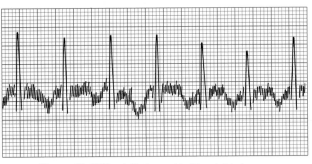

Figure 2-53 Artifact caused by 60-cycle interference.

ANALYZING A RHYTHM STRIP

[OBJECTIVE 21]
A systematic approach to rhythm analysis that is consistently applied when analyzing a rhythm strip is essential. If you do not develop such an approach, you are more likely to miss something important. Begin analyzing the rhythm strip from left to right.

Assess Rhythm/Regularity

The term rhythm is used to indicate the site of origin of an electrical impulse (such as a sinus rhythm or junctional rhythm) and to describe the regularity or irregularity of waveforms. The waveforms on an ECG strip are evaluated for regularity by measuring the distance between the P waves and QRS complexes. If the rhythm is regular, the R-R intervals (or P-P intervals, if assessing atrial rhythm) are the same. Generally, a variation of plus or minus 10% is acceptable. For example, if there are 10 small boxes in an R-R interval, an R wave could be "off" by 1 small box and still be considered regular.

Ventricular Rhythm

To determine if the ventricular rhythm is regular or irregular, measure the distance between two consecutive R-R intervals. Place one point of a pair of calipers (or make a mark on a piece of paper) on the beginning of an R wave. Place the other point of the calipers (or make a second mark on the paper) on the beginning of the R wave of the next QRS complex.

Without adjusting the calipers, evaluate each succeeding R-R interval. (If paper is used, lift the paper and move it across the rhythm strip.) Compare the distance measured with the other R-R intervals. If the ventricular rhythm is regular, the R-R intervals will measure the same. Rhythm and regularity also may be determined by counting the small squares between intervals and comparing the intervals.

Atrial Rhythm

To determine if the atrial rhythm is regular or irregular, follow the same procedure previously described for evaluation of ventricular rhythm but measure the distance between two consecutive P-P intervals (instead of R-R intervals) and compare that distance with the other P-P intervals. The P-P intervals will measure the same if the atrial rhythm is regular. For accuracy, the R-R or P-P intervals should be evaluated across an entire 6-second rhythm strip.

Terminology

Various terms may be used to describe an irregular rhythm, which may be normal, fast, or slow. If the variation between the shortest and longest R-R intervals (or P-P intervals) is less than four small boxes (0.16 sec), the rhythm is termed *essentially regular*. For example, the underlying rhythm may be regular but the pattern may be periodically interrupted by ectopic beats that arise from a part of the heart other than the SA node.

If the shortest and longest R-R intervals vary by more than 0.16 second, the rhythm is considered *irregular*. A *regularly irregular rhythm* is one in which the R-R intervals are not the same, the shortest and longest R-R intervals vary by more than 0.16 second, and there is a repeating pattern of irregularity. A regularly irregular rhythm may be due to grouped beating (a repeating pattern of irregularity). An *irregularly irregular rhythm* is one in which the R-R intervals are not the same, there is no repeating pattern of irregularity, and the shortest and longest R-R intervals vary by more than 0.16 second. An irregularly irregular rhythm may also be called a grossly or totally irregular rhythm.

Assess the Rate

A **tachycardia** exists if the rate is more than 100 beats/min. A **bradycardia** exists if the rate is less than 60 beats/min. There are several methods used for calculating heart rate (Figure 2-54). A discussion of each method follows.

Method 1: Six-Second Method

Most ECG paper is printed with 1-second or 3-second markers on the top or bottom of the paper. On ECG paper, 5 large boxes = 1 second, 15 large boxes = 3 seconds, and 30 large boxes = 6 seconds. To determine the ventricular rate, count the number of complete QRS complexes within a period of 6 seconds and multiply that number by 10 to find the number of complexes in 1 minute (Figure 2-54). This method may be used for regular and irregular rhythms. This is the

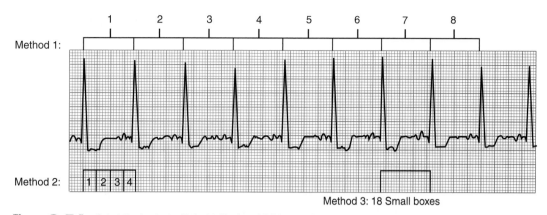

Figure 2-54   Calculating heart rate. Method 1: Number of R-R intervals in 6 seconds × 10 (e.g., 8 × 10 = 80/min). Method 2: Number of large boxes between QRS complexes divided into 300 (e.g., 300 divided by 4 = 75/min). Method 3: Number of small boxes between QRS complexes divided into 1500 (e.g., 1500 divided by 18 = 84/min).

simplest, quickest, and most commonly used method of rate measurement, but it also is the most inaccurate.

Method 2: Large Boxes

To determine the ventricular rate, count the number of large boxes between the R-R interval and divide into 300. To determine the atrial rate, count the number of large boxes between the P-P interval and divide into 300 (Table 2-8). This method is best used if the rhythm is regular; however, it may be used if the rhythm is irregular and a rate range (slowest [longest R-R interval] and fastest [shortest R-R interval] rate) is given.

A variation of the large box method is called the sequence method. To determine ventricular rate, select an R wave that falls on a dark vertical line. Number the next six consecutive dark vertical lines as follows: 300, 150, 100, 75, 60, and 50 (Figure 2-55). Note where the next R wave falls in relation to the six dark vertical lines already marked. This is the heart rate.

Method 3: Small Boxes

Each 1-mm box on the graph paper represents 0.04 second. A total of 1500 boxes represents 1 minute (60 sec/min divided by 0.04 sec/box = 1500 boxes/min). To calculate the ventricular rate, count the number of small boxes between the R-R interval and divide into 1500. To determine the atrial rate, count the number of small boxes between the P-P interval and divide into 1500. This method is time consuming but accurate. If the rhythm is irregular, a rate range should be given.

TABLE 2-8	Heart Rate Determination Based on the Number of Large Boxes		
Number of Large Boxes	Heart Rate (beats/min)	Number of Large Boxes	Heart Rate (beats/min)
1	300	6	50
2	150	7	43
3	100	8	38
4	75	9	33
5	60	10	30

Identify and Examine P Waves

To locate P waves, look to the left of each QRS complex. Normally one P wave precedes each QRS complex; they occur regularly; and they look similar in size, shape, and position. If no P wave is present, the rhythm originated in the AV junction or the ventricles. If one P wave is present before each QRS and the QRS is *narrow*, consider the following:

- Is the P wave positive? If so, the rhythm probably began in the SA node.
- Is the P wave negative or absent? If so, and the QRS complexes occur regularly, the rhythm probably started in the AV junction.

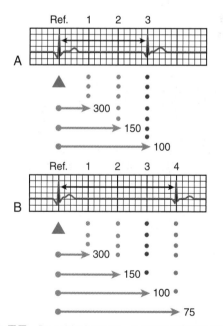

Figure 2-55   Determining heart rate—sequence method. To measure the ventricular rate, find a QRS complex that falls on a heavy dark line. Count 300, 150, 100, 75, 60, and 50 until a second QRS complex occurs. This will be the heart rate. **A,** Heart rate = 100. **B,** Heart rate = 75.

Assess Intervals (Evaluate Conduction)

PR Interval

Measure the PR interval. The PR interval is measured from the point where the P wave leaves the baseline to the beginning of the QRS complex. The normal PR interval is 0.12 to 0.20 second. If the PR intervals are the same, they are said to be constant. If the PR intervals are different, is a pattern present? In some dysrhythmias, the duration of the PR interval will increase until a P wave appears with no QRS after it. This is referred to as *lengthening* of the PR interval. PR intervals that vary in duration and have no pattern are said to be *variable*.

QRS Duration

Identify the QRS complexes and measure their duration. The beginning of the QRS is measured from the point where the first wave of the complex begins to deviate from the baseline. The point at which the last wave of the complex begins to level out at, above or below the baseline, marks the end of the QRS complex. The QRS is considered narrow (normal) if it measures 0.10 second or less and wide if it measures more than 0.10 second. A QRS complex of 0.10 second or less (narrow) is presumed to be supraventricular in origin.

QT Interval

Measure the QT interval in the leads that show the largest amplitude T waves. The QT interval is measured from the beginning of the QRS complex to the end of the T wave. If no Q wave is present, measure the QT interval from the beginning of the R wave to the end of the T wave. If the measured QT interval is less than half the R-R interval, it probably is normal. This method of QT interval measurement works well as a general guideline until the ventricular rate exceeds 100 beats/min.

Evaluate the Overall Appearance of the Rhythm

ST-Segment

Determine the presence of ST-segment elevation or depression. The TP- and PR-segments are used as the baseline from which to evaluate the degree of displacement of the ST-segment from the isoelectric line. The ST-segment is considered elevated if the segment is deviated above the baseline and is considered depressed if the segment deviates below it.

T Wave

Evaluate the T waves. Are the T waves upright and of normal height? The T wave following an abnormal QRS complex usually is opposite in direction of the QRS. Negative T waves may be an indicator of myocardial ischemia. Tall, pointed (peaked) T waves commonly are seen in hyperkalemia.

Interpret the Rhythm and Evaluate Its Clinical Significance

Interpret the rhythm, specifying the site of origin (pacemaker site) of the rhythm (sinus), the mechanism (bradycardia), and the ventricular rate. For example, "sinus bradycardia at 38 beats/min." Assess the patient to find out how he or she is tolerating the rate and rhythm.

REFERENCES

1. Chou T, Knilans TK: Electrocardiography in clinical practice: adult and pediatric, Philadelphia, 1996, WB Saunders.
2. Conover MB: The 12 electrocardiogram leads. In Understanding electrocardiography, ed 7, St Louis, 1996, Mosby, pp 3-11.
3. Guyton AC, Hall JE: The normal electrocardiogram. In Textbook of medical physiology, ed 9, Philadelphia, 1996, WB Saunders, pp 129-134.
4. Lipman BC, Cascio T: ECG assessment and interpretation, Philadelphia, 1994, FA Davis.
5. Mirvis DM, Goldberger AL: Electrocardiography. In: Zipes D, Libby P, Bonow RO et al (eds). Braunwald's heart disease: A textbook of cardiovascular medicine, ed 7, Philadelphia, 2004, WB Saunders.
6. Phalen T, Aehlert B: The 12-lead ECG in acute coronary syndromes, ed 2, St Louis, 2006 Elsevier.

STOP & REVIEW

Multiple Choice

In the space provided, identify the letter of the choice that best completes each statement or answers each question.

____ 1. In the normal heart, the primary pacemaker is the
a. AV node.
b. SA node.
c. AV junction.
d. Purkinje fibers.

____ 2. The PR interval is considered prolonged if it is more than _____ in duration.
a. 0.06 second
b. 0.12 second
c. 0.18 second
d. 0.20 second

____ 3. Which part of the conduction system receives an impulse from the bundle of His and relays it to the Purkinje fibers?
a. SA node
b. AV node
c. Right and left atria
d. Right and left bundle branches

____ 4. On the ECG, the time necessary for the spread of an electrical impulse through the AV node, bundle of His, right and left bundle branches, and the Purkinje fibers reflected by the
a. TP-segment
b. PR-segment
c. QT interval
d. QRS duration

____ 5. The normal duration of the QRS complex is
a. 0.10 second or less.
b. 0.20 second or less.
c. 0.04 to 0.14 second.
d. 0.20 to 0.38 second.

____ 6. The portion of the ECG tracing used to determine the degree of ST-segment displacement is the
a. PR interval.
b. QT interval.
c. TP- or PR-segment.
d. QRS complex or TP-segment.

____ 7. Which part of the conduction system receives an impulse from the SA node but delays relaying that impulse to the bundle of His, allowing time for the atria to empty their contents into the ventricles before the onset of ventricular contraction?
a. AV node
b. Right atrium
c. Left bundle branch
d. Right bundle branch

____ 8. Which of the following correctly reflects examples of escape pacemakers?
a. The SA node and AV junction
b. The AV junction and ventricles
c. The SA node and right bundle branch
d. The AV junction and left bundle branch

____ 9. Five large boxes, each consisting of five small boxes, represent _____ on ECG paper.
a. 1 second
b. 3 seconds
c. 6 seconds
d. 10 seconds

____ 10. Which of the following surfaces of the heart are not directly viewed when using a standard 12-lead ECG?
a. Anterior and lateral surfaces of the left ventricle
b. Lateral and inferior surfaces of the left ventricle
c. Inferior and posterior surfaces of the left ventricle
d. Right ventricle and posterior surface of the left ventricle

Completion

In the blanks provided, write the words that best complete each sentence.

11. The appearance of coved ("frowny face") ST-segment elevation is called a(n) _____ _____ _____.

12. A line between waveforms is called a(n) _____ _____.

13. _____ is the spread of an impulse through tissue already stimulated by that same impulse.

14. The cells of the heart that contain contractile filaments are called _____ cells.

15. Distortion of an ECG tracing by electrical activity that is noncardiac in origin is called _____ _____.

Matching

Match the key terms in the left column with the definitions in the right column by placing the letter of each correct answer in the space provided.

_____ **16.** Negative

_____ **17.** Electrolyte

_____ **18.** Repolarization

_____ **19.** Atrial

_____ **20.** Millimeters

_____ **21.** Polarized

_____ **22.** Epinephrine

_____ **23.** Anterior

_____ **24.** QT

_____ **25.** Membrane potential

_____ **26.** Complex

_____ **27.** Voltmeter

_____ **28.** Sodium

_____ **29.** Horizontal

_____ **30.** Potassium

_____ **31.** Interval

_____ **32.** Reentry

_____ **33.** Augmented

_____ **34.** Chemical

_____ **35.** Pericarditis

_____ **36.** Positive

_____ **37.** Ventricular

_____ **38.** Supernormal

_____ **39.** Vulnerable

_____ **40.** Escape

_____ **41.** Excitability

a. A waveform and a segment

b. The relative refractory period is also called the _____ period.

c. The T wave represents ventricular _____.

d. An ECG machine is a sophisticated _____.

e. The QRS complex represents _____ depolarization.

f. This condition causes ST-segment elevation in all or virtually all leads.

g. An important electrolyte that affects cardiac function.

h. The difference in electrical charges across the cell membrane.

i. The amplitude of a waveform is measured in _____.

j. The ability of cardiac muscle cells to respond to an outside stimulus

k. The "a" in aVR, aVL, and aVF.

l. The P wave represents _____ depolarization.

m. In leads I and II, the right arm is _____.

n. This medication will increase the heart rate and force of contraction.

o. On ECG paper, each _____ 1-mm box represents 0.04 second.

p. A(n) _____ pacemaker is a pacemaker site other than the SA node.

q. One of the directions in the horizontal plane

r. Several waveforms

s. The spread of an impulse through tissue already stimuated by that same impulse.

t. When the inside of a cell is more negative than the outside it is said to be _____.

u. The stimulus that alters the electrical charges across the cell membrane may be electrical, mechanical, or _____.

v. Depolarization is caused by the movement of _____ into the cell.

w. Element or compound that, when melted or dissolved in water or another solvent, breaks into ions

x. Each electrode placed in a "V" position is a _____ electrode.

y. During this period, a weaker than normal stimulus can cause depolarization of cardiac cells.

z. The _____ interval represents total ventricular activity.

Short Answer

42. Indicate the inherent rates for each of the following pacemaker sites:

Sinoatrial (SA) node: _____

Atrioventricular (AV) junction: _____

Ventricles: _____

43. List four (4) properties of cardiac cells.
1.

2.

3.

4.

44. List three (3) uses for ECG monitoring.
1.

2.

3.

45. Complete the following chart:

Lead	Positive electrode	Negative electrode	Heart surface viewed
Lead I	_____	_____	_____
Lead II	_____	_____	_____
Lead III	_____	_____	_____

46. List three (3) causes of artifact on an ECG tracing.
1.

2.

3.

47. List six (6) steps used in ECG rhythm analysis.
1.

2.

3.

4.

5.

6.

48. List the six (6) leads that view the heart in the frontal plane.

49. Is depolarization the same as contraction? Explain your answer.

50. What are the R-R and P-P intervals used for in ECG monitoring?

BASIC ELECTROPHYSIOLOGY—*PRACTICE RHYTHM STRIPS*

For each of the following rhythm strips determine the atrial and ventricular rates; label the P wave, QRS complex, and T wave; and measure the PR interval, QRS duration, and QT interval. Determine if the atrial and ventricular rhythm for each strip is regular or irregular. *Not all waveforms will be present in each of the following rhythm strips.*

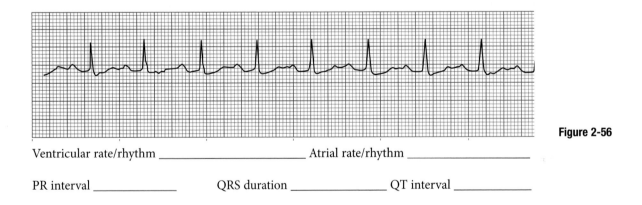

Figure 2-56

Ventricular rate/rhythm _____ Atrial rate/rhythm _____

PR interval _____   QRS duration _____ QT interval _____

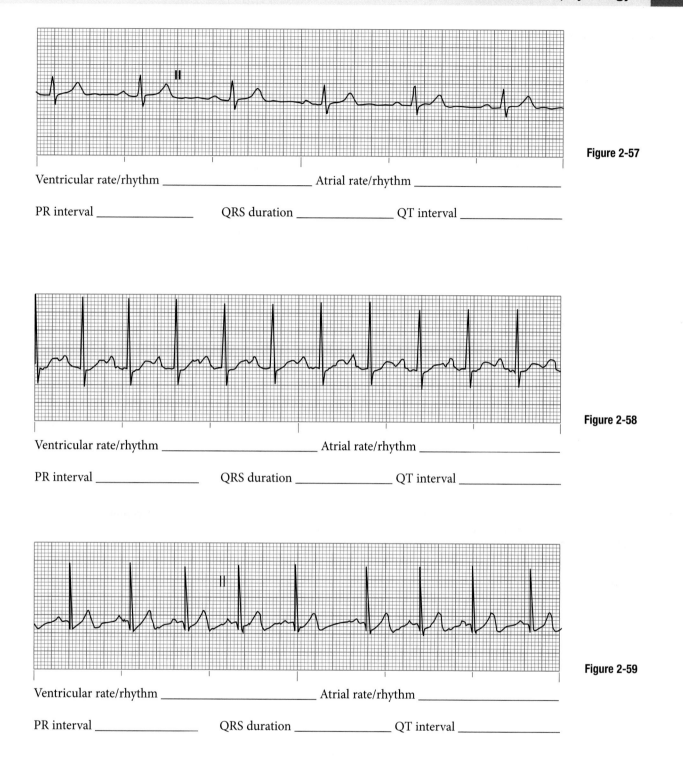

Figure 2-57

Ventricular rate/rhythm _____ Atrial rate/rhythm _____

PR interval _____ QRS duration _____ QT interval _____

Figure 2-58

Ventricular rate/rhythm _____ Atrial rate/rhythm _____

PR interval _____ QRS duration _____ QT interval _____

Figure 2-59

Ventricular rate/rhythm _____ Atrial rate/rhythm _____

PR interval _____ QRS duration _____ QT interval _____

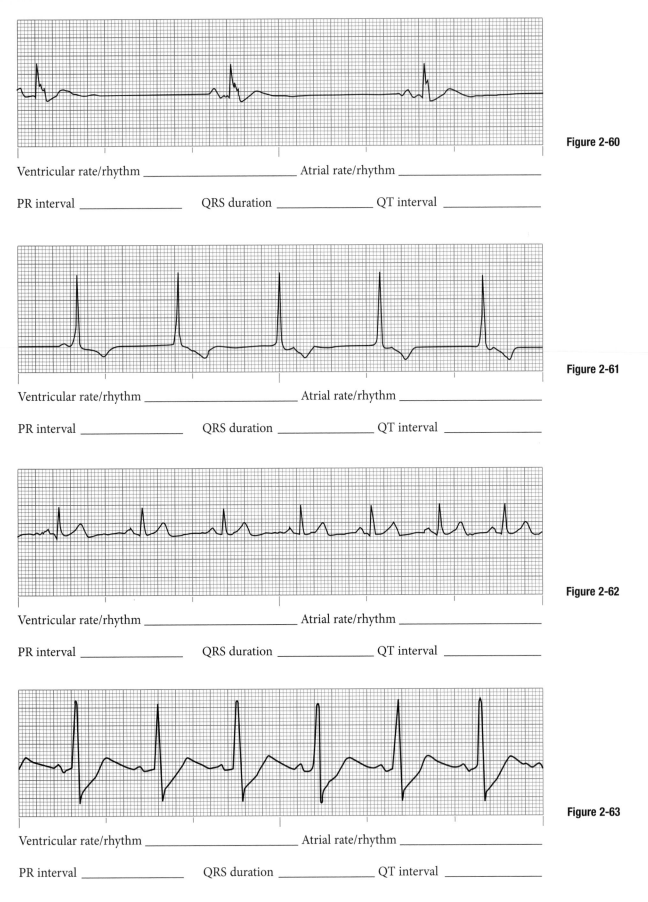

Figure 2-60

Ventricular rate/rhythm _____ Atrial rate/rhythm _____

PR interval _____ QRS duration _____ QT interval _____

Figure 2-61

Ventricular rate/rhythm _____ Atrial rate/rhythm _____

PR interval _____ QRS duration _____ QT interval _____

Figure 2-62

Ventricular rate/rhythm _____ Atrial rate/rhythm _____

PR interval _____ QRS duration _____ QT interval _____

Figure 2-63

Ventricular rate/rhythm _____ Atrial rate/rhythm _____

PR interval _____ QRS duration _____ QT interval _____

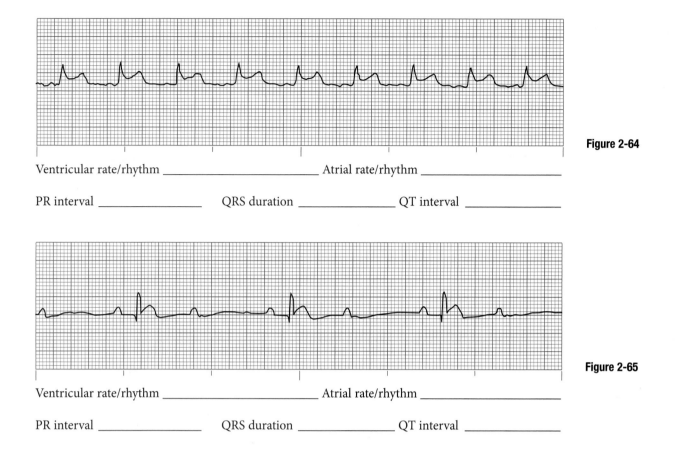

Figure 2-64

Ventricular rate/rhythm _____ Atrial rate/rhythm _____

PR interval _____ QRS duration _____ QT interval _____

Figure 2-65

Ventricular rate/rhythm _____ Atrial rate/rhythm _____

PR interval _____ QRS duration _____ QT interval _____

STOP & REVIEW ANSWERS

Multiple Choice

1. b
2. d
3. d
4. b
5. a

6. c
7. a
8. b
9. a
10. d

Completion

11. The appearance of coved ("frowny face") ST-segment elevation is called an *acute injury pattern*.
12. A line between waveforms is called a *segment*.
13. *Reentry* is the spread of an impulse through tissue already stimulated by that same impulse.

14. The cells of the heart that contain contractile filaments are called *myocardial* (or mechanical or working) cells.
15. Distortion of an ECG tracing by electrical activity that is noncardiac in origin is called *artifact*.

Matching

16. m
17. w
18. c
19. l
20. i
21. t
22. n
23. q
24. z
25. h
26. r
27. d
28. v

29. o
30. g
31. a
32. s
33. k
34. u
35. f
36. x
37. e
38. y
39. b
40. p
41. j

Short Answer

42. SA node: 60 to 100 beats/min
    AV junction: 40 to 60 beats/min
    Ventricles: 20 to 40 beats/min
43. The four properties of cardiac cells are: (1) automaticity, (2) excitability (or irritability), (3) conductivity, and (4) contractility.
44. ECG monitoring may be used to: (1) monitor a patient's heart rate; (2) evaluate the effects of disease or injury on heart function; (3) evaluate pacemaker function; (4) evaluate the response to medications (e. g., antiarrhythmics); and (5) to obtain a baseline recording before, during, and after a medical procedure.
45.

Lead	Positive electrode	Negative electrode	Heart surface viewed
Lead I	Left arm	Right arm	Lateral
Lead II	Left leg	Right arm	Inferior
Lead III	Left leg	Left arm	Inferior

46. Artifact may be due to loose electrodes, broken wires or ECG cables, muscle tremor, patient movement, external chest compressions, or 60-cycle interference.
47. 1. Assess rhythm/regularity.
    2. Assess the rate.
    3. Identify and examine P waves.
    4. Assess intervals; evaluate conduction (PR interval, QRS duration, QT interval).
    5. Evaluate the overall appearance of the rhythm (ST-segments, T waves).
    6. Interpret the rhythm and evaluate its clinical significance.
48. Six leads view the heart in the frontal plane: three bipolar leads and three unipolar leads. The bipolar leads are leads I, II, and III. The unipolar leads are aVR, aVL, and aVF.

49. Depolarization is not the same as contraction. Depolarization (an electrical event) is expected to result in contraction (a mechanical event). It is possible to see organized electrical activity on the cardiac monitor, yet evaluation of the patient reveals no palpable pulse. This clinical situation is called pulseless electrical activity (PEA).

50. The R-R (R wave-to-R wave) and P-P (P wave-to-P wave) intervals are used to determine the rate and regularity of a cardiac rhythm.

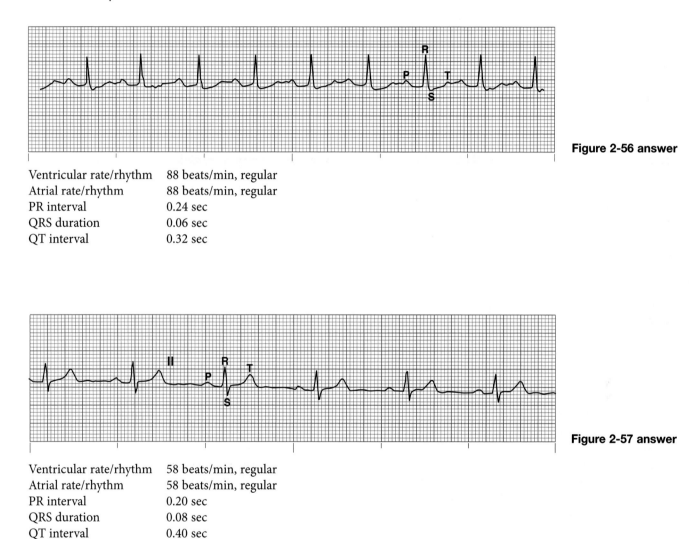

Figure 2-56 answer

Ventricular rate/rhythm	88 beats/min, regular
Atrial rate/rhythm	88 beats/min, regular
PR interval	0.24 sec
QRS duration	0.06 sec
QT interval	0.32 sec

Figure 2-57 answer

Ventricular rate/rhythm	58 beats/min, regular
Atrial rate/rhythm	58 beats/min, regular
PR interval	0.20 sec
QRS duration	0.08 sec
QT interval	0.40 sec

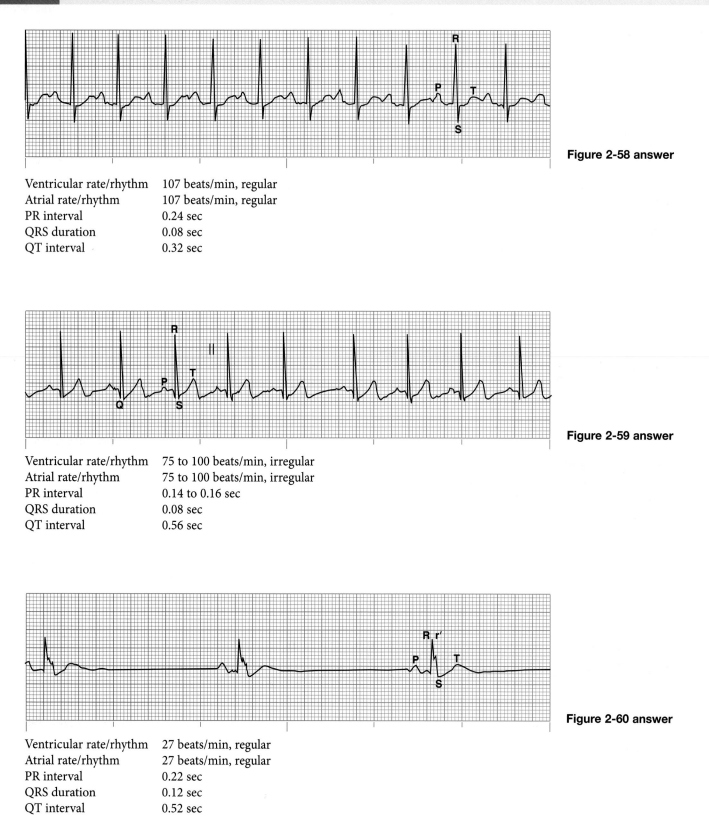

Figure 2-58 answer

Ventricular rate/rhythm	107 beats/min, regular
Atrial rate/rhythm	107 beats/min, regular
PR interval	0.24 sec
QRS duration	0.08 sec
QT interval	0.32 sec

Figure 2-59 answer

Ventricular rate/rhythm	75 to 100 beats/min, irregular
Atrial rate/rhythm	75 to 100 beats/min, irregular
PR interval	0.14 to 0.16 sec
QRS duration	0.08 sec
QT interval	0.56 sec

Figure 2-60 answer

Ventricular rate/rhythm	27 beats/min, regular
Atrial rate/rhythm	27 beats/min, regular
PR interval	0.22 sec
QRS duration	0.12 sec
QT interval	0.52 sec

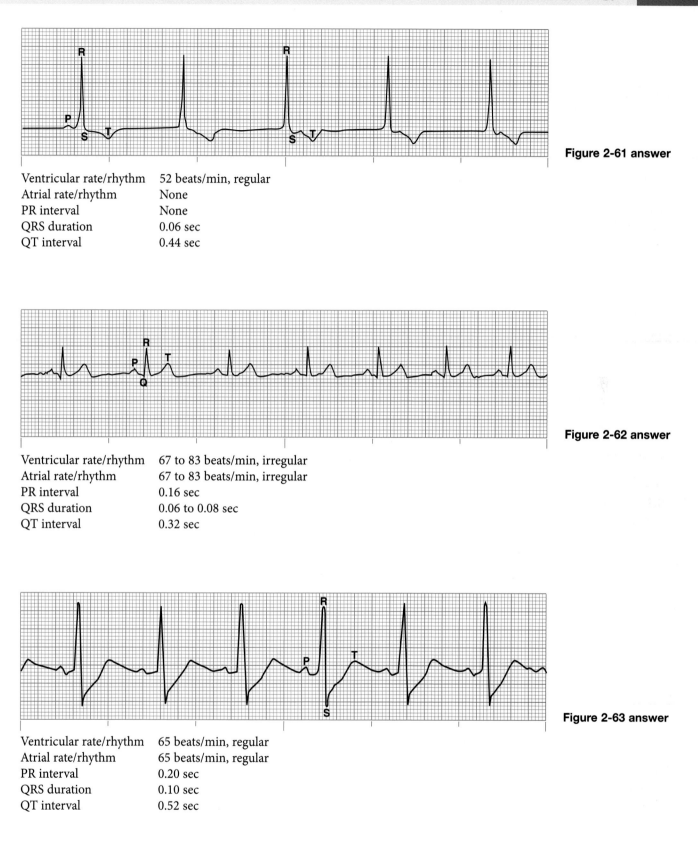

Figure 2-61 answer

Ventricular rate/rhythm	52 beats/min, regular
Atrial rate/rhythm	None
PR interval	None
QRS duration	0.06 sec
QT interval	0.44 sec

Figure 2-62 answer

Ventricular rate/rhythm	67 to 83 beats/min, irregular
Atrial rate/rhythm	67 to 83 beats/min, irregular
PR interval	0.16 sec
QRS duration	0.06 to 0.08 sec
QT interval	0.32 sec

Figure 2-63 answer

Ventricular rate/rhythm	65 beats/min, regular
Atrial rate/rhythm	65 beats/min, regular
PR interval	0.20 sec
QRS duration	0.10 sec
QT interval	0.52 sec

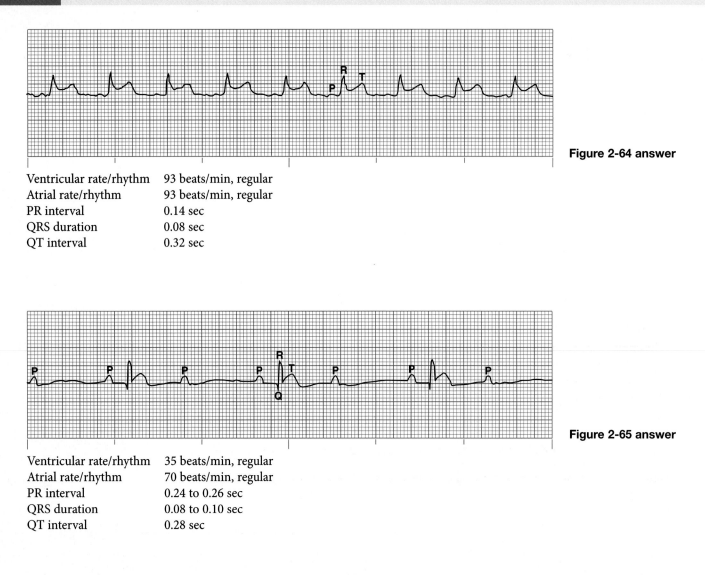

Figure 2-64 answer

Ventricular rate/rhythm	93 beats/min, regular
Atrial rate/rhythm	93 beats/min, regular
PR interval	0.14 sec
QRS duration	0.08 sec
QT interval	0.32 sec

Figure 2-65 answer

Ventricular rate/rhythm	35 beats/min, regular
Atrial rate/rhythm	70 beats/min, regular
PR interval	0.24 to 0.26 sec
QRS duration	0.08 to 0.10 sec
QT interval	0.28 sec

Sinus Mechanisms

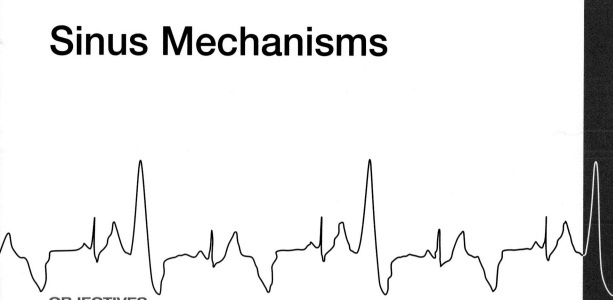

OBJECTIVES

After reading this chapter, you should be able to:

1. Describe the ECG characteristics of a sinus rhythm.
2. Describe the ECG characteristics, possible causes, signs and symptoms, and emergency management of sinus bradycardia.
3. Describe the ECG characteristics, possible causes, signs and symptoms, and emergency management of sinus tachycardia.
4. Describe the ECG characteristics, possible causes, signs and symptoms, and emergency management of sinus arrhythmia.
5. Describe the ECG characteristics, possible causes, signs and symptoms, and emergency management of sinoatrial block.
6. Describe the ECG characteristics, possible causes, signs and symptoms, and emergency management of sinus arrest.

INTRODUCTION

The normal heartbeat is the result of an electrical impulse that starts in the sinoatrial (SA) node. Normally, pacemaker cells within the SA node spontaneously depolarize more rapidly than other cardiac cells. As a result the SA node usually dominates other areas that may be depolarizing at a slightly slower rate. The impulse is sent to cells at the outside edge of the SA node and then to the myocardial cells of the surrounding atrium.

A rhythm that begins in the SA node has the following characteristics:

- A positive (upright) P wave before each QRS complex
- P waves that look alike
- A constant PR interval
- A regular atrial and ventricular rhythm (usually)

ECG Pearl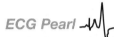

Most (but not all) rhythms that begin in the SA node are regular.

An electrical impulse that begins in the SA node may be affected by the following:

- Medications
- Diseases or conditions that cause the heart rate to speed up, slow down, or beat irregularly
- Diseases or conditions that delay or block the impulse from leaving the SA node
- Diseases or conditions that prevent an impulse from being generated in the SA node

SINUS RHYTHM

[OBJECTIVE 1]

Sinus rhythm is the name given to a normal heart rhythm. Sinus rhythm is sometimes called a *regular sinus rhythm* (RSR) or *normal sinus rhythm* (NSR). Sinus rhythm reflects normal electrical activity—that is, the rhythm starts in the SA node and then heads down the normal conduction pathway through the atria, AV junction, bundle branches, and ventricles. This results in depolarization of the atria and ventricles. The SA node normally produces electrical impulses faster than any other part of the heart's conduction system. As a result, the SA node is normally the heart's primary pacemaker. A person's heart rate varies with age (Table 3-1). In adults and adolescents, the SA node normally fires at a regular rate of 60 to 100 beats/min.

How Do I Recognize It?

Figure 3-1 is an example of a sinus rhythm. Let's look at this rhythm strip closely. A sinus rhythm has a regular atrial and ventricular rhythm. Find the QRS complexes on

TABLE 3-1	Normal Heart Rates by Age
Age	**Beats/min***
Infant (1-12 months)	100-160
Toddler (1-3 years)	90-150
Preschooler (4-5 years)	80-140
School-age (6-12 years)	70-120
Adolescent (13-18 years)	60-100
Adult	60-100

*Pulse rates for a sleeping child may be 10% lower than the low rate listed in age group.

ECG Pearl

In this chapter, you will begin learning the characteristics of specific ECG rhythms. Study these characteristics carefully and commit them to memory. Throughout this text, all ECG characteristics pertain to the adult patient unless otherwise noted.

the rhythm strip. Place one point of your calipers (or make a mark on a piece of paper) on the beginning of an R wave. Place the other point of the calipers (or make a second mark on the paper) on the beginning of the R wave of the next QRS complex. Without adjusting the calipers, evaluate each succeeding R-R interval. (If you are using paper, lift the paper and move it across the rhythm strip). Remember, a variation of plus or minus 10% is acceptable and the rhythm is still considered regular. The R-R intervals in this example are regular. Since you have already identified the R waves, determine the ventricular rate. In this rhythm strip, the ventricular rate is 75 beats/min. Remember, the built-in (intrinsic) rate for a rhythm that begins in the SA node is 60 to 100 beats/min. Therefore the rate of the rhythm in our example fits within the criteria for a sinus rhythm.

Now look to the left of the QRS complexes to find the P waves on the rhythm strip. A rhythm that begins in the SA node should have a positive (upright) P wave (in lead II) before each QRS complex. When you look at this rhythm strip, you can see one upright P wave before each QRS complex. Every P wave looks alike. Measure the P-P interval to see if the P waves occur regularly. Then determine the atrial rate. You will find that the P waves occur regularly at a rate of 75 beats/min.

Now measure the PR interval and QRS duration. In a sinus rhythm, the PR interval measures 0.12 to 0.20 second and is constant from beat to beat. In this example, the PR interval is 0.16 second. The QRS complex normally measures 0.10 second or less. If there is a delay in conduction through the bundle branches, the QRS may be wide (< 0.10 second). In our example, the QRS measures 0.08 second. Note the ST-segment depression. Now interpret the rhythm, specifying the site of origin (pacemaker site) of the rhythm

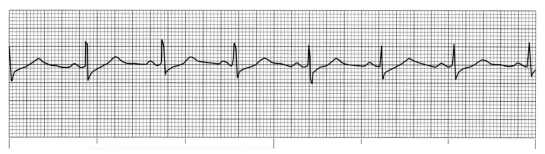

Figure 3-1 Sinus rhythm at 75 beats/min, ST-segment depression.

and the ventricular rate. Since the rhythm shown in Figure 3-1 fits the ECG criteria for a sinus rhythm, your identification should be "Sinus rhythm at 75 beats/min with ST-segment depression." A summary of the ECG characteristics of a sinus rhythm are shown in Table 3-2.

ECG Pearl

A **dysrhythmia** (also called an arrhythmia) is a sign of abnormal electrical activity.

SINUS BRADYCARDIA

[OBJECTIVE 2]

If the SA node fires at a rate slower than normal for the patient's age, the rhythm is called **sinus bradycardia** (brady = slow). The rhythm starts in the SA node and then travels the normal pathway of conduction through the atria, AV junction, bundle branches, and ventricles. This results in atrial and ventricular depolarization. In adults and adolescents, a sinus bradycardia has a heart rate of less than 60 beats/min. The term *severe sinus bradycardia* is sometimes used to describe a sinus bradycardia with a rate of less than 40 beats/min.

How Do I Recognize It?

Figure 3-2 is an example of sinus bradycardia. Table 3-3 lists the ECG characteristics of sinus bradycardia. You will note they are the same as the characteristics of a sinus rhythm

TABLE 3-2	Characteristics of Sinus Rhythm
Rate	60-100 beats/min
Rhythm	P-P interval regular, R-R interval regular
P waves	Positive (upright) in lead II, one precedes each QRS complex, P waves look alike
PR interval	0.12-0.20 sec and constant from beat to beat
QRS duration	0.10 sec or less unless an intraventricular conduction delay exists

with one exception—the rate. The rate of a sinus rhythm is 60 to 100 beats/min. The rate of a sinus bradycardia is less than 60 beats/min.

Examine this rhythm strip using the same format you previously used. Begin by locating the QRS complexes on the rhythm strip. Evaluate each succeeding R-R interval. The R-R intervals in this example are regular. Now determine the ventricular rate. In this rhythm strip, the ventricular rate is 46 beats/min. Now find the P waves on the rhythm strip. Remember that a rhythm that begins in the SA node should have a positive P wave (in lead II) before each QRS complex. In our example, you can see one upright P wave before each QRS complex and every P wave looks alike. Now measure the P-P interval to see if the P waves occur regularly and determine the atrial rate. The P waves occur regularly at a rate of 46 bpm. Now measure the PR interval and QRS duration. In this example, the PR interval is 0.14 second and the QRS complex measures 0.10 second. Now interpret the rhythm, specifying the pacemaker site of the rhythm and the ventricular rate. In our example, ST-segment depression is present and must be noted in our interpretation of the rhythm. Correct identification of this rhythm would be "Sinus bradycardia at 46 beats/min with ST-segment depression."

ECG Pearl

In sinus bradycardia, the QT interval may be longer than normal because of the slower heart rate.

What Causes It?

Sinus bradycardia occurs in adults during sleep and in well-conditioned athletes. It is also present in up to 35% of people under 25 years of age while at rest. Sinus bradycardia is common in some myocardial infarctions. Prolonged standing and stimulation of the vagus nerve can also result in slowing of the heart rate. For example, coughing, vomiting, straining to have a bowel movement, or sudden exposure of the face to cold water can result in slowing of the heart rate. Carotid sinus pressure can also slow the heart rate. In people who have a sensitive carotid sinus, slowing of the heart rate can occur when a tight collar is worn or with the impact of the stream of water on the neck while in the shower. Other causes of sinus bradycardia are shown in the first ECG Pearl below.

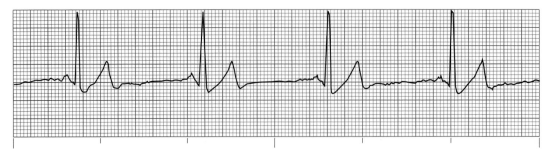

Figure 3-2 Sinus bradycardia at 46 bpm, ST-segment depression.

TABLE **3-3**	Characteristics of Sinus Bradycardia
Rate	Less than 60 beats/min
Rhythm	P-P interval regular, R-R interval regular
P waves	Positive (upright) in lead II, one precedes each QRS complex, P waves look alike
PR interval	0.12-0.20 sec and constant from beat to beat
QRS duration	0.10 sec or less unless an intraventricular conduction delay exists

ECG Pearl

Causes of Sinus Bradycardia
- Inferior myocardial infarction
- Posterior myocardial infarction
- Disease of the SA node
- Vagal stimulation
- Hypoxia
- Hypothermia
- Increased intracranial pressure
- Hypothyroidism
- Hypokalemia
- Post heart transplant
- Hyperkalemia
- Obstructive sleep apnea
- Medications such as calcium channel blockers, digitalis, Beta-blockers, amiodarone, and sotalol

ECG Pearl

Signs and Symptoms of Hemodynamic Compromise
- Changes in mental status
- Low blood pressure
- Chest pain
- Shortness of breath
- Signs of shock
- Congestive heart failure
- Pulmonary congestion
- Fall in urine output
- Cold, clammy skin

Remember that cardiac output = stroke volume × heart rate. Therefore a decrease in either stroke volume or heart rate may result in a decrease in cardiac output. A patient with an unusually slow heart may complain of weakness and/or dizziness. Fainting (syncope) can occur. Decreasing cardiac output will

eventually produce hemodynamic compromise. Signs and symptoms of hemodynamic compromise are shown in the second ECG Pearl below.

What Do I Do About It?

Assess how the patient tolerates the rhythm at rest and with activity. Many patients tolerate a heart rate of 50 to 60 beats/min but become symptomatic when the rate drops below 50. If the patient has no symptoms, no treatment is necessary. If the patient is symptomatic because of the slow rate, treatment may include oxygen, IV access, and administration of atropine and/or transcutaneous pacing. In the setting of a myocardial infarction, sinus bradycardia is often transient. A slow heart rate can be beneficial in the patient who has had an MI (and has no symptoms due to the slow rate). This is because the heart's demand for oxygen is less when the heart rate is slow.

 Atropine

Atropine is a vagolytic medication used to increase heart rate. *Vago* refers to the vagus nerves (right and left), which are main nerves of the parasympathetic division of the autonomic nervous system (ANS). *Lytic* refers to "lyse," which means to interfere with. Atropine works by blocking chemicals at the endings of the vagus nerves. This allows more activity from the sympathetic division of the ANS. As a result, the rate at which the SA node can fire is increased. Atropine also increases the rate at which an impulse is conducted through the AV node. It has little or no effect on the force of contraction, but may increase cardiac output due to its effect on heart rate (cardiac output = heart rate × stroke volume).

SINUS TACHYCARDIA

[OBJECTIVE 3]

If the SA node fires at a rate faster than normal for the patient's age, the rhythm is called **sinus tachycardia** (tachy = fast). Sinus tachycardia begins and ends gradually. The rhythm starts in the SA node and heads down the normal pathway of conduction through the atria, AV junction, bundle branches, and ventricles. This results in atrial and ventricular depolarization.

How Do I Recognize It?

A sinus tachycardia looks much like a sinus rhythm except that it is faster. At very fast rates, it may be hard to tell the difference between a P wave and T wave. Keep in mind that the QT interval normally shortens as heart rate increases.

Normal heart rates vary with age. In adults, the rate associated with sinus tachycardia is usually between 101 and 180 beats/min. Because an infant or child's heart rate can transiently increase during episodes of crying, pain, or in the presence of a fever, the term *tachycardia* is used to describe a significant and persistent increase in heart rate. In infants, a tachycardia is a heart rate of more than 200 beats/min. In a child over 5 years of age, a tachycardia is a heart rate of more than 160 beats/min.

Figure 3-3 is an example of sinus tachycardia. Table 3-4 lists the ECG characteristics of sinus tachycardia. Let us examine this rhythm strip more closely. By glancing at the strip from left to right, you can see that the rate is faster than that of a sinus rhythm. Locate the QRS complexes, evaluate the R-R intervals, and then determine the ventricular rate. The R-R intervals in this example are regular and the ventricular rate is 125 beats/min. Remember that the rate range for a sinus tachycardia is between 101 and 180 beats/min. Therefore the ventricular rate fits within the parameters of a sinus tachycardia.

Look at the P waves on the rhythm strip, evaluate the P-P intervals for regularity, and then determine the atrial rate. One upright P wave appears before each QRS complex, every P wave looks alike, and the P waves occur regularly at a rate of 125 beats/min. Now measure the PR interval and QRS duration. In this example, the PR interval is 0.16 second and the QRS complex measures 0.06 second. Now interpret the rhythm, noting the ST-segment depression that is present. The correct interpretation is "Sinus tachycardia at 125 beats/min with ST-segment depression."

TABLE 3-4	Characteristics of Sinus Tachycardia
Rate	101-180 beats/min
Rhythm	P-P interval regular, R-R interval regular
P waves	Positive (upright) in lead II, one precedes each QRS complex, P waves look alike. At very fast rates it may be hard to tell the difference between a P wave and a T wave
PR interval	0.12-0.20 sec (may shorten with faster rates) and constant from beat to beat
QRS duration	0.10 sec or less unless an intraventricular conduction delay exists

What Causes It?

Sinus tachycardia is a normal response to the body's demand for increased oxygen because of many conditions (see the ECG Pearl on the next page). The patient is often aware of an increase in heart rate. Some patients complain of palpitations, a racing heart, or "pounding" in their chest. This rhythm is seen in some patients with acute MI, especially those with an anterior infarction.

In a patient with coronary artery disease, sinus tachycardia can cause problems. The heart's demand for oxygen increases as the heart rate increases. As the heart rate increases, there is less time for the ventricles to fill and less blood for the ventricles to pump out with each contraction. This can lead to decreased cardiac output. Since the coronary arteries fill when the ventricles are at rest, rapid heart rates decrease the time for coronary artery filling. This decreases the heart's blood supply. Chest discomfort can result if the supply of blood and oxygen to the heart is inadequate. Sinus tachycardia in a patient who is having an acute MI may be an early warning signal for heart failure, cardiogenic shock, and more serious dysrhythmias.

What Do I Do About It?

Treatment for sinus tachycardia is directed at correcting the underlying cause (i.e., fluid replacement, relief of pain, removal of offending medications or substances, reducing fever, and/or anxiety). Sinus tachycardia in a patient experiencing an acute MI may be treated with medications to

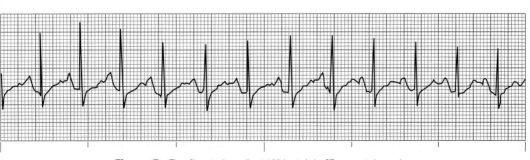
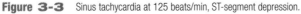

Figure 3-3 Sinus tachycardia at 125 beats/min, ST-segment depression.

slow the heart rate and decrease myocardial oxygen demand (such as beta-blockers), provided there are no signs of heart failure or other contraindications. Some dysrhythmias with very rapid ventricular rates (above 150 beats/min) require the delivery of medications or a shock to stop the rhythm. However, it is important to remember that shocking a sinus tachycardia is inappropriate—treat the reason for the tachycardia. Figure 3-4 shows the differences between sinus rhythm, sinus bradycardia, and sinus tachycardia.

SINUS ARRHYTHMIA

[OBJECTIVE 4]

As you have seen so far, the SA node fires quite regularly most of the time. When it fires irregularly, the resulting rhythm is called **sinus arrhythmia**. Sinus arrhythmia begins in the SA node and follows the normal pathway of conduction through the atria, AV junction, bundle branches, and ventricles, resulting in atrial and ventricular depolarization. Sinus arrhythmia that is associated with the phases of respiration and changes in intrathoracic pressure is called *respiratory sinus arrhythmia*. Sinus arrhythmia that is not related to the respiratory cycle is called *nonrespiratory sinus arrhythmia*.

How Do I Recognize It?

A sinus arrhythmia usually occurs at a rate of 60 to 100 beats/min. If sinus arrhythmia is associated with a slower than normal rate, it is called *sinus brady-arrhythmia*. If the rhythm

is associated with a faster than normal rate, it is known as *sinus tachy-arrhythmia*.

Let's look at the rhythm strip in Figure 3-5. How does this rhythm differ from the others we have discussed so far? Without using calipers or a piece of paper, you can see that it is irregular. Recognizing that, the rhythm can't be a sinus rhythm (because a sinus rhythm is regular). Now, let's determine the atrial and ventricular rate. Since the rhythm is irregular, it is best to give a rate range. To do that we will need to find the slowest part of the rhythm and calculate that rate. We will then need to find the fastest part of the rhythm and calculate that rate. Looking from left to right, the slowest part of this rhythm strip appears to be between the fifth and sixth beats (they have the longest R-R and P-P interval). The rate between these beats is 54 beats/min. The distance between the second and third beats and fourth and fifth beats appears to be the same. These beats are the fastest in this rhythm strip (they have the shortest R-R and P-P interval). The rate between these beats is 88 beats/min. This rhythm strip was obtained from a healthy 26-year-old adult at rest. If we were able to see the patient and watch his respiratory rate and ECG at the same time, you would see a pattern. The patient's heart rate increases gradually during inspiration (R-R intervals shorten) and decreases with expiration (R-R intervals lengthen). Looking closely at the rest of the rhythm strip, you can see one upright P wave before each QRS complex. The PR interval and QRS duration are within normal limits. To identify this rhythm, we will call it a sinus arrhythmia at 54 to 88 beats/min. Table 3-5 lists the characteristics of sinus arrhythmia.

What Causes It?

Respiratory sinus arrhythmia is a normal phenomenon that occurs with changes in intrathoracic pressure. The heart rate increases with inspiration (R-R intervals shorten) and decreases with expiration (R-R intervals lengthen). The changes in rhythm disappear when the patient holds his breath. Sinus arrhythmia is most commonly observed in children and adults less than 30 years of age.

Nonrespiratory sinus arrhythmia can be seen in people with normal hearts, but is more likely in older individuals and in those with heart disease. It is common after acute inferior wall MI and may be seen with increased intracranial pressure. Nonrespiratory sinus arrhythmia may be the result of effects of medications (such as digitalis and morphine) or carotid sinus pressure.

What Do I Do About It?

Sinus arrhythmia usually does not require treatment unless it is accompanied by a slow heart rate that causes hemodynamic compromise. If hemodynamic compromise is present, IV atropine may be indicated.

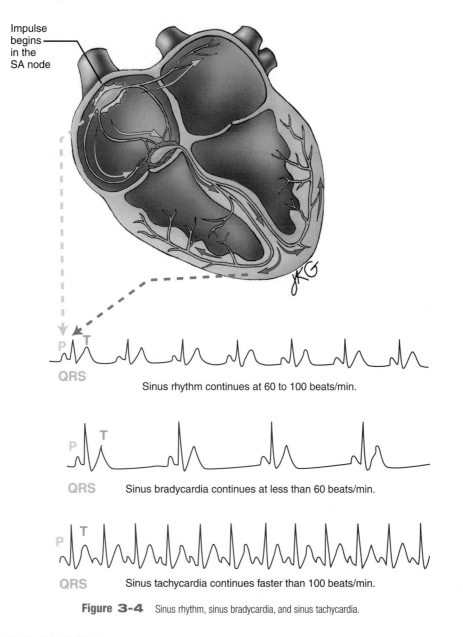

Impulse begins in the SA node

P T
QRS
Sinus rhythm continues at 60 to 100 beats/min.

P T
QRS
Sinus bradycardia continues at less than 60 beats/min.

P T
QRS
Sinus tachycardia continues faster than 100 beats/min.

Figure 3-4   Sinus rhythm, sinus bradycardia, and sinus tachycardia.

SINOATRIAL (SA) BLOCK

[OBJECTIVE 5]

In sinoatrial (SA) block (also called sinus exit block), the pacemaker cells within the SA node initiate an impulse but it is blocked as it exits the SA node. This results in periodically absent PQRST complexes. SA block is thought to occur because of failure of the transitional cells in the SA node to conduct the impulse from the pacemaker cells to the surrounding atrium. Thus SA block is a disorder of conductivity.

How Do I Recognize It?

The rhythm of the SA node is not affected by SA block because impulses are generated regularly. However, because an impulse is blocked as it exits the SA node, the atria are not activated. This appears on the ECG as a single missed beat (a P wave, QRS complex, and T wave are missing). The pause caused by the missed beat is the same as (or an exact multiple of) the distance between two P-P intervals of the underlying rhythm.

Look at the example of SA block in Figure 3-6. As you quickly scan the rhythm strip from left to right, the pause between the third and fourth beats should be obvious. The atrial and ventricular rhythm is irregular because of the pause. (It is also correct to say that the atrial and ventricular rhythms are regular except for the event; in this case, the pause is the event). Begin analyzing the rhythm strip by determining atrial and ventricular rate and regularity. Since there is a pause, it is best to give a rate range. In our example, the rate varies from 36 to 71 beats/min. You can see a positive P wave in front of each QRS complex. The P

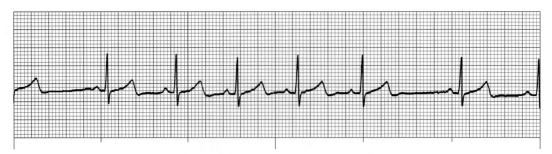

Figure 3-5 Sinus arrhythmia at 54 to 88 beats/min.

TABLE 3-5	Characteristics of Sinus Arrhythmia
Rate	Usually 60-100 beats/min, but may be slower or faster
Rhythm	Irregular, phasic with respiration; heart rate increases gradually during inspiration (R-R intervals shorten) and decreases with expiration (R-R intervals lengthen)
P waves	Positive (upright) in lead II, one precedes each QRS complex, P waves look alike
PR interval	0.12-0.20 sec and constant from beat to beat
QRS duration	0.10 sec or less unless an intraventricular conduction delay exists

waves look alike. The PR interval is 0.16 second and constant from beat to beat. The QRS complex is 0.08 second, which is within normal limits. Because the P waves are upright and each P wave is associated with a QRS complex, we know that the underlying rhythm came from the SA node. So far, we can identify this rhythm as a sinus rhythm with a ventricular rate of 36 to 71 beats/min.

Now we need to figure out what caused the pause between beats 3 and 4. First, look to the left of the pause and examine the waveforms of the beat that comes before the pause. Compare these waveforms to the others in the rhythm strip. It is important to do this because sometimes waveforms "hide" on top of other waveforms and distort their shape. In our example, nothing seems to be amiss.

Now use your calipers or paper and plot P waves and R waves from left to right across the strip. When you do this, make a mark on the rhythm strip where the next PQRST cycle should have occurred. You will find that exactly one PQRST cycle is missing. The P-P interval is an exact multiple of the distance between two P-P intervals of the underlying sinus rhythm. This occurred because impulses were generated regularly but failed to exit the SA node between beats 3 and 4. To complete our identification of this rhythm, we will explain the pause as an SA block. Putting it all together, we have a sinus rhythm at a rate of 36 to 71 beats/min with an episode of SA block. Table 3-6 lists the ECG characteristics of SA block.

What Causes It?

SA block is rather uncommon. Causes of SA block are shown in the ECG Pearl below. If episodes of SA block are frequent and/or accompanied by a slow heart rate, the patient may show signs and symptoms of hemodynamic compromise.

What Do I Do About It?

If the episodes of SA block are transient and there are no significant signs or symptoms, the patient is observed. If signs of hemodynamic compromise are present and are the result of medication toxicity, the offending agents should be withheld. If the episodes of SA block are frequent, IV atropine, temporary pacing, or insertion of a permanent pacemaker may be needed.

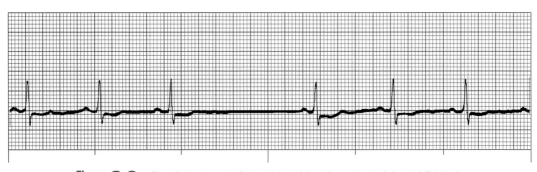

Figure 3-6 Sinus rhythm at a rate of 36 to 71 beats/min with an episode of sinoatrial (SA) block.

TABLE 3-6	Characteristics of Sinoatrial (SA) Block
Rate	Usually normal but varies because of the pause
Rhythm	Irregular due to the pause(s) caused by the SA block—the pause is the same as (or an exact multiple of) the distance between two other P-P intervals
P waves	Positive (upright) in lead II, P waves look alike. When present, one precedes each QRS complex.
PR interval	0.12-0.20 sec and constant from beat to beat
QRS duration	0.10 sec or less unless an intraventricular conduction delay exists

ECG Pearl

Causes of SA Block
- Acute MI
- Medications such as digitalis, quinidine, procainamide, or salicylates
- Coronary artery disease
- Myocarditis
- Congestive heart failure
- Carotid sinus sensitivity
- Increased vagal tone

SINUS ARREST

[OBJECTIVE 6]

Sinus arrest, also called sinus pause or sinoatrial (SA) arrest, is a disorder of the property of automaticity. In sinus arrest, the pacemaker cells of the SA node fail to initiate an electrical impulse for one or more beats. When the SA node fails to initiate an impulse, an escape pacemaker site (the AV junction or ventricles) should assume responsibility for pacing the heart. If they do not, you will see absent PQRST complexes on the ECG.

How Do I Recognize It?

Figure 3-7 shows an example of sinus arrest. Looking at the rhythm strip from left to right, you can see a period of no electrical activity between the third and fourth beats. Begin analyzing the rhythm strip by determining the atrial and ventricular rates and regularity. Because the rhythmicity of this dysrhythmia occurs as the result of a specific event and the remainder of the rhythm is regular, the regularity (rhythm) may be described as irregular or as regular except for the event. Since there is a pause, it is best to give a rate range. In our example, the rate varies from 24 to 81 beats/min. You can see a positive P wave in front of each QRS complex. The P waves look alike. The PR interval is 0.20 second and constant from beat to beat. The QRS complex is 0.10 second. Because the P waves are upright and each P wave is associated with a QRS complex, we know that the underlying rhythm came from the SA node. Therefore the underlying rhythm is a sinus rhythm with a ventricular rate of 24 to 81 beats/min.

Now let's try to explain what caused the pause between beats 3 and 4. Look to the left of the pause and examine the waveforms of the beat that comes before the pause. Compare these waveforms to the others in the rhythm strip. There does not appear to be any distortion of the waveforms. Using your calipers or paper, plot P waves and R waves from left to right across the strip. When you do this, make a mark on the rhythm strip where the next PQRST cycles should have occurred. You will find that more than one PQRST cycle is missing. Because the SA node periodically failed to produce impulses, the P-P intervals are not exact multiples of other P-P intervals. This is characteristic of a sinus arrest. To complete our identification of this rhythm strip, we must add this explanation for the pause we saw. Therefore our final identification is a sinus rhythm at a rate of 24 to 81 beats/min with an episode of sinus arrest. Table 3-7 lists the ECG characteristics of sinus arrest.

What Causes It?

Causes of sinus arrest include hypoxia, myocardial ischemia or infarction, hyperkalemia, digitalis toxicity, reactions to medications such as beta-blockers and calcium channel blockers, carotid sinus sensitivity, or increased vagal tone. Signs of hemodynamic compromise such as weakness, lightheadedness, dizziness, or syncope may be associated with this dysrhythmia.

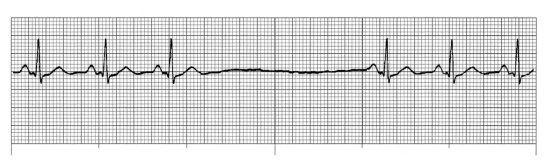

Figure 3-7 Sinus rhythm at a rate of 24 to 81 beats/min with an episode of sinus arrest.

TABLE **3-7**	Characteristics of Sinus Arrest
Rate	Usually normal but varies because of the pause
Rhythm	Irregular—the pause is of undetermined length (more than one PQRST complex is missing) and is not the same distance as other P-P intervals
P waves	Positive (upright) in lead II, P waves look alike. When present, one precedes each QRS complex.
PR interval	0.12-0.20 sec and constant from beat to beat
QRS duration	0.10 sec or less unless an intraventricular conduction delay exists

What Do I Do About It?

If the episodes of sinus arrest are transient and there are no significant signs or symptoms, observe the patient. If hemodynamic compromise is present, IV atropine may be indicated. If the episodes of sinus arrest are frequent and/or prolonged (more than 3 sec), temporary pacing or insertion of a permanent pacemaker may be warranted.

A summary of the characteristics of sinus mechanisms can be found in Table 3-8.

TABLE **3-8**	Sinus Mechanisms—Summary of Characteristics					
Characteristic	Sinus Rhythm	Sinus Bradycardia	Sinus Tachycardia	Sinus Arrhythmia	SA Block	Sinus Arrest
Rate (beats/min)	60-100	Less than 60	101-180	Usually 60-100	Varies	Varies
Rhythm	Regular	Regular	Regular	Irregular, typically phasic with respiration	Regular except for the event; pause is the same (or an exact multiple of) as the distance between two P-P intervals of underlying rhythm	Regular except for the event; pause of undetermined length—not a multiple of other P-P intervals
P Waves (lead II)	Positive, one precedes each QRS	Positive, one precedes each QRS	Positive, one precedes each QRS	Positive, one precedes each QRS	When present, positive, one precedes each QRS	When present, positive, one precedes each QRS
PR Interval	0.12-0.20 sec	0.12-0.20 sec	0.12-0.20 sec	0.12-0.20 sec	When present, 0.12-0.20 sec	When present, 0.12-0.20 sec
QRS	0.10 sec or less unless abnormally conducted	0.10 sec or less unless abnormally conducted	0.10 sec or less unless abnormally conducted	0.10 sec or less unless abnormally conducted	0.10 sec or less unless abnormally conducted	0.10 sec or less unless abnormally conducted

STOP & REVIEW

Multiple Choice

In the space provided, identify the letter of the choice that best completes each statement or answers each question.

____ 1. The normal duration of the PR interval is _____ second.
   a. 0.04 to 0.10
   b. 0.06 to 0.14
   c. 0.12 to 0.20
   d. 0.16 to 0.24

____ 2. Which of the following is commonly associated with an inferior or posterior myocardial infarction?
   a. Sinus tachycardia
   b. Sinus bradycardia
   c. SA block
   d. Sinus arrhythmia

____ 3. The portion of the ECG tracing between the QRS complex and the T wave is called the:
   a. ST-segment.
   b. PR interval.
   c. PR-segment
   d. QT interval.

____ 4. On an ECG, what is the first negative deflection seen after the P wave?
   a. Q wave
   b. R wave
   c. S wave
   d. T wave

____ 5. A 50-year-old man presents with chest pain that begins in the center of his chest and radiates to his jaw. On a 0 to 10 scale, he rates his pain 8/10. His blood pressure is 166/84, pulse 146, respirations 16. The cardiac monitor shows a sinus tachycardia with ST-segment elevation in leads I and aVL. The patient denies any allergies. Oxygen is being administered and intravenous (IV) access has been established. Which of the following should you do first?
   a. Give atropine.
   b. Give dopamine.
   c. Give aspirin and epinephrine.
   d. Give aspirin, nitroglycerin, and morphine if needed.

____ 6. The period during the cardiac cycle when cells cannot respond to a stimulus, no matter how strong, is called the _____ period.
   a. supernormal
   b. depolarized
   c. relative refractory
   d. absolute refractory

____ 7. In the heart's conduction system, the _____ receive(s) an electrical impulse from the bundle of His and relays it to the Purkinje fibers in ventricular myocardium.
   a. sinoatrial (SA) node
   b. atrioventricular (AV) node
   c. atrioventricular (AV) junction
   d. right and left bundle branches

____ 8. Leads II, III, and aVF view the _____ surface of the heart.
   a. anterior
   b. inferior
   c. posterior
   d. lateral

Matching

Match each item with the correct item below.

____ **9.** Normal QRS duration in an adult

____ **10.** Sinus arrest is a disorder of _____.

____ **11.** Dysrhythmia with a pause of undetermined length that is not the same distance as other P-P intervals

____ **12.** Rate associated with a sinus bradycardia

____ **13.** SA block is a disorder of _____.

____ **14.** Dysrhythmia that originates from the SA node and has a ventricular rate of 101 to 180 beats/min

____ **15.** Appearance of P waves that originate from the SA node

____ **16.** Cardiac output

____ **17.** Pacemaker with an intrinsic rate of 20 to 40 beats/min

____ **18.** Normal rate for a sinus rhythm

____ **19.** This medication may be used to increase heart rate if the QRS is narrow and the patient is symptomatic because the rate is slow.

____ **20.** Dysrhythmia with a pause that is the same as (or an exact multiple of) the distance between two other P-P intervals

____ **21.** Medications that may be administered to slow the heart rate and decrease myocardial oxygen demand

____ **22.** Common dysrhythmia associated with respiratory rate

____ **23.** If the SA node fails to generate an impulse, the next (escape) pacemaker that should generate an impulse

____ **24.** Any disturbance or abnormality in a normal rhythmic pattern

a. beta-blockers

b. Sinus arrhythmia

c. Purkinje fibers/ventricles

d. 60-100 beats/min

e. Atropine

f. Sinus arrest

g. Dysrhythmia

h. AV junction

i. Conductivity

j. 0.06-0.10 sec

k. Automaticity

l. SA block

m. Less than 60 beats/min

n. Stroke volume × heart rate

o. Sinus tachycardia

p. Smooth, rounded, upright

Short Answer

25. Without looking back in the chapter, see if you can answer the following questions about the characteristics of a sinus rhythm.

Rate: _____

Rhythm: _____

P waves: _____

PR interval (PRI): _____

QRS duration: _____

Keep the ECG characteristics of sinus rhythm in mind as you answer the following questions.

26. What is the most important difference between sinus rhythm and sinus bradycardia?

27. What is the most important difference between sinus rhythm and sinus tachycardia?

28. What is the most important difference between sinus rhythm and sinus arrhythmia?

29. List five (5) signs or symptoms of hemodynamic compromise.
   1.

   2.

   3.

   4.

   5.

30. List five (5) causes of sinus tachycardia.
   1.

   2.

   3.

   4.

   5.

SINUS MECHANISMS—*PRACTICE RHYTHM STRIPS*

For each of the following rhythm strips, determine the atrial and ventricular rate and rhythm, measure the PR interval and QRS duration, and then identify the rhythm. All strips were recorded in lead II unless otherwise noted.

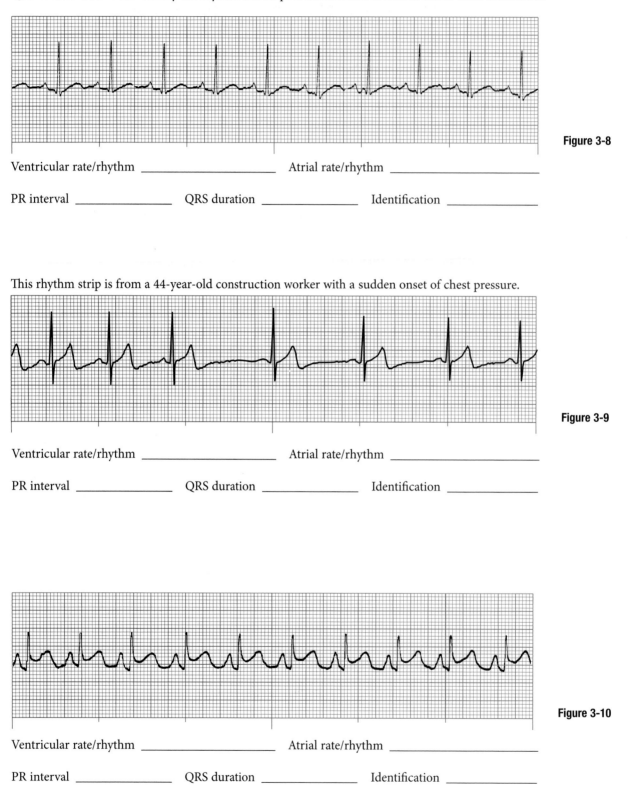

Figure 3-8

Ventricular rate/rhythm _____   Atrial rate/rhythm _____

PR interval _____   QRS duration _____   Identification _____

This rhythm strip is from a 44-year-old construction worker with a sudden onset of chest pressure.

Figure 3-9

Ventricular rate/rhythm _____   Atrial rate/rhythm _____

PR interval _____   QRS duration _____   Identification _____

Figure 3-10

Ventricular rate/rhythm _____   Atrial rate/rhythm _____

PR interval _____   QRS duration _____   Identification _____

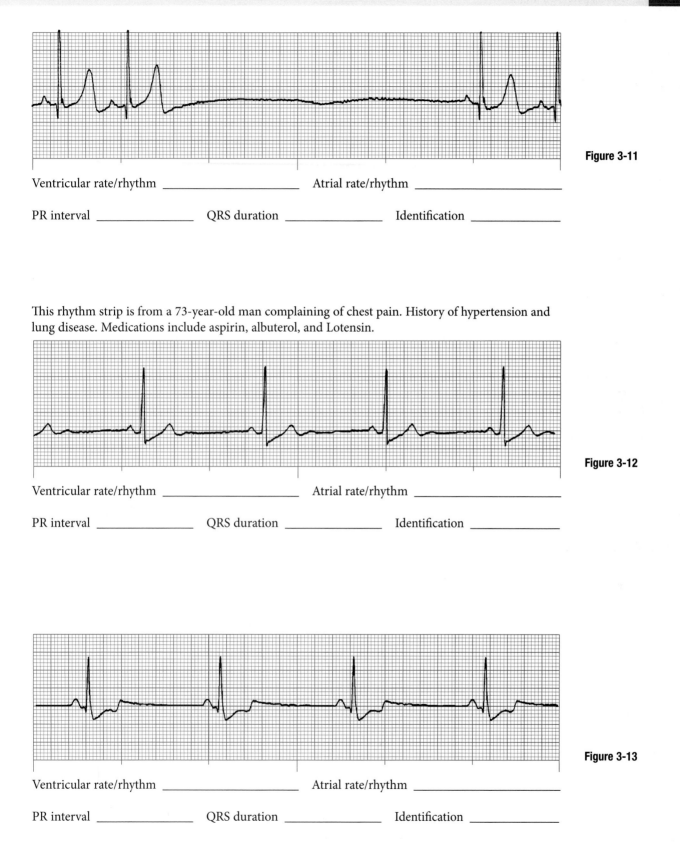

Figure 3-11

Ventricular rate/rhythm _____   Atrial rate/rhythm _____

PR interval _____   QRS duration _____   Identification _____

This rhythm strip is from a 73-year-old man complaining of chest pain. History of hypertension and lung disease. Medications include aspirin, albuterol, and Lotensin.

Figure 3-12

Ventricular rate/rhythm _____   Atrial rate/rhythm _____

PR interval _____   QRS duration _____   Identification _____

Figure 3-13

Ventricular rate/rhythm _____   Atrial rate/rhythm _____

PR interval _____   QRS duration _____   Identification _____

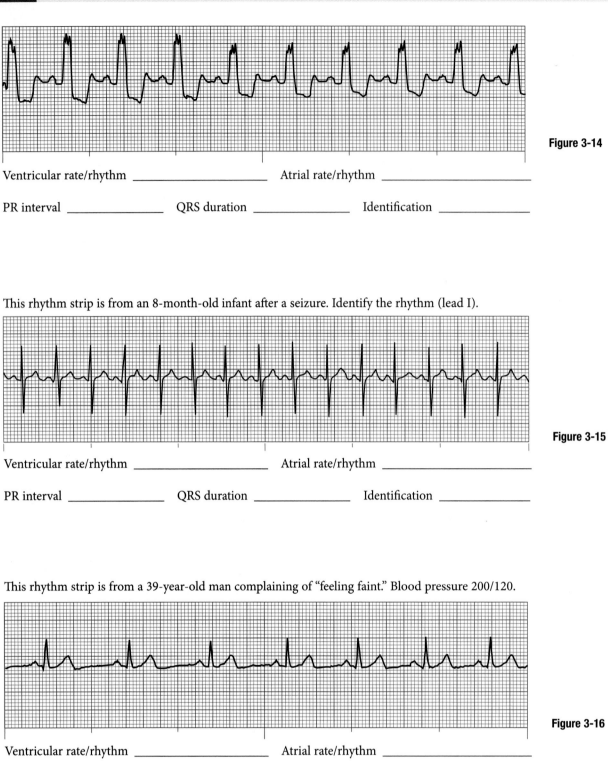

Figure 3-14

Ventricular rate/rhythm _____   Atrial rate/rhythm _____

PR interval _____   QRS duration _____   Identification _____

This rhythm strip is from an 8-month-old infant after a seizure. Identify the rhythm (lead I).

Figure 3-15

Ventricular rate/rhythm _____   Atrial rate/rhythm _____

PR interval _____   QRS duration _____   Identification _____

This rhythm strip is from a 39-year-old man complaining of "feeling faint." Blood pressure 200/120.

Figure 3-16

Ventricular rate/rhythm _____   Atrial rate/rhythm _____

PR interval _____   QRS duration _____   Identification _____

These rhythm strips are from a 35-year-old man complaining of a sudden onset of severe substernal chest pain. He has no significant past medical history and takes no medications. His initial blood pressure is 56/0.

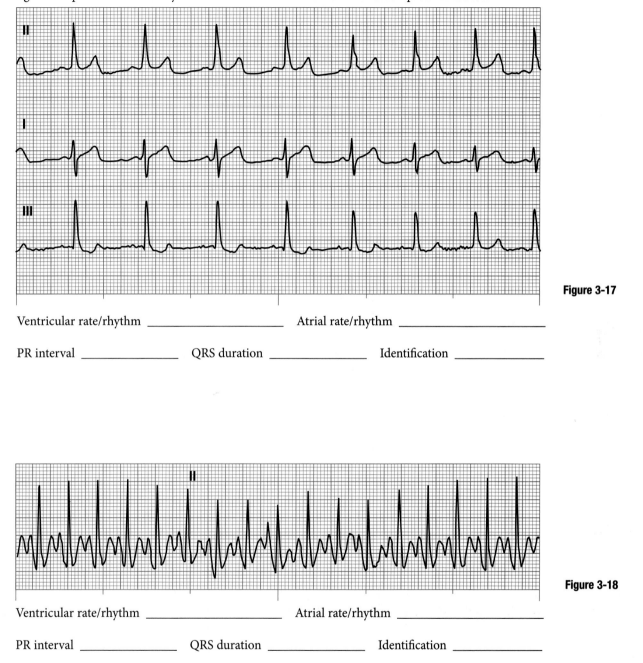

Figure 3-17

Ventricular rate/rhythm _____   Atrial rate/rhythm _____

PR interval _____   QRS duration _____   Identification _____

Figure 3-18

Ventricular rate/rhythm _____   Atrial rate/rhythm _____

PR interval _____   QRS duration _____   Identification _____

This rhythm strip is from a 61-year-old woman with an altered level of responsiveness. Blood pressure is 112/62. Blood sugar is 42.

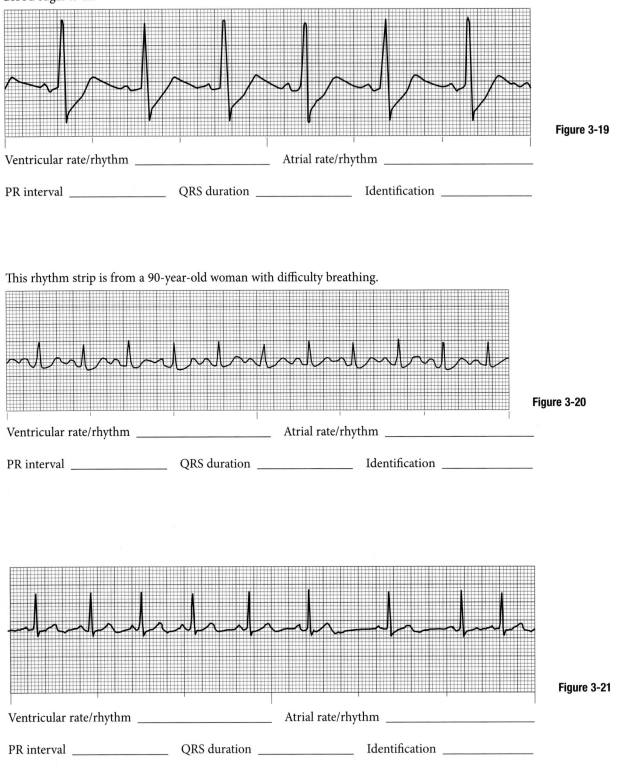

Figure 3-19

Ventricular rate/rhythm _____   Atrial rate/rhythm _____

PR interval _____   QRS duration _____   Identification _____

This rhythm strip is from a 90-year-old woman with difficulty breathing.

Figure 3-20

Ventricular rate/rhythm _____   Atrial rate/rhythm _____

PR interval _____   QRS duration _____   Identification _____

Figure 3-21

Ventricular rate/rhythm _____   Atrial rate/rhythm _____

PR interval _____   QRS duration _____   Identification _____

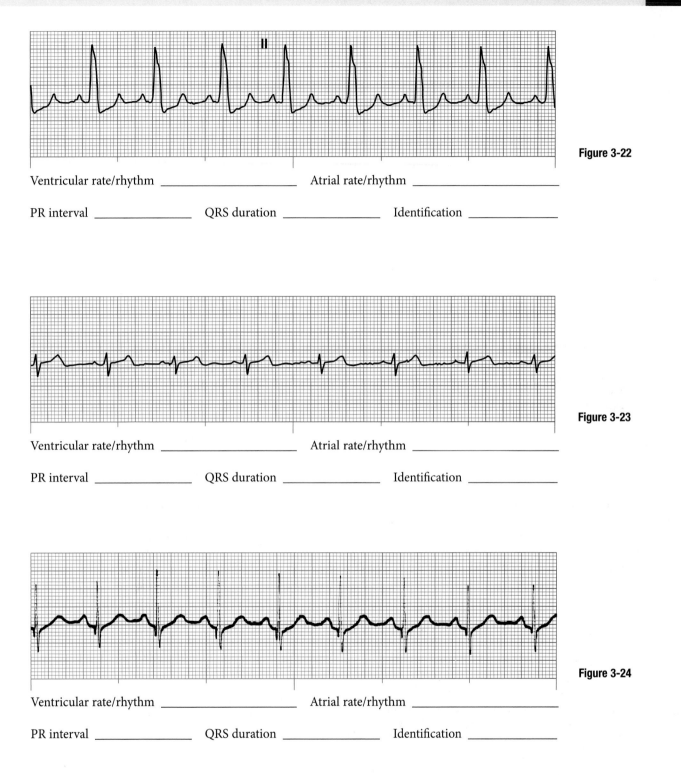

Figure 3-22

Ventricular rate/rhythm _____   Atrial rate/rhythm _____

PR interval _____   QRS duration _____   Identification _____

Figure 3-23

Ventricular rate/rhythm _____   Atrial rate/rhythm _____

PR interval _____   QRS duration _____   Identification _____

Figure 3-24

Ventricular rate/rhythm _____   Atrial rate/rhythm _____

PR interval _____   QRS duration _____   Identification _____

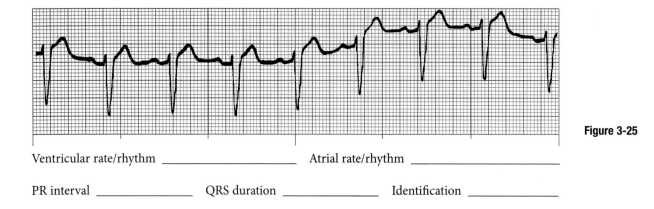

Figure 3-25

Ventricular rate/rhythm _____ Atrial rate/rhythm _____

PR interval _____ QRS duration _____ Identification _____

STOP & REVIEW ANSWERS

Multiple Choice

1. c	**5.** d
2. b	**6.** d
3. a	**7.** d
4. a	**8.** b

Matching

9. j	**17.** c
10. k	**18.** d
11. f	**19.** e
12. m	**20.** l
13. i	**21.** a
14. o	**22.** b
15. p	**23.** h
16. n	**24.** g

Short Answer

25.

Rate	Rhythm	P waves	PR interval	QRS duration
60-100 beats/ min	Regular	Uniform in appearance, positive (upright) in lead II, one precedes each QRS complex	0.12-0.20 sec and constant from beat to beat	0.10 sec or less

26. A sinus rhythm has a rate of 60 to 100 beats/min. A sinus bradycardia has a rate of less than 60 beats/min.

27. A sinus rhythm has a rate of 60 to 100 beats/min. A sinus tachycardia has a rate of 101 to 180 beats/min.

28. A sinus rhythm has a regular atrial and ventricular rhythm. A sinus arrhythmia occurs when the SA node fires irregularly, resulting in an irregular atrial and ventricular rhythm.

29. Signs and symptoms of hemodynamic compromise
- Changes in mental status (restlessness, confusion, possible loss of consciousness)
- Low blood pressure
- Chest pain
- Shortness of breath
- Signs of shock
- Congestive heart failure
- Pulmonary congestion
- Fall in urine output
- Cold, clammy skin

30. Causes of sinus tachycardia
- Exercise
- Fever
- Pain
- Fear and anxiety
- Hypoxia
- Congestive heart failure
- Acute myocardial infarction
- Infection
- Sympathetic stimulation
- Shock
- Dehydration, hypovolemia
- Pulmonary embolism
- Hyperthyroidism
- Medications such as epinephrine, atropine, and dopamine
- Caffeine-containing beverages
- Nicotine
- Drugs such as cocaine, amphetamines

Figure 3-8 answer

Ventricular rate/rhythm	95 beats/min, regular
Atrial rate/rhythm	95 beats/min, regular
PR interval	0.16 sec
QRS duration	0.08 sec
Identification	Sinus rhythm at 95 beats/min

Figure 3-9 answer

Ventricular rate/rhythm	52 to 94 beats/min, irregular
Atrial rate/rhythm	52 to 94 beats/min, irregular
PR interval	0.12 sec
QRS duration	0.08 sec
Identification	Sinus arrhythmia at 52 to 94 beats/min

Figure 3-10 answer

Ventricular rate/rhythm	98 beats/min, regular
Atrial rate/rhythm	98 beats/min, regular
PR interval	0.16 sec
QRS duration	0.04 to 0.06 sec
Identification	Sinus rhythm at 98 bpm; ST-segment elevation

Figure 3-11 answer

Ventricular rate/rhythm	0 to 75 beats/min, irregular
Atrial rate/rhythm	0 to 75 beats/min, irregular
PR interval	0.16 sec
QRS duration	0.08 sec
Identification	Sinus rhythm at about 75 beats/min with an episode of sinus arrest; tall T waves

Figure 3-12 answer

Ventricular rate/rhythm	44 beats/min, regular
Atrial rate/rhythm	44 beats/min, regular
PR interval	0.16 sec
QRS duration	0.06 sec
Identification	Sinus bradycardia at 44 beats/min, ST-segment depression. Note the upright U waves following each T wave.

Figure 3-13 answer

Ventricular rate/rhythm	40 beats/min, regular
Atrial rate/rhythm	40 beats/min, regular
PR interval	0.16 sec
QRS duration	0.08 sec
Identification	Sinus bradycardia at 40 beats/min; ST-segment depression, inverted T waves.

Figure 3-14 answer

Ventricular rate/rhythm	94 beats/min, regular
Atrial rate/rhythm	94 beats/min, regular
PR interval	0.18 sec
QRS duration	0.12 sec
Identification	Sinus rhythm at 94 beats/min with a wide (and notched) QRS, ST-segment depression

Figure 3-15 answer

Ventricular rate/rhythm	150 beats/min, regular
Atrial rate/rhythm	150 beats/min, regular
PR interval	0.12 sec
QRS duration	0.06 to 0.08 sec
Identification	Sinus tachycardia at 150 beats/min

Figure 3-16 answer

Ventricular rate/rhythm	67 to 83 beats/min, irregular
Atrial rate/rhythm	67 to 83 beats/min, irregular
PR interval	0.16 sec
QRS duration	0.06 to 0.08 sec
Identification	Sinus arrhythmia at 67 to 83 beats/min

Figure 3-17 answer

Ventricular rate/rhythm	75 beats/min, regular
Atrial rate/rhythm	75 beats/min, regular
PR interval	0.14 sec
QRS duration	0.08 sec
Identification	Sinus rhythm at 75 beats/min, ST-segment depression

Figure 3-18 answer

Ventricular rate/rhythm	167 beats/min, regular
Atrial rate/rhythm	167 beats/min, regular
PR interval	0.12 sec
QRS duration	0.06 sec
Identification	Sinus tachycardia at 167 beats/min

Figure 3-19 answer

Ventricular rate/rhythm	65 beats/min, regular
Atrial rate/rhythm	65 beats/min, regular
PR interval	0.20 sec
QRS duration	0.10 sec
Identification	Sinus rhythm at 65 beats/min with ST-segment depression

Figure 3-20 answer

Ventricular rate/rhythm	111 beats/min, regular
Atrial rate/rhythm	111 beats/min, regular
PR interval	0.16 sec
QRS duration	0.04 to 0.06 sec
Identification	Sinus tachycardia at 111 beats/min

Figure 3-21 answer

Ventricular rate/rhythm	64 to 94 beats/min, irregular
Atrial rate/rhythm	64 to 94 beats/min, irregular
PR interval	0.16 sec
QRS duration	0.06 to 0.08 sec
Identification	Sinus arrhythmia at 64 to 94 beats/min

Figure 3-22 answer

Ventricular rate/rhythm	71 beats/min, regular
Atrial rate/rhythm	71 beats/min, regular
PR interval	0.16 to 0.20 sec
QRS duration	0.12 to 0.14 sec
Identification	Sinus rhythm at 71 beats/min with a wide QRS, ST-segment depression

Figure 3-23 answer

Ventricular rate/rhythm	71 beats/min, regular
Atrial rate/rhythm	71 beats/min, regular
PR interval	0.12 sec
QRS duration	0.08 sec
Identification	Sinus rhythm at 71 beats/min

Figure 3-24 answer

Ventricular rate/rhythm	85 beats/min, regular
Atrial rate/rhythm	85 beats/min, regular
PR interval	0.16 sec
QRS duration	0.08 sec
Identification	Sinus rhythm at 85 beats/min

Figure 3-25 answer

Ventricular rate/rhythm	83 beats/min, regular
Atrial rate/rhythm	83 beat/min, regular
PR interval	0.18 sec
QRS duration	0.12 sec
Identification	Sinus rhythm with a wide QRS at 83 beats/min

Atrial Rhythms

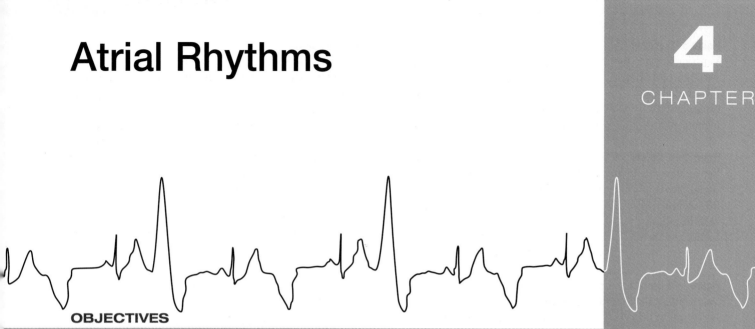

OBJECTIVES

After reading this chapter, you should be able to:

1. Explain the concepts of altered automaticity, triggered activity, and reentry.
2. Explain the terms bigeminy, trigeminy, quadrigeminy, and run when used to describe premature complexes.
3. Describe the ECG characteristics, possible causes, signs and symptoms, and initial emergency care for premature atrial complexes (PACs).
4. Explain the difference between a compensatory and noncompensatory pause.
5. Explain the terms wandering atrial pacemaker and multifocal atrial tachycardia.
6. Describe the ECG characteristics, possible causes, signs and symptoms, and initial emergency care for wandering atrial pacemaker (multiformed atrial rhythm).
7. Describe the ECG characteristics, possible causes, signs and symptoms, and initial emergency care for multifocal atrial tachycardia (MAT).
8. List four examples of vagal maneuvers.
9. Describe the ECG characteristics, possible causes, signs and symptoms, and initial emergency care for atrial tachycardia (AT).
10. Explain the terms paroxysmal atrial tachycardia (PAT) and paroxysmal supraventricular tachycardia (PSVT).
11. Discuss the indications and procedure for synchronized cardioversion.
12. Describe the ECG characteristics, possible causes, signs and symptoms, and initial emergency care for atrioventricular nodal reentrant tachycardia (AVNRT).
13. Describe the ECG characteristics, possible causes, signs and symptoms, and initial emergency care for atrioventricular reentrant tachycardia (AVRT).
14. Describe the ECG characteristics, possible causes, signs and symptoms, and initial emergency care for atrial flutter.
15. Describe the ECG characteristics, possible causes, signs and symptoms, and initial emergency care for atrial fibrillation (AFib).

INTRODUCTION

The atria are thin-walled, low-pressure chambers that receive blood from the systemic circulation and lungs. There is normally a continuous flow of blood from the superior and inferior vena cavae into the atria. Approximately 70% of this blood flows directly through the atria and into the ventricles before the atria contract. When the atria contract, an additional 30% is added to filling of the ventricles. This additional contribution of blood because of atrial contraction is called **atrial kick**.

P waves reflect atrial depolarization. A rhythm that begins in the SA node has one positive (upright) P wave before each QRS complex. A rhythm that begins in the atria will have a positive P wave that is shaped differently than P waves that begin in the SA node. This difference in P wave configuration occurs because the impulse begins in the atria and follows a different conduction pathway to the AV node.

ATRIAL DYSRHYTHMIAS: MECHANISMS

[OBJECTIVE 1]

Atrial dysrhythmias reflect abnormal electrical impulse formation and conduction in the atria. They result from altered automaticity, triggered activity, or reentry. Altered automaticity and triggered activity are disorders in impulse *formation*. Reentry is a disorder in impulse *conduction*. Dysrhythmias that result from disorders of impulse formation are often referred to as automatic. Dysrhythmias that result from a disorder in impulse conduction are referred to as reentrant.

Altered Automaticity

Altered automaticity occurs in normal pacemaker cells and in myocardial working cells that do not normally function as pacemaker sites. In altered automaticity, these cells fire and initiate impulses before a normal SA node impulse. If the rapid firing rate occurs for more than 50% of the day, it is said to be incessant. The rapid firing rate may also occur periodically. In these cases it is said to be episodic. Atrial dysrhythmias associated with altered automaticity include premature atrial complexes and atrial fibrillation.

ECG Pearl

Causes of Altered Automaticity
- Ischemia
- Drug toxicity
- Hypocalcemia
- Imbalance of electrolytes across the cardiac cell membrane

Triggered Activity

Triggered activity results from abnormal electrical impulses that sometimes occur during repolarization (afterdepolarizations), when cells are normally quiet. Triggered activity occurs when escape pacemaker and myocardial working cells fire more than once after stimulation by a single impulse. Triggered activity can result in atrial or ventricular beats that occur alone, in pairs, in "runs" (three or more beats), or as a sustained ectopic rhythm.

ECG Pearl

Causes of Triggered Activity
- Hypoxia
- Catecholamine increase
- Hypomagnesemia
- Myocardial ischemia and injury
- Medications that prolong repolarization (e.g., quinidine)

Reentry

Reentry (reactivation) is a condition in which an impulse returns to stimulate tissue that was previously depolarized. Reentry requires[3] (Figure 4-1):
- A potential conduction circuit or circular conduction pathway
- A block within part of the circuit
- Delayed conduction within the remainder of the circuit

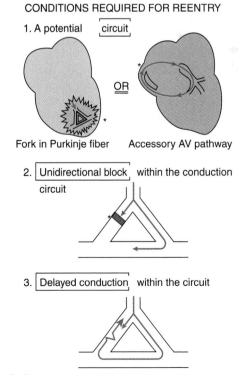

CONDITIONS REQUIRED FOR REENTRY

1. A potential circuit

Fork in Purkinje fiber   Accessory AV pathway

2. Unidirectional block within the conduction circuit

3. Delayed conduction within the circuit

Figure 4-1   Reentry requires (1) a potential conduction circuit or circular conduction pathway, (2) a block within part of the circuit, and (3) delayed conduction with the remainder of the circuit.

Normally, an impulse spreads through the heart only once after it is initiated by pacemaker cells. In reentry, an electrical impulse is delayed or blocked (or both) in one or more areas of the conduction system while being conducted normally through the rest of the system. This results in the delayed electrical impulse entering cardiac cells that have just been depolarized by the normally conducted impulse. If the delayed impulse stimulates a relatively refractory area, the impulse can cause those cells to fire. This can produce a single early (premature) beat or repetitive electrical impulses, resulting in short periods of rapid rhythms (tachydysrhythmias).

Macroreentry circuits and microreentry circuits are two main types of reentry circuits. If the reentry circuit involves conduction through a large area of the heart, such as the entire right or left atrium, it is called a macroreentry circuit. A reentry circuit involving conduction within a small area is called a microreentry circuit. Atrial rhythms associated with reentry include atrial flutter, AV nodal reentrant tachycardia (AVNRT), and AV reentrant tachycardia (AVRT).

ECG Pearl

Common Causes of Reentry
- Hyperkalemia
- Myocardial ischemia
- Some antiarrhythmic medications

Most atrial dysrhythmias are not life-threatening, but some may be associated with extremely fast ventricular rates. Increases in heart rate shorten all phases of the cardiac cycle, but the most important is a decrease in the length of time spent in diastole. Remember that as the heart rate increases, there is less time for the ventricles to fill and less blood for the ventricles to pump out with each contraction. Thus an excessively fast heart rate can lead to decreased cardiac output. Factors that influence heart rate include hormone levels (e.g., thyroxin, epinephrine, norepinephrine), medications, stress, anxiety, fear, and body temperature.

PREMATURE ATRIAL COMPLEXES (PACs)

[OBJECTIVE 2]
Premature beats appear early, that is, they occur before the next expected beat. Premature beats are identified by their site of origin:
- Premature atrial complexes (PACs)
- Premature junctional complexes (PJCs)
- Premature ventricular complexes (PVCs)

The term *complex* is used instead of *contraction* to correctly identify an early beat because the ECG depicts electrical activity, not mechanical function of the heart. Some areas prefer the term "conduction" instead of complex.

Premature beats may occur in patterns:
- Pairs (coupled): Two premature beats in a row
- "Runs" or "bursts": Three or more premature beats in a row
- Bigeminy: Every other beat is a premature beat
- Trigeminy: Every third beat is a premature beat
- Quadrigeminy: Every fourth beat is a premature beat

How Do I Recognize It?

[OBJECTIVE 3]
A **premature atrial complex** (PAC) occurs when an irritable site (focus) within the atria fires before the next SA node impulse is due to fire. This interrupts the sinus rhythm. If the irritable site is close to the SA node, the atrial P wave will look very similar to the P waves initiated by the SA node. The P wave of a PAC may be biphasic (partly positive, partly negative), flattened, notched, pointed, or lost in the preceding T wave.

ECG Pearl

A PAC has a positive P wave before the QRS complex. Sometimes the P waves are clearly seen and sometimes they are not. If the P wave of an early beat isn't obvious, look for it in the T wave of the preceding beat. The T wave of the preceding beat may be of higher amplitude than other T waves or have an extra "hump." This suggests the presence of a hidden P wave.

When compared with the P-P intervals of the underlying rhythm, a PAC is premature—occurring before the next expected sinus P wave. PACs are identified by:
- Early (premature) P waves
- Positive (upright) P waves (in lead II) that differ in shape from sinus P waves
- Early P waves that may or may not be followed by a QRS complex

Look closely at the rhythm strip in Figure 4-2. Begin by locating the QRS complexes on the rhythm strip. Evaluate each succeeding R-R interval. The R-R intervals in this example occur regularly except for three beats. Determine the ventricular rate between the regular R-R intervals. The ventricular rate between the regular R-R intervals is 111 beats/min.

Now find the P waves on the rhythm strip. Remember that P waves that begin in the SA node are normally smooth and rounded. Atrial P waves will look different. Using a pen or pencil, mark an "S" (for SA node) above each normal looking P wave. Mark an "A" above those P waves that look different. When you are finished, you should have an "A" marked over the P waves in beats 2, 7, and 10. The rest of the P waves should be marked with an "S."

Notice that the waveforms marked with an "S" above them occur regularly except when they are interrupted by the three atrial beats. Using the sinus beats as your guide, determine the

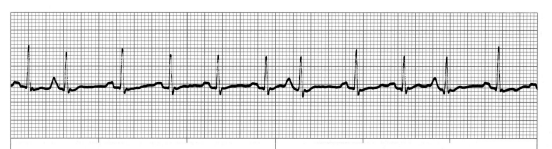

Figure 4-2 Sinus tachycardia with three PACs. From the left, beats 2, 7, and 10 are PACs.

atrial rate. The atrial rate between the regular P-P intervals is 111 beats/min. Based on the rate (more than 100 beats/min) and an upright P wave before each QRS, we know that the underlying rhythm is a sinus tachycardia. Using your calipers (or a piece of paper), find two sinus beats that appear next to each other (such as beats 4 and 5). Now move your calipers (or paper) to the right. If beat 6 occurred on time, it will line up with your calipers (or paper). It is on time. Now move your calipers to the right again. The right point of your calipers shows where the next sinus beat should have occurred. You can see that beat 7 occurred earlier than expected. This is a premature beat. When you continue this process you will find that beat 10 is also early. Working backward (and without adjusting your calipers), if you place the left point of your calipers on beat 1 in the rhythm strip, you'll see that beat 2 is also early. So far we can identify this rhythm as a sinus tachycardia at 111 beats/min with three premature beats.

Measure the PR interval and QRS duration. The PR interval is 0.16 second and the QRS is 0.08 second in duration. Since premature beats can start from more than one area of the heart, we must identify where the premature beats came from. To do this, we must examine the premature beats more closely. Look carefully at beats 2, 7, and 10. The QRS complexes look the same as those of the underlying rhythm. This is because the impulse is conducted normally through the AV junction, bundle branches, and ventricles. Now look to the left of the QRS complex in each of these early beats and look at the P waves. Each P wave is positive (upright) but looks different than the P waves of the sinus beats. This is an important finding and one that tells you that the P waves came from the atria. The early beats are premature atrial complexes. A PAC is not an entire rhythm—it is a single beat. Therefore you must identify the underlying rhythm and the ectopic beat(s). To complete our identification of this rhythm, we have a sinus tachycardia at 111 beats/min with three premature atrial complexes. The ECG characteristics of PACs are shown in Table 4-1.

Noncompensatory vs. Compensatory Pause

[OBJECTIVE 4]

A **noncompensatory (incomplete)** pause often follows a PAC. This represents the delay during which the SA node resets its rhythm for the next beat. A **compensatory (complete)** pause

TABLE 4-1	Characteristics of Premature Atrial Complexes (PACs)
Rate	Usually within normal range, but depends on underlying rhythm
Rhythm	Regular with premature beats
P waves	Premature (occurring earlier than the next expected sinus P wave), positive (upright) in lead II, one before each QRS complex, often differ in shape from sinus P waves—may be flattened, notched, pointed, biphasic, or lost in the preceding T wave
PR interval	May be normal or prolonged depending on the prematurity of the beat
QRS duration	Usually 0.10 sec or less but may be wide (aberrant) or absent, depending on the prematurity of the beat; the QRS of the PAC is similar in shape to those of the underlying rhythm unless the PAC is abnormally conducted

often follows premature ventricular complexes (PVCs). To find out whether or not the pause following a premature complex is compensatory or noncompensatory, measure the distance between three normal beats. Then compare that measurement to the distance between three beats, one of which includes the premature complex. The pause is *noncompensatory* if the normal beat following the premature complex occurs before it was expected (i.e., the period between the complex before and after the premature beat is less than two normal R-R intervals). The pause is *compensatory* if the normal beat following the premature complex occurs when expected (i.e., the period between the complex before and after the premature beat is the same as two normal R-R intervals).

Aberrantly Conducted PACs

If a PAC occurs very early, the right bundle branch can be slow to respond to the impulse (refractory). The impulse travels down the left bundle branch with no problem. Stimulation of the left bundle branch subsequently results in stimulation of the right bundle branch. The QRS will appear wide (greater than 0.10 sec) because of this delay in ventricular depolarization. PACs associated with a wide QRS complex are called **aberrantly conducted PACs**. This indicates that conduction through the ventricles is abnormal. Figure 4-3 shows a rhythm strip with two PACs. The first PAC (arrow) was conducted abnormally, producing a wide QRS complex. The second PAC (arrow) was conducted normally. Compare the T waves before each PAC with those of the underlying sinus bradycardia.

Nonconducted PACs

Sometimes, when a PAC occurs very early and close to the T wave of the preceding beat, only a P wave may be seen with no QRS after it (appearing as a pause) (Figure 4-4). This type of PAC is called a *nonconducted* or *blocked* PAC because the P wave occurred too early to be conducted. Nonconducted PACs occur because the AV junction is still refractory to stimulation and unable to conduct the impulse to the ventricles (thus no QRS complex). Look for the early P wave in the T wave of the preceding beat.

What Causes Them?

[OBJECTIVE 3]

PACs may be due to altered automaticity or reentry. PACs are very common and can occur at any age. They are very frequent in the elderly. Their presence does not necessarily imply underlying cardiac disease. Causes of PACs include:
- Emotional stress
- Congestive heart failure
- Acute coronary syndromes
- Mental and physical fatigue
- Atrial enlargement
- Valvular heart disease
- Digitalis toxicity

- Electrolyte imbalance
- Hyperthyroidism
- Stimulants: caffeine, tobacco, cocaine

What Do I Do About It?

[OBJECTIVE 3]

PACs usually do not require treatment if they are infrequent. The patient may complain of a "skipped beat" or occasional "palpitations" (if PACs are frequent) or may be unaware of their occurrence. In susceptible individuals, frequent PACs may set off episodes of atrial fibrillation, atrial flutter, or PSVT. Frequent PACs are treated by correcting the underlying cause:
- Reducing stress
- Reducing or eliminating stimulants
- Treating congestive heart failure
- Correcting electrolyte imbalances

If needed, frequent PACs may be treated with beta-blockers, calcium channel blockers, and/or antianxiety medications.

WANDERING ATRIAL PACEMAKER

How Do I Recognize It?

[OBJECTIVES 5, 6]

Multiformed atrial rhythm is an updated term for the rhythm formerly known as **wandering atrial pacemaker**. With this rhythm, the size, shape, and direction of the P waves vary, sometimes from beat to beat. The difference in the look of the P waves is a result of the gradual shifting of the dominant pacemaker between the SA node, the atria, and/or the AV junction (Figure 4-5). Wandering atrial pacemaker is associated with a normal or slow rate and irregular P-P, R-R,

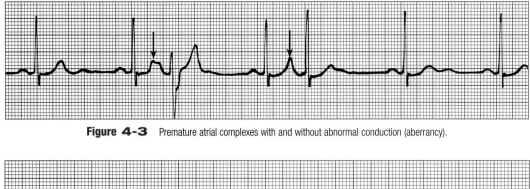

Figure 4-3   Premature atrial complexes with and without abnormal conduction (aberrancy).

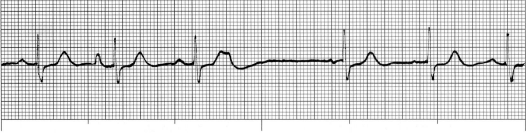

Figure 4-4   Sinus rhythm with a nonconducted (blocked) PAC.

Lead II (continuous)

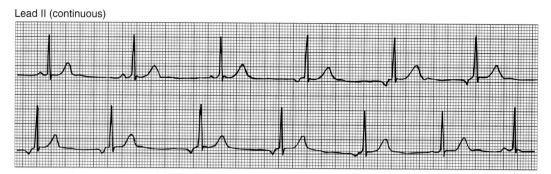

Figure 4-5   Wandering atrial pacemaker. Continuous strip (lead II).

and PR intervals because of the different sites of impulse formation. The QRS duration is normally 0.10 second or less because conduction through the ventricles is usually normal. The ECG characteristics of wandering atrial pacemaker are shown in Table 4-2.

ECG Pearl ⟋ᴎ⟍

At least three different P wave configurations, seen in the same lead, are required for a diagnosis of wandering atrial pacemaker or multifocal atrial tachycardia.

TABLE 4-2	Characteristics of Wandering Atrial Pacemaker (Multiformed Atrial Rhythm)
Rate	Usually 60-100 beats/min, but may be slow; if the rate is greater than 100 beats/min, the rhythm is termed *multifocal* (or *chaotic*) *atrial tachycardia*
Rhythm	May be irregular as the pacemaker site shifts from the SA node to ectopic atrial locations and the AV junction
P waves	Size, shape, and direction may change from beat to beat; at least three different P wave configurations (seen in the same lead) are required for a diagnosis of wandering atrial pacemaker or multifocal atrial tachycardia
PR interval	Variable
QRS duration	0.10 sec or less unless an intraventricular conduction delay exists

What Causes It?

Wandering atrial pacemaker may be observed in normal, healthy hearts (particularly in athletes) and during sleep. It may also occur with some types of underlying heart disease and with digitalis toxicity. This dysrhythmia usually produces no signs and symptoms unless it is associated with a slow rate.

What Do I Do About It?

Wandering atrial pacemaker is usually a transient rhythm that resolves on its own when the firing rate of the SA node increases and the sinus resumes pacing responsibility. If the rhythm occurs because of digitalis toxicity, the drug should be withheld.

MULTIFOCAL ATRIAL TACHYCARDIA

How Do I Recognize It?

[OBJECTIVE 7]
When the wandering atrial pacemaker is associated with a ventricular rate greater than 100 beats/min, the rhythm is called **multifocal atrial tachycardia (MAT)** or *chaotic atrial tachycardia* (Figure 4-6). In MAT, multiple ectopic sites stimulate the atria. MAT may be confused with atrial fibrillation since both rhythms are irregular; however, P waves (although varying in size, shape, and direction) are clearly visible in MAT.

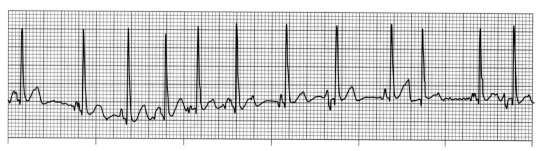

Figure 4-6   Multifocal atrial tachycardia (MAT), also known as chaotic atrial tachycardia.

What Causes It?

Multifocal atrial tachycardia is most often seen in the following:
- Severe chronic obstructive pulmonary disease (COPD)
- Hypoxia
- Acute coronary syndromes
- Digoxin toxicity
- Rheumatic heart disease
- Theophylline toxicity
- Electrolyte imbalances

What Do I Do About It?

Treatment of MAT is directed at the underlying cause. If the patient is stable and symptomatic but you are uncertain if the rhythm is MAT, you can try a vagal maneuver. If vagal maneuvers are ineffective, you can try adenosine IV. Remember that MAT is the result of random and chaotic firing of multiple sites in the atria. MAT does not involve reentry through the AV node. Therefore it is unlikely that vagal maneuvers or giving adenosine will terminate the rhythm. However, they may momentarily slow the rate enough so that you can look at the P waves and determine the specific type of tachycardia. By determining the type of tachycardia, treatment specific to that rhythm can be given.

If you know the rhythm is MAT and the patient is symptomatic, it is best to consult a cardiologist before starting treatment. Calcium channel blockers, such as diltiazem, may be ordered to control the ventricular rate.

Vagal Maneuvers

[OBJECTIVE 8]

Vagal maneuvers are methods used to stimulate baroreceptors located in the internal carotid arteries and the aortic arch. Stimulation of these receptors results in reflex stimulation of the vagus nerve and release of acetylcholine. Acetylcholine slows conduction through the AV node, resulting in slowing of the heart rate. Although there is some overlap of the right and left vagus nerves, it is thought that the right vagus nerve has more fibers to the SA node and atrial muscle and the left vagus more fibers to the AV node and some ventricular muscle.

Examples of vagal maneuvers include:
- Coughing
- Squatting
- Breath-holding
- Carotid sinus massage. This procedure is performed with the patient's neck extended. Firm pressure is applied just underneath the angle of the jaw for up to 5 seconds (Figure 4-7). Carotid pressure should be avoided in older patients and in patients with carotid artery bruits. Simultaneous, bilateral carotid pressure should *never* be performed.
- Application of a cold stimulus to the face (e.g., a washcloth soaked in iced water, cold pack, or crushed ice mixed with water in a plastic bag or glove) for up to 10 seconds. This technique is often effective in infants and young children.

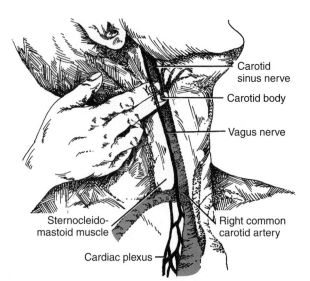

Figure 4-7   Carotid sinus massage. The carotid sinus (carotid body) is located at the bifurcation of the carotid artery at the angle of the jaw.

When using this method, do not obstruct the patient's mouth or nose or apply pressure to the eyes.
- Valsalva's maneuver. Instruct the patient to blow through an occluded straw or take a deep breath and bear down as if having a bowel movement for up to 10 seconds. This strains the abdominal muscles and increases intrathoracic pressure.
- Gagging. Use a tongue depressor or culturette swab to briefly touch the back of the throat.

The procedure for performing carotid sinus massage is shown in Skill 4-1.

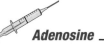

Adenosine

- Adenosine is found naturally in all body cells and is rapidly metabolized in the blood vessels. Adenosine slows the rate of the SA node, slows conduction time through the AV node, can interrupt reentry pathways that involve the AV node, and can restore sinus rhythm in SVT.
- Reentry circuits are the underlying mechanism for many episodes of SVT. Adenosine acts at specific receptors to cause a temporary block of conduction through the AV node, interrupting these reentry circuits.
- Adenosine has an onset of action of 10 to 40 seconds and duration of 1 to 2 minutes. Because of its short half-life (10 sec), and to boost delivery of the drug to its site of action in the heart, select the injection port on the IV tubing that is nearest the patient. Administer the drug using a two-syringe technique. Prepare one syringe with the drug, and the other with a 20-mL normal saline flush. Insert both syringes into the injection port in the IV tubing. Administer the medication IV as rapidly as possible (i.e., over a period of seconds) and *immediately* follow with the saline flush. If the patient has a central line in place, the dosages of adenosine should be reduced to avoid prolonged bradycardia or severe side effects.
- Adenosine may cause facial flushing because the drug causes mild dilation of blood vessels in the skin. Coughing, dyspnea, and bronchospasm may occur because it

(cont'd next page)

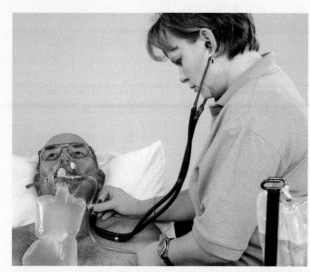

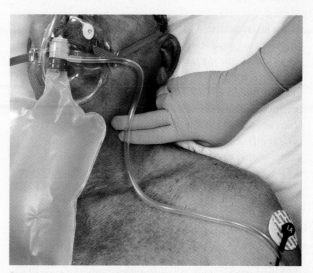

Step 1 Before performing this procedure, take appropriate standard precautions. Make sure suction, a defibrillator, and emergency medications are available and that you have a physician's order to perform the procedure. Place the patient on oxygen, assess the patient's vital signs, establish IV access, and apply ECG electrodes. Explain the procedure to the patient. Gently palpate each carotid artery separately to assess pulse quality. If the pulses are markedly unequal, consult a physician before performing the procedure. Check for carotid bruits by listening to each carotid artery with a stethoscope. A bruit is a blowing or wishing sound created by the turbulence within the vessel. If a bruit is heard, do not perform this procedure.

Step 2 If no bruit is heard and no contraindications are present, turn the patient's head to one side. Press print or record on the cardiac monitor to run a continuous ECG strip during the procedure. With two fingers, locate the carotid pulse just underneath the angle of the jaw. With firm pressure, press the carotid artery toward the cervical vertebrae. Begin an up-and-down motion for no longer than 10 seconds. Never massage both carotid arteries at the same time. Visually monitor the patient and ECG throughout the procedure.

Note the onset and end of the vagal maneuver on the rhythm strip.

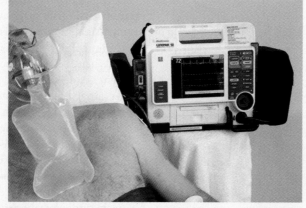

Step 3 After the procedure, reassess the patient's vital signs and the ECG rhythm.

is a mild bronchoconstrictor. Adenosine should be avoided in patients with severe asthma.
- A 12-lead ECG recording is desirable when adenosine is used.
- Adenosine should be used with caution in patients with severe coronary artery disease because vasodilation of normal coronary vessels may produce ischemia in vulnerable territory. It should be used only with full resuscitative equipment available.[1]

SUPRAVENTRICULAR TACHYCARDIA (SVT)

Supraventricular arrhythmias begin above the bifurcation of the bundle of His. This means that supraventricular arrhythmias include rhythms that begin in the SA node, atrial tissue, or the AV junction. The term **supraventricular tachycardia** (**SVT**) includes three main types of fast rhythms, which are shown in Figure 4-8.

- Atrial tachycardia (AT). In AT, an irritable site in the atria fires automatically at a rapid rate.
- AV nodal reentrant tachycardia (AVNRT). AV nodal reentrant tachycardia is also called AV nodal reciprocating tachycardia. In AVNRT, fast and slow pathways in the AV node form an electrical circuit or loop. The impulse spins around the AV nodal (junctional) area.
- AV reentrant tachycardia (AVRT). AV reentrant tachycardia is also called AV reciprocating tachycardia. In AVRT, the impulse begins above the ventricles but travels via a pathway other than the AV node and bundle of His.

ECG Pearl

It is important to look closely for P waves in all dysrhythmias, but is very important when trying to figure out the origin of a tachycardia. If P waves are not visible in one lead, try looking in another before finalizing your rhythm diagnosis.

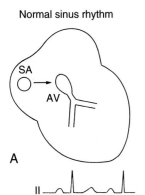

Normal sinus rhythm

Atrial tachycardia (AT)

A

B

Atrioventricular nodal reentrant tachycardia (AVNRT)

Atrioventricular reentrant tachycardia (AVRT)

C

D

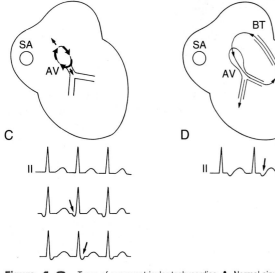

Figure 4-8   Types of supraventricular tachycardias. **A,** Normal sinus rhythm is presented here as a reference. **B,** Atrial tachycardia. **C,** AV nodal reentrant tachycardia (AVNRT). **D,** AV reentrant tachycardia (AVRT); BT = bypass tract.

Atrial Tachycardia

[OBJECTIVES 9, 10]
How Do I Recognize It?
Atrial tachycardia is usually the result of altered automaticity or triggered activity. An irritable site in the atria fires at a rate of 150 to 250 times per minute (Figures 4-9 and 4-10). This rapid atrial rate overrides the SA node and becomes the pacemaker. Conduction of the atrial impulse to the ventricles is often 1:1. This means that every atrial impulse is conducted through the AV node to the ventricles. This results in a P wave preceding each QRS complex. Although the P waves appear upright, they tend to look different from those seen when the impulse is initiated from the SA node. Because conducted impulses travel through the ventricles in the usual manner, the QRS complexes appear normal. The ECG characteristics of atrial tachycardia are shown in Table 4-3.

ECG Pearl

Atrial tachycardia is often precipitated by a PAC. When three or more PACs occur in a row at a rate of more than 100 beats/min, atrial tachycardia is present.

The term **paroxysmal** is used to describe a rhythm that starts or ends suddenly. Atrial tachycardia that starts or ends suddenly is called **paroxysmal atrial tachycardia** (**PAT**). PAT may last for minutes, hours, or days. With very rapid atrial rates, the AV node begins to filter some of the impulses coming to it. By doing so it protects the ventricles from excessively rapid rates. When the AV node selectively filters conduction of some of these impulses, the rhythm is called **paroxysmal atrial tachycardia with block**. PAT with block is often associated with disease of the AV node, medications that slow conduction through the AV node, or digitalis toxicity. When PAT with block exists, more than one P wave is present before each QRS. When the AV node blocks every other atrial impulse from traveling to the ventricles, the rhythm is called PAT with 2:1 block (Figure 4-11).

There is more than one type of atrial tachycardia. Multifocal atrial tachycardia has already been discussed.

- Atrial tachycardia that begins in a small area (focus) within the heart is called focal atrial tachycardia. There are several types of focal atrial tachycardia. Focal atrial tachycardia may be due to an automatic, triggered, or reentrant mechanism. A patient with focal atrial tachycardia often presents with paroxysmal atrial tachycardia. The atrial rate is usually between 100 and 250 beats/min and rarely 300 beats/min.
- Automatic atrial tachycardia (also called ectopic atrial tachycardia) is another type of AT in which a small cluster of cells with altered automaticity fire. The impulse is spread from the cluster of cells to the surrounding atrium and then to the ventricles via the AV node. This type of AT often has a "warm up" period. This means there is a progressive shortening of the P-P interval for the first few

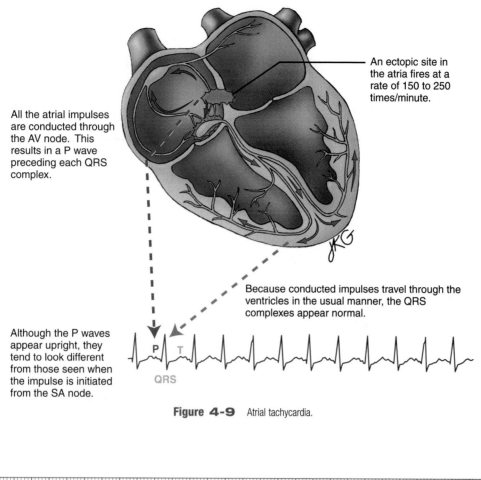

An ectopic site in the atria fires at a rate of 150 to 250 times/minute.

All the atrial impulses are conducted through the AV node. This results in a P wave preceding each QRS complex.

Because conducted impulses travel through the ventricles in the usual manner, the QRS complexes appear normal.

Although the P waves appear upright, they tend to look different from those seen when the impulse is initiated from the SA node.

Figure 4-9   Atrial tachycardia.

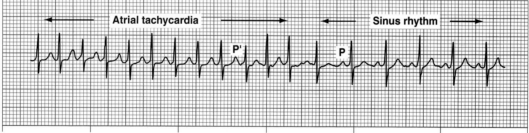

Figure 4-10   Atrial tachycardia (a type of supraventricular tachycardia) that ends spontaneously with the abrupt resumption of sinus rhythm. The P waves of the tachycardia (rate: about 150 beats/min) are superimposed on the preceding T waves.

TABLE 4-3	Characteristics of Atrial Tachycardia
Rate	100-250 beats/min
Rhythm	Regular
P waves	One positive P wave precedes each QRS complex in lead II; P waves differ in shape from sinus P waves; if the atrial rhythm originates in the low portion of the atrium, P waves will be negative in lead II. With rapid rates, it is difficult to distinguish P waves from T waves.
PR interval	May be shorter or longer than normal
QRS duration	0.10 sec or less unless an intraventricular conduction delay exists

beats of the arrhythmia. Automatic AT gradually slows down as it ends. This has been called a "cool down" period. The atrial rate is usually between 100 and 250 beats/min. P waves look different from sinus P waves but are still related to the QRS complex. Vagal maneuvers do not usually stop the tachycardia, but they may slow the ventricular rate.

What Causes It?

Atrial tachycardia can occur in persons with normal hearts or in patients with organic heart disease. Atrial tachycardia associated with automaticity or triggered activity is often related to an acute event including:

- Stimulant use (such as caffeine, albuterol, theophylline, cocaine)

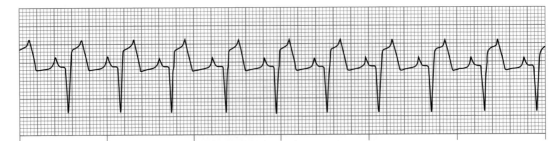

Figure 4-11   Atrial tachycardia with 2:1 block. P waves are clearly seen before the QRS complexes. Others are hidden in the T waves. Atrial rate is 180 beats/min. Ventricular rate is 90 beats/min.

- Infection
- Electrolyte imbalance
- Acute illness with excessive catecholamine release
- Myocardial infarction

What Do I Do About It?

[OBJECTIVE 9]

Signs and symptoms associated with atrial tachycardia vary widely and may include the following:

- Asymptomatic
- Palpitations
- Fluttering sensation in the chest
- Chest pressure
- Dyspnea
- Fatigue
- Dizziness or lightheadedness
- Syncope or near-syncope

When taking the patient's history, try to find out how often the episodes occur, how long they last, and possible triggers. If the patient complains of palpitations, it is important to find out if they are regular or irregular. Palpitations that occur regularly with a sudden onset and end are usually due to AVNRT or AVRT. Irregular palpitations may be due to premature complexes, atrial fibrillation, or multifocal atrial tachycardia.[1] Tachycardias may cause syncope because the rapid ventricular rate decreases cardiac output and blood flow to the brain. Syncope is most likely to occur just after the onset of a rapid atrial tachycardia or when the rhythm stops abruptly. Predisposed persons may experience angina or congestive heart failure.

ECG Pearl

The signs and symptoms experienced by a patient with a tachycardia depend on the following:
- Ventricular rate
- How long the tachycardia lasts
- General health, presence of underlying heart disease
The faster the heart rate, the more likely the patient is to have signs and symptoms resulting from the rapid rate.

If episodes of atrial tachycardia are short, the patient may be asymptomatic. A rhythm that lasts from three beats up to 30 seconds is a nonsustained rhythm. A sustained rhythm is one that lasts more than 30 seconds. If atrial tachycardia is sustained and the patient is symptomatic because of the rapid rate, treatment usually includes oxygen, intravenous (IV) access, and vagal maneuvers. Although AT will rarely stop with vagal maneuvers, they are used to try to stop the rhythm or slow conduction through the AV node. If this fails, antiarrhythmic medications should be tried. Adenosine is the drug of choice, except for patients with severe asthma. A significant percentage of ATs will terminate with administration of adenosine.[1] If needed, calcium channel blockers or beta-blockers or amiodarone may be used to slow the ventricular rate. Amiodarone is preferred for patients with poor ventricular function, such as signs of congestive heart failure. Synchronized cardioversion seldom stops automatic ATs, but may be successful for ATs due to reentry or triggered automaticity. Synchronized cardioversion should be considered for patients with drug-resistant arrhythmias.[1]

Atrial tachycardia with AV block often occurs because of excess digitalis. In these cases, the patient's ventricular rate is not excessively fast. The drug should be withheld and serum digoxin levels obtained. Long-term medication therapy may include the use of calcium channel blockers or beta-blockers. When atrial tachycardia is difficult to control and causes serious signs and symptoms, radiofrequency catheter ablation may be necessary. When catheter ablation is performed, electrophysiologic studies are done to locate the abnormal pathways and reentry circuits in the heart. Once localized, a special ablation catheter is placed at the site of the abnormal pathway. Low-energy, high-frequency current is delivered through this catheter. With each burst of energy from the catheter, an area of tissue is destroyed (ablated). The energy is applied in various areas until the unwanted pathway is no longer functional and the circuit is broken. Atrial tachycardias can occasionally recur at a different site following a successful ablation.

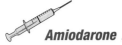

Amiodarone

- Amiodarone directly depresses the automaticity of the SA and AV nodes, slows conduction through the AV node and in the accessory pathway of patients with Wolff-Parkinson-White syndrome, inhibits alpha- and beta-adrenergic receptors, and possesses both vagolytic and calcium-channel blocking properties. Because of these properties, amiodarone is used for a wide range of both atrial and ventricular dysrhythmias in adults and children.
- Amiodarone prolongs the PR, QRS, and QT intervals, and has an additive effect with other medications that prolong the QT interval (e.g., procainamide, phenothiazines, some tricyclic antidepressants, thiazide diuretics, sotalol). Although prolongation of the QRS duration and QT interval may be beneficial in some patients, it may also increase the risk for Torsades de Pointes (a type of polymorphic VT associated with a long QT interval).
- Hypotension, bradycardia, and AV block are adverse effects of amiodarone administration. Slow the infusion rate or discontinue if seen.

Synchronized Cardioversion

[OBJECTIVE 11]

Synchronized cardioversion is the delivery of a shock to the heart by means of a defibrillator to terminate a rapid dysrhythmia. A synchronized shock means the shock is timed to avoid the vulnerable period during the cardiac cycle. On the ECG, this period occurs during the peak of the T wave to approximately the end of the T wave. When the "sync" control is pressed, the machine searches for the highest (R wave deflection) or deepest (QS deflection) part of the QRS complex. When a QRS complex is detected, the monitor places a "flag" or "sync marker" on that complex that may appear as an oval, square, line, or highlighted triangle on the ECG display, depending on the monitor used. When the shock controls are pressed while the defibrillator is charged in "sync" mode, the machine will discharge energy only if both discharge buttons are pushed and the monitor tells the defibrillator that a QRS complex has been detected.

Indications

Since the machine must be able to detect a QRS complex in order to "sync," synchronized cardioversion is used to treat tachycardias (except sinus tachycardia) with a ventricular rate greater than 150 beats/min that have a clearly identifiable QRS complex (such as some narrow-QRS tachycardias and ventricular tachycardia).

Procedure

The steps for performing synchronized cardioversion are shown in Skill 4-2.

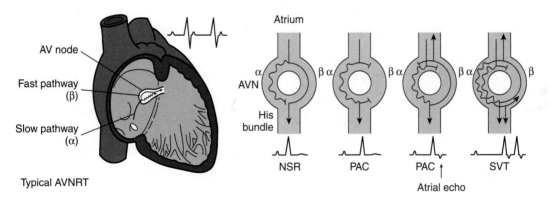

Figure 4-12   Schematic for SVT due to AV nodal reentry. AV = AV node, NSR = normal sinus rhythm, PAC = premature atrial complex, SVT = supraventricular tachycardia.

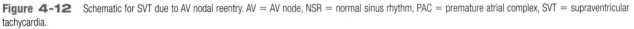
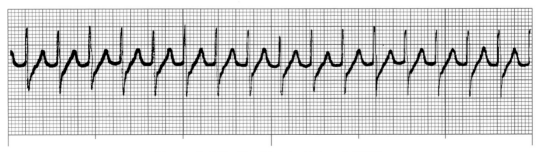

Figure 4-13   AV nodal reentrant tachycardia (AVNRT).

SKILL 4-2 Synchronized Cardioversion

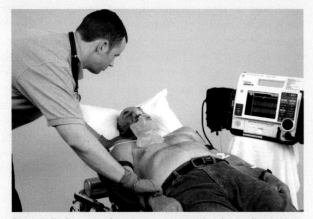

Step 1 Before performing synchronized cardioversion, take appropriate standard precautions and verify that the procedure is indicated. Identify the rhythm on the cardiac monitor. Print an ECG strip to document the patient's rhythm. Assess the patient for serious signs and symptoms from the tachycardia. Make sure suction and emergency medications are available. Give oxygen and start an IV. If the patient is awake, explain the procedure.

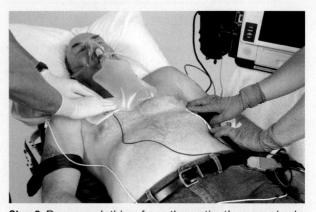

Step 2 Remove clothing from the patient's upper body. With gloves, remove nitroglycerin paste or patches from the patient's chest if present and quickly wipe away any medication residue. If present, remove excessive hair from the sites where the paddles or electrodes will be placed. Shave hair if necessary (and if time permits). Avoid cutting the skin. Do not apply alcohol, tincture of benzoin, or antiperspirant to the skin. Turn the power on to the defibrillator. If using standard paddles, you must use defibrillation gel or defibrillation gel pads between the paddle electrode surface and the patient's skin. Place pregelled defibrillation pads on the patient's chest at this time. If using multipurpose adhesive electrodes, place them in proper position on the patient's bare chest.

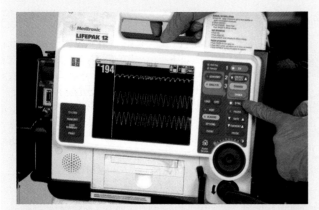

Step 3 Press the "sync" control on the defibrillator. Select a lead with an optimum QRS complex amplitude (positive or negative) and no artifact. If using adhesive electrodes, select the "paddles" lead. Make sure the machine is marking or flagging each QRS complex and no artifact is present. The sense marker should appear near the middle of each QRS complex. If sense markers do not appear or are seen in the wrong place (such as on a T wave), adjust the ECG size or select another lead.

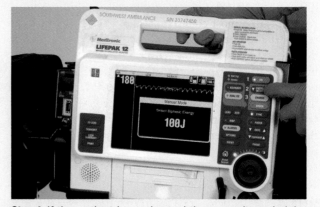

Step 4 If the patient is awake and time permits, administer sedation per agency protocol or physician orders unless contraindicated. Make sure the machine is in "sync" mode and then select the appropriate energy level on the defibrillator.

SKILL 4-2   Synchronized Cardioversion—cont'd

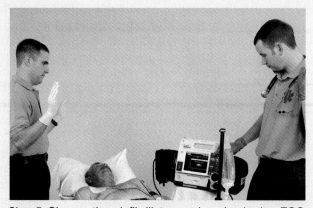

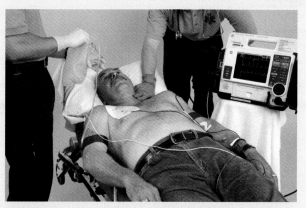

Step 5 Charge the defibrillator and recheck the ECG rhythm. If using standard paddles, place the paddles on the pregelled defibrillator pads on the patient's chest and apply firm pressure. If the rhythm is unchanged, call "Clear!" and look around you. Make sure everyone is clear of the patient, bed, and any equipment connected to the patient. Make sure oxygen is not flowing over the patient's chest.

Step 6 If the area is clear, press and *hold* both discharge buttons at the same time until the shock is delivered. A slight delay may occur while the machine detects the next QRS complex. Release the shock controls after the shock has been delivered. Reassess the rhythm and the patient. If the tachycardia persists, make sure the machine is in sync mode before delivering another shock. If the rhythm changes to ventricular fibrillation, make sure the patient has no pulse. If no pulse is present, make sure the sync control is off and defibrillate.

AV Nodal Reentrant Tachycardia (AVNRT)

[OBJECTIVES 10, 12]

AVNRT is the most common type of SVT. It is caused by reentry in the area of the AV node. Although AVNRT begins in the area of the AV node and could be discussed in the junctional rhythms chapter, it is discussed here because it was once thought to be a type of paroxysmal atrial tachycardia. In the normal AV node, there is only one pathway through which an electrical impulse is conducted from the SA node to the ventricles. Patients with AVNRT have two conduction pathways within the AV node that conduct impulses at different speeds and recover at different rates. The fast pathway conducts impulses rapidly but has a long refractory period (slow recovery time). The slow pathway conducts impulses slowly but has a short refractory period (fast recovery time) (Figure 4-12). Under the right conditions, the fast and slow pathways can form an electrical circuit or loop. As one side of the loop is recovering, the other is firing.

AVNRT is usually caused by a PAC that is spread by the electrical circuit. This allows the impulse to spin around in a circle indefinitely, reentering the normal electrical pathway with each pass around the circuit. The result is a very rapid and regular rhythm that ranges from 150 to 250 beats/min.

Look at the example of AVNRT in Figure 4-13. You can see narrow-QRS complexes that occur at a regular rate of 168 beats/min. P waves are not clearly seen. Because AVNRT begins in the area of the AV node, the impulse spreads to the atria and ventricles at almost the same time. This results in P waves that are usually hidden in the QRS complex. If the ventricles are stimulated first and then the atria, a negative

(inverted) P wave will appear after the QRS in leads II, III, and aVF. When the atria are depolarized after the ventricles, the P wave typically distorts the end of the QRS complex. Since P waves are not seen before the QRS complex the PR interval is not measurable. In our example of AVNRT, you can see ST-segment depression. ST-segment changes (usually depression) are common in patients with supraventricular tachycardias. In most patients, these ST-segment changes are thought to be the result of repolarization changes. However, in elderly patients and those with a high likelihood of ischemic heart disease, ST-segment changes may represent ECG changes consistent with an acute coronary syndrome. The patient should be watched closely. Appropriate laboratory tests and a 12-lead ECG should be obtained to rule out infarction as needed. The ECG characteristics of AVNRT are summarized in Table 4-4.

A regular, narrow-QRS tachycardia that starts or ends suddenly is called **paroxysmal supraventricular tachycardia** (PSVT) (Figure 4-14). PSVT is discussed here since most supraventricular tachycardias are due to AVNRT. P waves are seldom seen because they are hidden in T waves of preceding beats. The QRS is narrow unless there is a problem with conduction of the impulse through the ventricles, as in a bundle branch block.

What Causes It?

AVNRT can occur at any age. Whether a person is born with a tendency to have AVNRT or whether it develops later in life for an unknown reason has not been clearly determined. AVNRT is common in individuals with no structural heart disease but can be triggered by hypoxia, stress, anxiety,

TABLE 4-4	Characteristics of AV Nodal Reentrant Tachycardia (AVNRT)
Rate	150-250 beats/min (usually 180-200 beats/min in adults)
Rhythm	Ventricular rhythm is usually very regular
P waves	P waves are often hidden in the QRS complex. If the ventricles are stimulated first and then the atria, a negative (inverted) P wave will appear after the QRS in leads II, III, and aVF. When the atria are depolarized after the ventricles, the P wave typically distorts the end of the QRS complex.
PR interval	P waves are not seen before the QRS complex, therefore the PR interval is not measurable
QRS duration	0.10 sec or less unless an intraventricular conduction delay exists

caffeine, smoking, sleep deprivation, and many medications. In adults, AVNRT frequently presents in the third or fourth decade of life, occurring more often in women than in men. AVNRT also occurs in persons with COPD, coronary artery disease, valvular heart disease, congestive heart failure, and digitalis toxicity. AVNRT can cause angina or myocardial infarction in patients with coronary artery disease.

What Do I Do About It?

Treatment depends on the severity of the patient's signs and symptoms. Signs and symptoms that may be associated with rapid ventricular rates may include the following:

- Palpitations (common)
- Lightheadedness
- Neck vein pulsations
- Syncope or near-syncope
- Dyspnea
- Weakness
- Nausea
- Nervousness, anxiety
- Chest pain or pressure
- Signs of shock
- Congestive heart failure

If the patient is stable but symptomatic (and symptoms are due to the rapid heart rate), treatment usually includes oxygen, IV access, and vagal maneuvers. AVNRT is usually responsive to vagal maneuvers. However, if vagal maneuvers do not slow the rate or cause conversion of the tachycardia to a sinus rhythm, the first antiarrhythmic given is usually adenosine. An unstable patient is one who has signs and symptoms of hemodynamic compromise. Examples of these signs and symptoms include shock, chest pain, hypotension, shortness of breath, pulmonary congestion, congestive heart failure, acute MI, and/or decreased level of consciousness. If the patient is unstable, treatment usually includes oxygen, IV access, sedation (if the patient is awake and time permits), followed by synchronized cardioversion.

Recurrent AVNRT may require treatment with a long-acting calcium channel blocker or beta-blocker. Antiarrhythmics such as amiodarone may also be used. Recurrent episodes vary in frequency, duration, and severity from several times a day to every 2 to 3 years. Patients who are resistant to drug therapy or who do not wish to remain on life-long medications for the dysrhythmia are candidates for radiofrequency catheter ablation. Catheter ablation has become the treatment of choice in the management of patients with symptomatic recurrent episodes of AVNRT. It is successful in permanently interrupting the circuit and curing the dysrhythmia in most cases.

AV Reentrant Tachycardia (AVRT)

[OBJECTIVE 13]

The next most common type of SVT is AV reentrant tachycardia (AVRT). Remember that the AV node is normally the only electrical connection between the atria and ventricles. AVRT involves a pathway of impulse conduction outside the AV node and bundle of His. **Preexcitation** is a term used to describe rhythms that originate from above the ventricles but in which the impulse travels via a pathway other than the AV node and bundle of His. As a result, the supraventricular impulse excites the ventricles earlier than would be expected if the impulse traveled by way of the normal conduction system. Patients with preexcitation syndromes are prone to AVRT. The most common type of preexcitation syndrome is called **Wolff-Parkinson-White (WPW) syndrome.**

During fetal development, strands of myocardial tissue form connections between the atria and ventricles, outside the normal conduction system. These strands normally become nonfunctional shortly after birth. In patients with preexcitation syndrome, these connections persist as congenital malformations of working myocardial tissue. Because these connections bypass part or all of the normal conduction system,

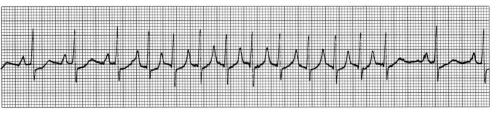

Figure 4-14   Paroxysmal supraventricular tachycardia (PSVT).

they are called **accessory pathways** (Figure 4-15). Some people have more than one accessory pathway. The term **bypass tract** is used when one end of an accessory pathway is attached to normal conductive tissue.

How Do I Recognize It?

The ECG characteristics of WPW described here are usually seen when the patient is *not* having a tachycardia. WPW syndrome usually goes undetected until it manifests in a patient as a tachycardia. In WPW associated with a sinus rhythm, the P wave looks normal. Remember that the AV node normally delays the impulse it receives from the SA node. If this delay did not occur, the atria and ventricles would contract at about the same time. The delay in conduction allows the atria to empty blood into the ventricles before the next ventricular contraction begins. The PR interval is short (less than 0.12 sec) because the impulse travels very quickly across the accessory pathway, bypassing the normal delay in the AV node (Figure 4-16).

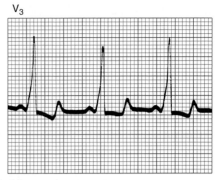

Figure 4-16 Lead V$_3$. Typical WPW pattern showing the short PR interval, delta wave, wide QRS complex, and secondary ST and T wave changes.

As the impulse crosses the insertion point of the accessory pathway in the ventricular muscle, that part of the ventricle is stimulated earlier (preexcited) than if the impulse had followed the normal conduction pathway through the bundle of His and Purkinje fibers. On the ECG, preexcitation of the

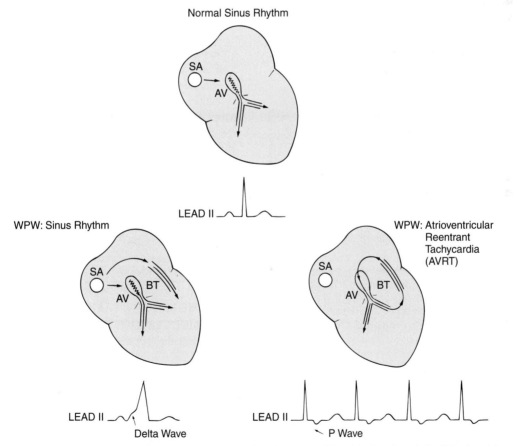

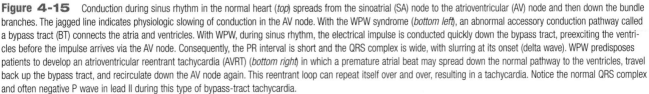

Figure 4-15 Conduction during sinus rhythm in the normal heart (*top*) spreads from the sinoatrial (SA) node to the atrioventricular (AV) node and then down the bundle branches. The jagged line indicates physiologic slowing of conduction in the AV node. With the WPW syndrome (*bottom left*), an abnormal accessory conduction pathway called a bypass tract (BT) connects the atria and ventricles. With WPW, during sinus rhythm, the electrical impulse is conducted quickly down the bypass tract, preexciting the ventricles before the impulse arrives via the AV node. Consequently, the PR interval is short and the QRS complex is wide, with slurring at its onset (delta wave). WPW predisposes patients to develop an atrioventricular reentrant tachycardia (AVRT) (*bottom right*) in which a premature atrial beat may spread down the normal pathway to the ventricles, travel back up the bypass tract, and recirculate down the AV node again. This reentrant loop can repeat itself over and over, resulting in a tachycardia. Notice the normal QRS complex and often negative P wave in lead II during this type of bypass-tract tachycardia.

ventricles can be seen as a **delta wave** in some leads. A delta wave is an initial slurring of the QRS complex (Figure 4-17). Delta waves are the result of initial activation of the ventricles by conduction over the accessory pathway.

ECG Pearl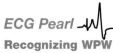

Recognizing WPW
- Short PR interval
- Delta wave
- Widening of the QRS

Normally, conduction through the Purkinje fibers is very fast. In WPW, the spread of the impulse is slow because it must spread from working cell to working cell in the ventricular muscle. This is because the accessory pathway bypasses the specialized cells of the heart's conduction system. Because the impulse spreads slowly through the working cells, the delay in conduction results in a QRS that is usually more than 0.12 second in duration. The QRS complex seen in WPW is actually a combination of the impulse that preexcites the ventricles through the accessory pathway and the impulse that follows the normal conduction pathway through the AV node. As a result, the end (terminal) portion of the QRS usually looks normal. However, since the ventricles are activated abnormally, they repolarize abnormally. This is seen on the

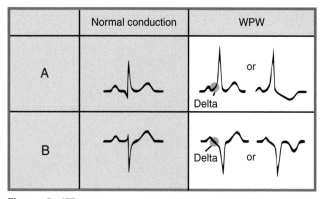

	Normal conduction	WPW
A		
B		

Figure 4-17 Delta waves may be positive or negative. **A,** The usual appearance of WPW in leads where the QRS complex is mainly upright. **B,** The usual appearance of WPW when the QRS is predominantly negative. Negative delta waves may simulate pathologic Q waves—mimicking myocardial infarction.

ECG as ST-segment and T wave changes. The direction of the ST-segment and T wave changes are usually opposite the direction of the delta wave and QRS complex, which can mimic myocardial ischemia or injury. An example of WPW is shown in Figure 4-18. The ECG characteristics of WPW are summarized in Table 4-5.

What Causes It?

WPW is one of the most common causes of tachydysrhythmias in infants and children (Figure 4-19). Although it is likely that the accessory pathway in WPW is congenital in origin, symptoms associated with preexcitation often do not appear until young adulthood.

What Do I Do About It?

Some people with WPW never have symptoms. Common signs and symptoms associated with WPW and a rapid ventricular rate include the following:
- Palpitations
- Lightheadedness
- Shortness of breath
- Anxiety
- Weakness
- Dizziness
- Chest discomfort
- Signs of shock

If the patient is symptomatic because of the rapid ventricular rate, treatment will depend on how unstable the patient is. Consultation with a cardiologist is recommended. A stable but symptomatic patient is usually treated with oxygen, IV access, and IV medications such as amiodarone. Do not give drugs that slow or block conduction through the AV node, such as adenosine, digoxin, diltiazem, or verapamil. They may speed up conduction through the accessory pathway. This can result in a further *increase* in heart rate. If the patient is unstable, preparations should be made for synchronized cardioversion.

Atrial Flutter

[OBJECTIVE 14]

Atrial flutter is an ectopic atrial rhythm in which an irritable site fires regularly at a very rapid rate (Figure 4-20).

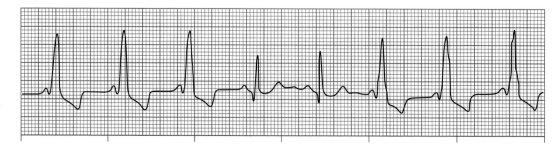

Figure 4-18 This rhythm strip shows an example of intermittent preexcitation. The first three beats show preexcitation. This is followed by abrupt normalization of the QRS complex in the next two beats. The preexcitation pattern returns for the final three beats.

TABLE 4-5	Characteristics of Wolff-Parkinson-White (WPW) Syndrome
Rate	Usually 60-100 beats/min, if the underlying rhythm is sinus in origin
Rhythm	Regular, unless associated with atrial fibrillation
P waves	Normal and positive in lead II unless WPW is associated with atrial fibrillation
PR interval	If P waves are observed, less than 0.12 sec
QRS duration	Usually greater than 0.12 sec; slurred up-stroke of the QRS complex (delta wave) may be seen in one or more leads.

How Do I Recognize It?

Atrial flutter has been classified into two types.
- Type I atrial flutter (also called *typical atrial flutter*) is caused by reentry. In this type of atrial flutter, an impulse circles around a large area of tissue, such as the entire right atrium. The atrial rate ranges from 250 to 350 beats/min.
- Type II atrial flutter is called *atypical* or *very rapid atrial flutter*. The precise mechanism of type II atrial flutter has not been defined. Patients with this type of atrial flutter often develop atrial fibrillation. In type II atrial flutter, the atrial rate ranges from 350 to 450 beats/min.

In atrial flutter, an irritable focus within the atrium typically depolarizes at a rate of 300/min. If each impulse were transmitted to the ventricles, the ventricular rate would equal 300/min. The healthy AV node protects the ventricles from these extremely fast atrial rates. Normally, the AV node cannot conduct faster than about 180 impulses/min. Thus, at

an atrial rate of 300/min, every other impulse arrives at the AV node while it is still refractory. The resulting ventricular response of 150 beats/min is called 2:1 conduction. (The ratio of the atrial rate [300/min] to the ventricular rate [150/min] is 2 to 1). Conduction ratios in atrial flutter are usually even (2:1, 4:1, 6:1) but can vary. In individuals with an accessory pathway, atrial flutter may be associated with 1:1 conduction (because the AV node is bypassed), producing extremely rapid ventricular rates.

In atrial flutter, atrial waveforms are produced that resemble the teeth of a saw, or a picket fence, called "flutter" waves. Flutter waves are best observed in leads II, III, aVF, and V_1. Because P waves are not observed in atrial flutter, the PR interval is not measurable. The QRS complex is usually 0.10 second or less because atrial flutter is a supraventricular rhythm, and the impulse is conducted normally through the AV junction and ventricles. However, if flutter waves are buried in the QRS complex or if an intraventricular conduction delay exists, the QRS will appear wide (greater than 0.10 sec). If the AV node blocks the impulses coming to it at a regular rate, the resulting ventricular rhythm will be regular. If the AV node blocks the impulses at an irregular rate, the resulting ventricular rhythm will be irregular.

When atrial flutter is present with 2:1 conduction, it may be difficult to tell the difference between atrial flutter and sinus tachycardia, atrial tachycardia, AVNRT, AVRT, or PSVT. Vagal maneuvers may help identify the rhythm by temporarily slowing AV conduction and revealing the underlying flutter waves. When vagal maneuvers are used in atrial flutter, the response is usually sudden slowing and then a return to the former rate. Vagal maneuvers will not usually convert atrial flutter because the reentry circuit is located in the atria, not the AV node. An example of atrial flutter is

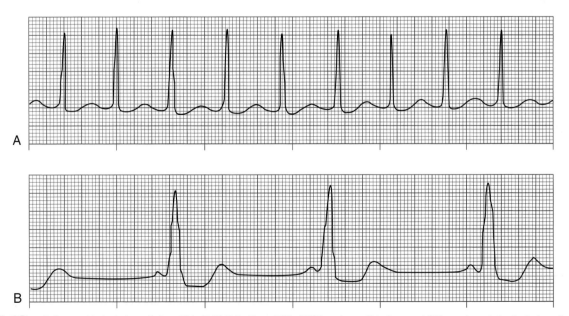

Figure 4-19   **A,** Supraventricular tachycardia in a child with Wolff-Parkinson-White (WPW) syndrome. Note the normal QRS complexes during the tachycardia. **B,** Later, the typical features of WPW syndrome are visible (short PR interval, delta wave, and wide QRS).

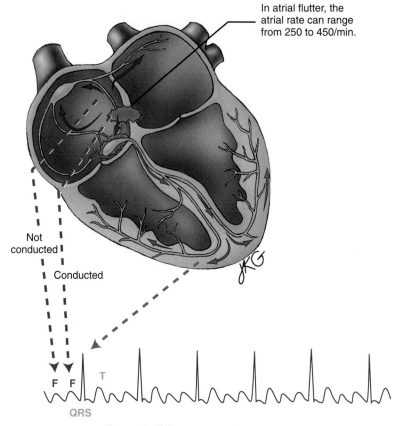

In atrial flutter, the atrial rate can range from 250 to 450/min.

Not conducted

Conducted

F F   T

QRS

Figure 4-20   Atrial flutter. F = flutter wave.

ECG Pearl

Atrial flutter or atrial fibrillation that has a ventricular rate of more than 100 beats/min is described as "uncontrolled." The ventricular rate is considered "rapid" when it is 150 beats/min or more. New-onset atrial flutter or fibrillation is often associated with a rapid ventricular rate. Atrial flutter or atrial fibrillation with a rapid ventricular response is commonly called "Afib with RVR" or "Aflutter with RVR."

Atrial flutter or atrial fibrillation that has a ventricular rate of less than 100 beats/min is described as "controlled." A controlled ventricular rate may be the result of:
- A healthy AV node protecting the ventricles from very fast atrial impulses
- Medications used to control (block) conduction through the AV node, decreasing the number of impulses reaching the ventricles

shown in Figure 4-21. The ECG characteristics of atrial flutter are shown in Table 4-6.

What Causes It?

Atrial flutter is usually caused by a reentry circuit in which an impulse circles around a large area of tissue, such as the entire right atrium. It is usually a paroxysmal rhythm that is precipitated by a PAC. It may last for seconds to hours

and occasionally 24 hours or more. Chronic atrial flutter is unusual. This is because the rhythm usually converts to sinus rhythm or atrial fibrillation, either on its own or with treatment.

ECG Pearl

Conditions Associated with Atrial Flutter
- Hypoxia
- Pulmonary embolism
- Chronic lung disease
- Mitral or tricuspid valve stenosis or regurgitation
- Pneumonia
- Ischemic heart disease
- Complication of myocardial infarction
- Cardiomyopathy
- Hyperthyroidism
- Digitalis or quinidine toxicity
- Cardiac surgery
- Pericarditis/myocarditis

What Do I Do About It?

Patients with atrial flutter commonly present with complaints of palpitations, difficulty breathing, fatigue, or chest discomfort. The severity of signs and symptoms associated with atrial flutter vary, depending on the ventricular rate, how long the rhythm has been present, and the patient's cardiovascular

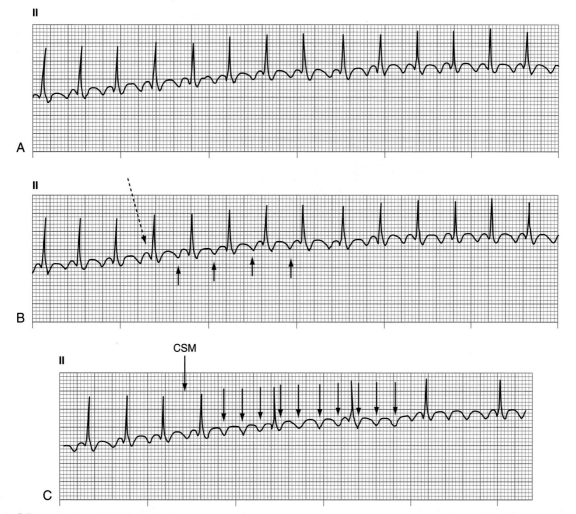

Figure 4-21   Atrial flutter. **A,** This rhythm strip shows a narrow-QRS tachycardia with a ventricular rate just under 150 beats/min. **B,** The same rhythm shown in **A** with arrows added indicating possible atrial activity. **C,** When carotid sinus massage (CSM) is performed, the rate of conduction through the AV node slows, revealing atrial flutter.

status. The faster the ventricular rate, the more likely the patient is to be symptomatic with this rhythm.

It is best to consult a cardiologist when considering treatment options. If atrial flutter is associated with a rapid ventricular rate and the patient is stable but symptomatic,

TABLE 4-6	Characteristics of Atrial Flutter
Rate	Atrial rate 250-450 beats/min, typically 300 beats/min; ventricular rate variable—determined by AV blockade; the ventricular rate will usually not exceed 180 beats/min due to the intrinsic conduction rate of the AV junction
Rhythm	Atrial regular, ventricular regular or irregular depending on AV conduction/blockade
P waves	No identifiable P waves; saw-toothed "flutter" waves are present
PR interval	Not measurable
QRS Duration	0.10 sec or less but may be widened if flutter waves are buried in the QRS complex or an intraventricular conduction delay exists

treatment is usually aimed at controlling the ventricular rate with medications such as diltiazem or beta-blockers. Beta-blockers should generally be avoided in the presence of severe underlying pulmonary disease or heart failure.

Synchronized cardioversion should be considered for any patient in atrial flutter that has serious signs and symptoms because of the rapid ventricular rate (such as hypotension, signs of shock, or heart failure). If synchronized cardioversion is performed, atrial flutter can be successfully converted to a sinus rhythm using low energy levels.

Atrial Fibrillation

[OBJECTIVE 15]

Atrial fibrillation (AFib) occurs because of altered automaticity in one or several rapidly firing sites in the atria or reentry involving one or more circuits in the atria (Figure 4-22). Irritable sites in the atria fire at a rate of 400 to 600 times per minute. These rapid impulses cause the muscles of the atria to quiver (fibrillate). This results in ineffectual atrial contraction,

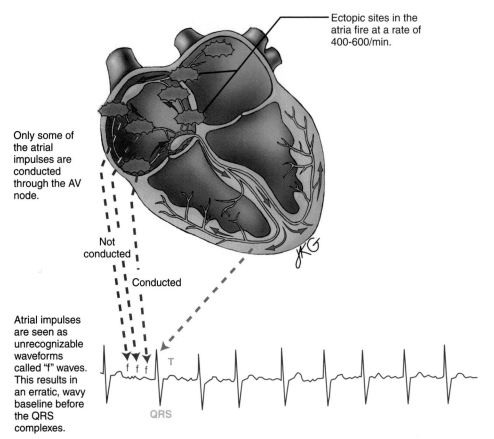

Ectopic sites in the atria fire at a rate of 400-600/min.

Only some of the atrial impulses are conducted through the AV node.

Not conducted

Conducted

Atrial impulses are seen as unrecognizable waveforms called "f" waves. This results in an erratic, wavy baseline before the QRS complexes.

Figure 4-22   Atrial fibrillation. f = fibrillatory wave

decreased stroke volume, a subsequent decrease in cardiac output, and loss of atrial kick.

How Do I Recognize It?

In atrial fibrillation, the AV node attempts to protect the ventricles from the hundreds of impulses bombarding it per minute. It does this by blocking many of the impulses generated by the irritable sites in the atria. The ventricular rate and rhythm are determined by the degree of blocking by the AV node of these rapid impulses.

Look at the example of atrial fibrillation in Figure 4-23. One of the first things you notice is that the ventricular rhythm is irregular. In AFib, atrial depolarization occurs very irregularly. This results in an irregular ventricular rhythm. The ventricular

rhythm associated with AFib is described as irregularly irregular. Since the ventricular rhythm is irregular, we should give a ventricular rate range when describing the rhythm. In our example, the ventricular rate ranges from 67 to 120 beats/min.

Because of the quivering of the atrial muscle and because there is no uniform wave of atrial depolarization in AFib, there is no P wave. Instead, you see a baseline that looks erratic (wavy). This corresponds with the rapid atrial rate. These wavy deflections are called "fibrillatory waves." Since there is no P wave, we cannot measure a PR interval. The QRS complex is narrow because the impulse started above the bifurcation of the bundle of His and was conducted normally through the AV junction and ventricles.

Suspect toxicity due to digitalis, beta-blockers, or calcium channel blockers if AFib occurs with a slow, regular ventricular

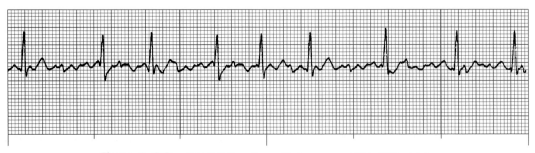

Figure 4-23   Atrial fibrillation with a ventricular response of 67 to 120 beats/min.

rate. This can occur when a patient who has AFib is prescribed medications to slow the ventricular rate. Excess medication can cause complete AV block (Figure 4-24). The ECG characteristics of AF are shown in Table 4-7.

What Causes It?

Atrial fibrillation can occur in patients with or without detectable heart disease or related symptoms.

Patients who experience AFib are at increased risk of having a stroke. Because the atria do not contract effectively and expel all of the blood within them, blood may pool within them and form clots. A stroke can result if a clot moves from the atria and lodges in an artery in the brain. A clot may dislodge on its own or because of conversion to a sinus rhythm.

ECG Pearl

Conditions Associated With Atrial Fibrillation

- Idiopathic (no clear cause)
- Hypertension
- Ischemic heart disease
- Advanced age
- Rheumatic heart disease (especially mitral valve disease)
- Cardiomyopathy
- Congestive heart failure
- Congenital heart disease
- Sick sinus syndrome/degenerative conduction system disease
- Wolff-Parkinson-White syndrome
- Pericarditis
- Pulmonary embolism
- Chronic lung disease
- After surgery
- Diabetes
- Stress
- Sympathomimetics
- Excessive caffeine
- Hypoxia
- Hypokalemia
- Hypoglycemia
- Systemic infection
- Hyperthyroidism
- Electrocution

TABLE 4-7	Characteristics of Atrial Fibrillation
Rate	Atrial rate usually 400-600 beats/min; ventricular rate variable
Rhythm	Ventricular rhythm usually irregularly irregular
P waves	No identifiable P waves, fibrillatory waves present; erratic, wavy baseline
PR interval	Not measurable
QRS duration	0.10 sec or less but may be widened if an intraventricular conduction delay exists

What Do I Do About It?

Atrial fibrillation may occur as a self-limiting episode, come and go, or exist as a sustained rhythm. The severity of signs and symptoms associated with AFib vary. Treatment decisions are based on the ventricular rate, the duration of the rhythm, the patient's general health, and how he is tolerating the rhythm. It is best to consult a cardiologist when considering treatment options. AFib with a rapid ventricular response may produce signs and symptoms that include lightheadedness, palpitations, dyspnea, chest discomfort, and hypotension.

If AFib is associated with a rapid ventricular rate and the patient is stable but symptomatic, treatment is usually aimed at controlling the ventricular rate with medications such as diltiazem or beta-blockers. Beta-blockers should generally be avoided in the presence of severe underlying pulmonary disease or heart failure.

Synchronized cardioversion should be considered if the patient in Afib has serious signs and symptoms because of the rapid ventricular rate (such as hypotension, signs of shock, or heart failure). Anticoagulation is recommended before attempting to convert AFib to a sinus rhythm if AFib has been present for 48 hours or longer. Catheter ablation is recommended for selected patients with AFib, such as those who have AFib with WPW syndrome and a history of syncope due to the rapid heart rate. A summary of atrial rhythm characteristics can be found in Tables 4-8 and 4-9.

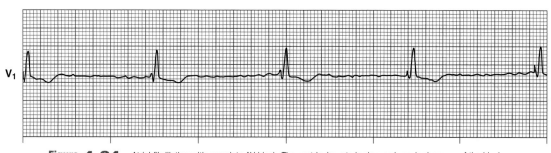

Figure 4-24 Atrial fibrillation with complete AV block. The ventricular rate is slow and regular because of the block.

TABLE **4-8**	Atrial Rhythms—Summary of Characteristics			
	PACs	Wandering Atrial Pacemaker	Atrial Tachycardia	AVNRT
Rate	Usually within normal range, but depends on underlying rhythm	Usually 60-100 beats/min; if rate greater than 100 beats/min, rhythm is called multifocal atrial tachycardia	100-250 beats/min	150-250 beats/min
Rhythm	Regular with premature beats	May be irregular as pacemaker site shifts from SA node to ectopic atrial locations and AV junction	Regular	Ventricular rhythm is usually very regular
P Waves (lead II)	Premature, positive in lead II, one precedes each QRS, differ from sinus P waves, may be lost in preceding T wave	Size, shape, and direction may change from beat to beat	Atrial P waves differ from sinus P waves; isoelectric baseline usually present between P waves	P waves often hidden in QRS complex
PR Interval	May be normal or prolonged	Varies	May be shorter or longer than normal	If P waves are seen, the PRI will usually measure 0.12-0.20 sec
QRS	0.10 sec or less unless abnormally conducted	0.10 sec or less unless abnormally conducted	0.10 sec or less unless abnormally conducted	0.10 sec or less unless abnormally conducted

TABLE **4-9**	Atrial Rhythms—Summary of Characteristics		
	Atria Flutter	Atrial Fibrillation (AFib)	WPW
Rate	Atrial rate 250-450 beats/min, typically 300 beats/min; ventricular rate variable—determined by AV blockade	Atrial rate 400-600 beats/min; ventricular rate variable	60-100 beats/min, if the underlying rhythm is sinus in origin
Rhythm	Atrial regular, ventricular regular or irregular	Ventricular rhythm usually irregularly irregular	Regular, unless associated with atrial fibrillation
P Waves (lead II)	No identifiable P waves; saw-toothed "flutter" waves present	No identifiable P waves; fibrillatory waves present; erratic, wavy baseline	Normal and positive in lead II unless WPW is associated with AFib
PR Interval	Not measurable	Not measurable	If P waves are seen, less than 0.12 sec
QRS	0.10 sec or less unless abnormally conducted	0.10 sec or less unless abnormally conducted	Usually greater than 0.12 sec. Delta wave may be seen in one or more leads.

REFERENCES

1. Blomström-Lundqvist C, Scheinman MM, Aliot EM, Campbell WB, Haines DE, Kuck KH, Lerman BB et al: ACC/AHA/ESC guidelines for the management of patients with supraventricular arrhythmias—executive summary: a report of the American College of Cardiology/American Heart Association Task Force on Practice Guidelines, and the European Society of Cardiology Committee for Practice Guidelines (Writing Committee to Develop Guidelines for the Management of Patients With Supraventricular Arrhythmias.), *J Am Coll Cardiol* 2003;42:1493-1531.
2. Crawford MV, Spence MI: Electrical complications in coronary artery disease: Arrhythmias. In: Common sense approach to coronary care, ed 6, St Louis, 1995, Mosby, pp 208-274.

STOP & REVIEW

True/False

Decide whether each statement is true or false. In the space provided, write T for true or F for false.

____ 1. A macroreentrant circuit is one that involves a small area of heart tissue, usually a few centimeters or less.

____ 2. Most patients with type I atrial flutter develop atrial fibrillation.

____ 3. In atrial fibrillation, the PR interval is usually less than 0.20 second in duration.

____ 4. Atrial tachycardia is a form of supraventricular tachycardia.

Multiple Choice

In the space provided, identify the letter of the choice that best completes each statement or answers each question.

____ 5. Which of the following dysrhythmias is most likely to be associated with a reduction in cardiac output and loss of atrial kick?
   a. Premature atrial complexes
   b. Atrial fibrillation
   c. Sinus tachycardia
   d. Wandering atrial pacemaker

____ 6. On the ECG, an impulse that begins in the atria and occurs earlier than the next expected sinus beat will appear as:
   a. A QRS measuring more than 0.10 second in duration.
   b. A P wave that may appear in the T wave of the preceding beat.
   c. A P wave that appears after the QRS complex.
   d. A P wave with a PR interval measuring more than 0.20 second.

____ 7. A 77-year-old woman is complaining of a sudden onset of palpitations. The cardiac monitor reveals atrial fibrillation with a ventricular response of 144 to 210 beats/min while the patient is at rest. In this situation, the ventricular rate associated with this rhythm is considered to be:
   a. Controlled
   b. Uncontrolled

____ 8. A compensatory pause is a:
   a. Period during the cardiac cycle during which cardiac cells cannot be stimulated to conduct an electrical impulse, no matter how strong the stimulus.
   b. Delay that occurs following a premature beat that resets the SA node.
   c. Series of waveforms.
   d. Period during the cardiac cycle during which cardiac cells can be stimulated to conduct an electrical impulse, if exposed to a stronger than normal stimulus.

Matching

____ **9.** Medications that should be avoided in the presence of severe underlying pulmonary disease

____ **10.** Early

____ **11.** Usual cause of atrial flutter

____ **12.** Before elective cardioversion, prophylactic treatment with a(n) ___ is recommended for the patient in atrial flutter or fibrillation.

____ **13.** Irregularly irregular ventricular rhythm, no identifiable P waves

____ **14.** The most common preexcitation syndrome

____ **15.** Updated term for wandering atrial pacemaker

____ **16.** This often follows a PAC and represents the delay during which the SA node resets its rhythm for the next beat

____ **17.** Common complaint in a patient with a rapid heart rate

____ **18.** Medication often used to slow the ventricular rate in atrial flutter and atrial fibrillation

____ **19.** Baseline appearance in atrial fibrillation

____ **20.** Early beat initiated by an irritable atrial site

____ **21.** Sudden onset or cessation of a dysrhythmia

____ **22.** The name given a PAC associated with a wide QRS complex

____ **23.** Nonconducted PAC

____ **24.** Atrial flutter or atrial fibrillation that has a ventricular rate of more than 100 beats/min

____ **25.** Atrial rate associated with atrial fibrillation

____ **26.** Patients who experience AFib are at increased risk of having this

____ **27.** Drug of choice for AVRNT

____ **28.** Consequence of decreased ventricular filling time

____ **29.** Multifocal atrial tachycardia is also called ___ atrial tachycardia

____ **30.** Every third beat comes from somewhere other than the SA node

____ **31.** Atrial rate associated with Type I atrial flutter

____ **32.** Cardiac glycoside

____ **33.** Waveforms resemble the teeth of a saw or picket fence before the QRS

____ **34.** Every fourth beat comes from somewhere other than the SA node

a. Diltiazem

b. Aberrantly conducted PAC

c. Stroke

d. Uncontrolled

e. Digoxin

f. Anticoagulant

g. Atrial flutter

h. Noncompensatory pause

i. Paroxysmal

j. Premature

k. Decreased stroke volume

l. 400-600/min

m. Atrial fibrillation

n. Multiformed atrial rhythm

o. Adenosine

p. Wolff-Parkinson-White syndrome

q. Chaotic

r. Palpitations

s. Reentry

t. Premature atrial complex

u. Trigeminy

v. Early P wave with no QRS following it

w. Beta-blockers

x. Erratic

y. Quadrigeminy

z. 250-350/min

Short Answer

35. Why do some patients experience syncope with a tachycardia?

36. What is the most common type of supraventricular tachycardia (SVT)?

37. Paroxysmal atrial tachycardia is visible on a patient's cardiac monitor. What does "paroxysmal" mean?

38. List the three (3) main ECG findings associated with Wolff-Parkinson-White (WPW) syndrome.
  1.

  2.

  3.

39. List the three (3) dysrhythmias that most commonly occur in WPW syndrome.
  1.

  2.

  3.

40. Explain why patients who experience atrial fibrillation are at increased risk of having a stroke.

For each of the following rhythm strips, determine the atrial and ventricular rate and rhythm, measure the PR interval and QRS duration, and then identify the rhythm. All strips were recorded in lead II unless otherwise noted. Note: These rhythm strips include sinus and atrial rhythms.

This rhythm strip is from a 74-year-old woman with difficulty breathing.

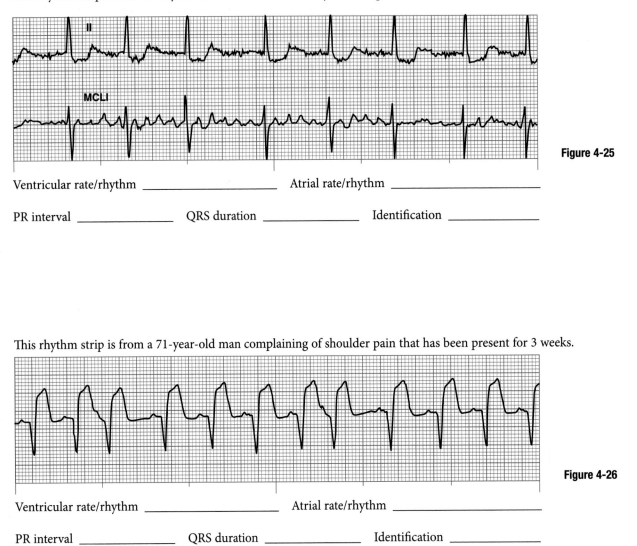

Figure 4-25

Ventricular rate/rhythm _____   Atrial rate/rhythm _____

PR interval _____   QRS duration _____   Identification _____

This rhythm strip is from a 71-year-old man complaining of shoulder pain that has been present for 3 weeks.

Figure 4-26

Ventricular rate/rhythm _____   Atrial rate/rhythm _____

PR interval _____   QRS duration _____   Identification _____

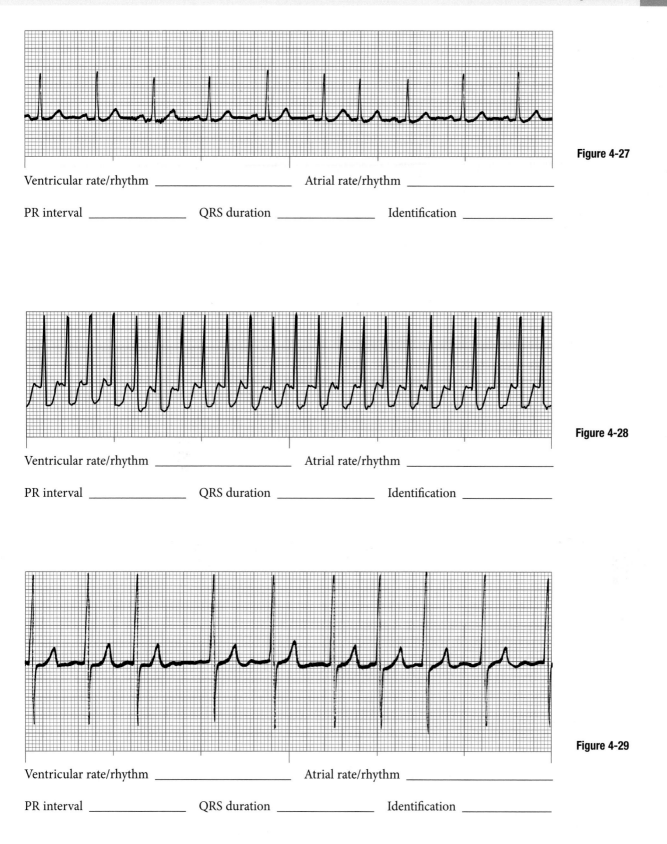

Figure 4-27

Ventricular rate/rhythm _____   Atrial rate/rhythm _____

PR interval _____   QRS duration _____   Identification _____

Figure 4-28

Ventricular rate/rhythm _____   Atrial rate/rhythm _____

PR interval _____   QRS duration _____   Identification _____

Figure 4-29

Ventricular rate/rhythm _____   Atrial rate/rhythm _____

PR interval _____   QRS duration _____   Identification _____

This rhythm strip is from an 82-year-old man complaining of back pain. Top = lead II, bottom = MCL₁.

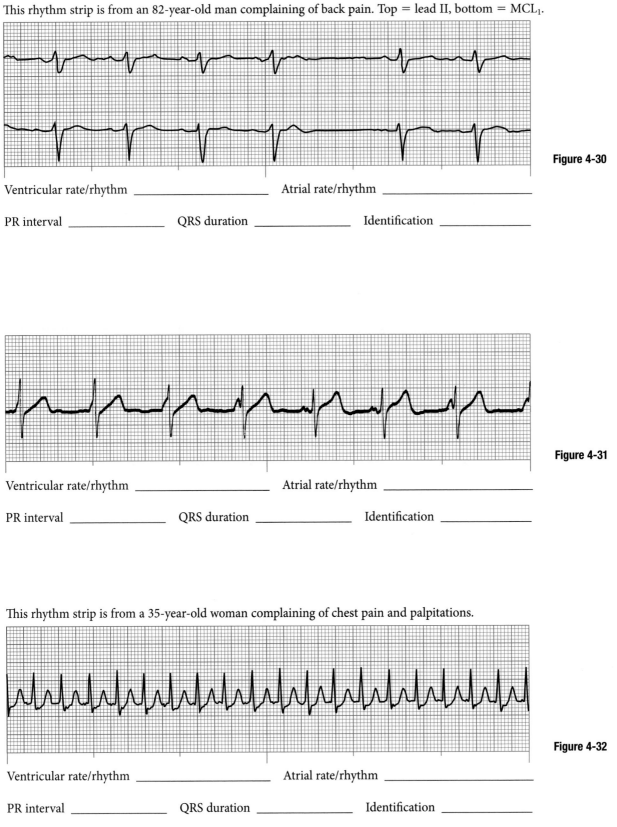

Figure 4-30

Ventricular rate/rhythm _____   Atrial rate/rhythm _____

PR interval _____   QRS duration _____   Identification _____

Figure 4-31

Ventricular rate/rhythm _____   Atrial rate/rhythm _____

PR interval _____   QRS duration _____   Identification _____

This rhythm strip is from a 35-year-old woman complaining of chest pain and palpitations.

Figure 4-32

Ventricular rate/rhythm _____   Atrial rate/rhythm _____

PR interval _____   QRS duration _____   Identification _____

This rhythm strip is from an 82-year-old woman who had a ground level fall. Blood pressure 110/72. Blood sugar is 156.

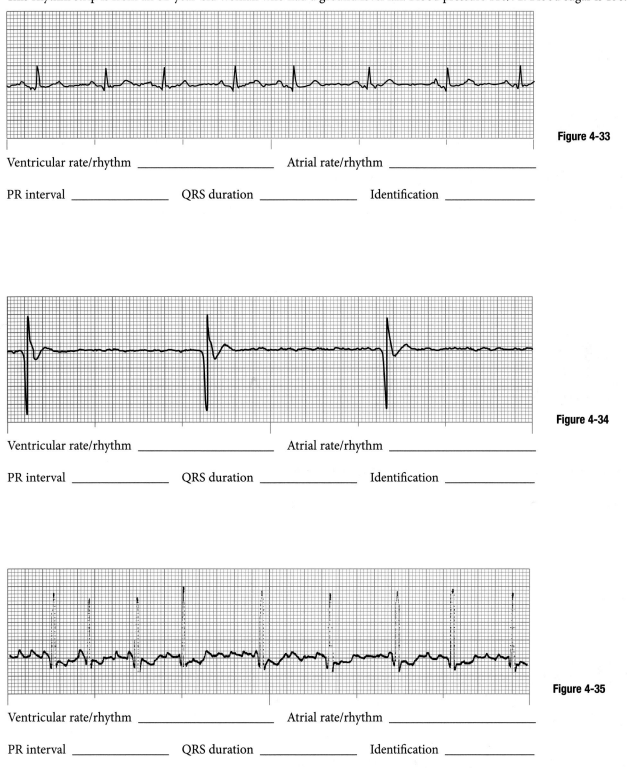

Figure 4-33

Ventricular rate/rhythm _____   Atrial rate/rhythm _____

PR interval _____   QRS duration _____   Identification _____

Figure 4-34

Ventricular rate/rhythm _____   Atrial rate/rhythm _____

PR interval _____   QRS duration _____   Identification _____

Figure 4-35

Ventricular rate/rhythm _____   Atrial rate/rhythm _____

PR interval _____   QRS duration _____   Identification _____

This rhythm strip is from a 57-year-old man with no cardiac history.

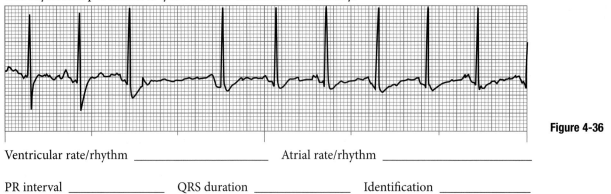

Figure 4-36

Ventricular rate/rhythm _____   Atrial rate/rhythm _____

PR interval _____   QRS duration _____   Identification _____

This rhythm strip is from a 67-year-old woman complaining of dizziness and a "funny feeling" in her chest. She denies chest pain and is not short of breath.

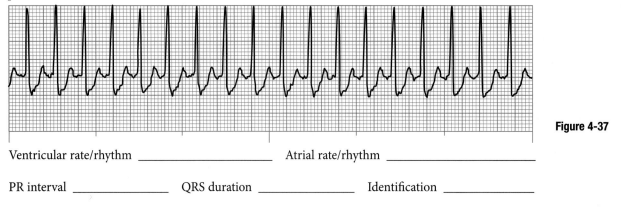

Figure 4-37

Ventricular rate/rhythm _____   Atrial rate/rhythm _____

PR interval _____   QRS duration _____   Identification _____

These rhythm strips are from a 78-year-old man complaining of shortness of breath. He has a history of COPD, coronary artery disease, and hypertension.

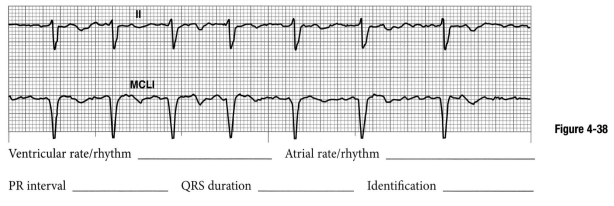

Figure 4-38

Ventricular rate/rhythm _____   Atrial rate/rhythm _____

PR interval _____   QRS duration _____   Identification _____

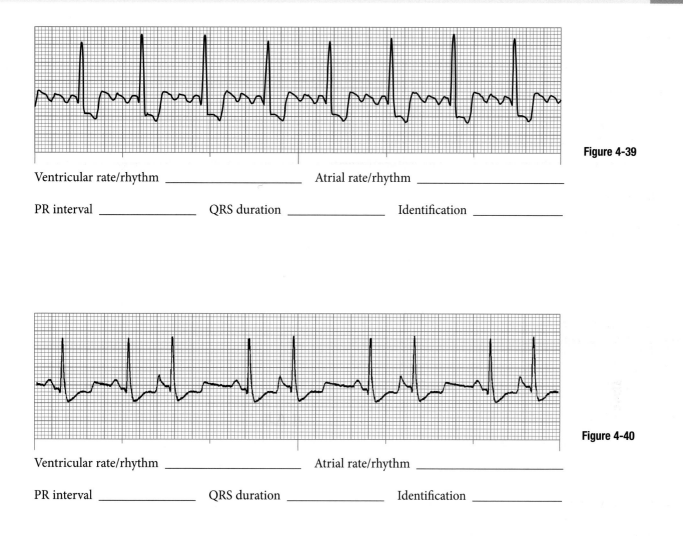

Figure 4-39

Ventricular rate/rhythm _____ Atrial rate/rhythm _____

PR interval _____ QRS duration _____ Identification _____

Figure 4-40

Ventricular rate/rhythm _____ Atrial rate/rhythm _____

PR interval _____ QRS duration _____ Identification _____

This rhythm strip is from an 89-year-old man complaining of weakness and nausea for 3 to 4 days. BP is 122/82. He has a history of diabetes.

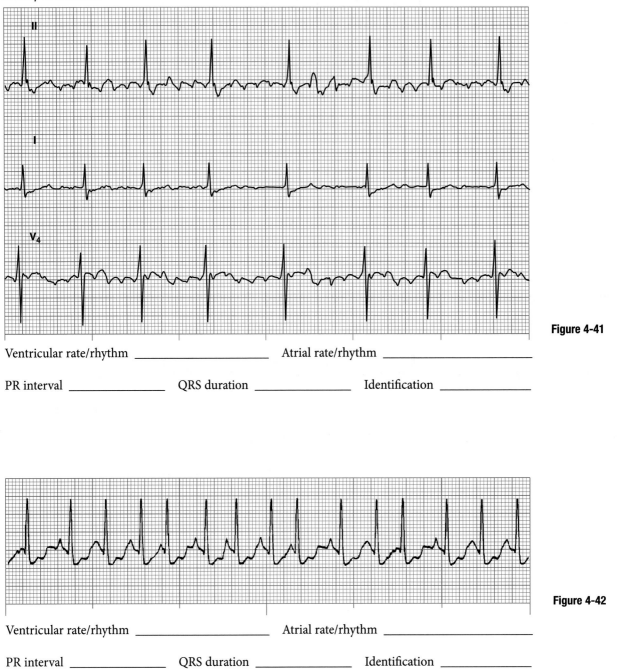

Figure 4-41

Ventricular rate/rhythm _____   Atrial rate/rhythm _____

PR interval _____   QRS duration _____   Identification _____

Figure 4-42

Ventricular rate/rhythm _____   Atrial rate/rhythm _____

PR interval _____   QRS duration _____   Identification _____

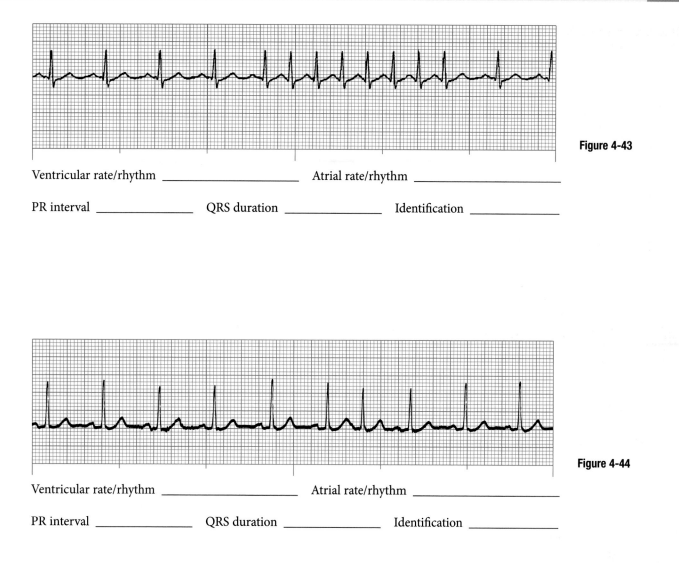

Figure 4-43

Ventricular rate/rhythm _____ Atrial rate/rhythm _____

PR interval _____ QRS duration _____ Identification _____

Figure 4-44

Ventricular rate/rhythm _____ Atrial rate/rhythm _____

PR interval _____ QRS duration _____ Identification _____

STOP & REVIEW ANSWERS

True/False

1. F

2. F

3. F

4. T

Multiple Choice

5. b

6. b

7. b

8. b

Matching

9. w

10. j

11. s

12. f

13. m

14. p

15. n

16. h

17. r

18. a

19. x

20. t

21. i

22. b

23. v

24. d

25. l

26. c

27. o

28. k

29. q

30. u

31. z

32. e

33. g

34. y

Short Answer

35. Tachycardias may cause syncope because the rapid ventricular rate decreases cardiac output and blood flow to the brain. Syncope is most likely to occur just after the onset of a rapid atrial tachycardia or when the rhythm stops abruptly.

36. AV nodal reentrant tachycardia (AVNRT) is the most common type of SVT.

37. The term *paroxysmal* is used to describe a rhythm that starts or ends suddenly. Some physicians use this term to describe the sudden onset or end of a patient's symptoms.

38. **1.** Short PR interval

2. Delta wave

3. Widening of the QRS

39. Different types of dysrhythmias occur in WPW syndrome. The most common is AVRT, followed by atrial fibrillation and atrial flutter.

40. Because the atria do not contract effectively and expel all of the blood within them, blood may pool within them and form clots. A clot may dislodge on its own or because of conversion to a sinus rhythm. A stroke can result if a clot moves from the atria and lodges in an artery in the brain.

Figure 4-25 answer

Ventricular rate/rhythm	75 to 107 beats/min, irregular
Atrial rate/rhythm	Unable to determine
PR interval	Unable to determine
QRS duration	0.08 sec
Identification	Atrial flutter at 75 to 107 beats/min

Figure 4-26 answer

Ventricular rate/rhythm	115 beats/min , regular except for events
Atrial rate/rhythm	115 beats/min, regular except for events
PR interval	0.12 sec (sinus beats)
QRS duration	0.08 sec (sinus beats)
Identification	Sinus tachycardia at 115 beats/min with PACs and ST-segment elevation

Figure 4-27 answer

Ventricular rate/rhythm	93 beats/min, regular except for the event
Atrial rate/rhythm	93 beats/min, regular except for the event
PR interval	0.16 sec
QRS duration	0.04 sec
Identification	Sinus rhythm at 93 beats/min with a PAC (PAC is the seventh complex from the left)

Figure 4-28 answer

Ventricular rate/rhythm	231 beats/min, regular
Atrial rate/rhythm	Unable to determine
PR interval	Unable to determine
QRS duration	0.06 sec
Identification	AV nodal reentrant tachycardia (AVNRT) at 231 beats/min with ST-segment depression

Figure 4-29 answer

Ventricular rate/rhythm	68 to 115 beats/min, irregular
Atrial rate/rhythm	Unable to determine
PR interval	Unable to determine
QRS duration	0.06 sec
Identification	Atrial fibrillation at 68 to 115 beats/min

Figure 4-30 answer

Ventricular rate/rhythm	75 beats/min, regular except for event
Atrial rate/rhythm	75 beats/min, regular except for event
PR interval	0.20 sec
QRS duration	0.12 sec
Identification	Sinus rhythm at 75 beats/min with a wide QRS and a nonconducted PAC

Figure 4-31 answer

Ventricular rate/rhythm	70 beats/min, regular
Atrial rate/rhythm	70 beats/min (sinus beats), unable to determine
PR interval	Varies
QRS duration	Varies
Identification	Underlying rhythm is sinus with delta waves present; ventricular rate approximately 70 beats/min; patient with know WPW

Figure 4-32 answer

Ventricular rate/rhythm	188 beats/min, regular
Atrial rate/rhythm	Unable to determine
PR interval	Unable to determine
QRS duration	0.06 sec
Identification	AVNRT at 188 beats/min with ST-segment depression

Figure 4-33 answer

Ventricular rate/rhythm	79 beats/min, regular except for event
Atrial rate/rhythm	79 beats/min, regular except for event
PR interval	0.16 sec
QRS duration	0.06 sec
Identification	Sinus rhythm at 79 beats/min with PACs

Figure 4-34 answer

Ventricular rate/rhythm	29 beats/min, regular
Atrial rate/rhythm	Unable to determine
PR interval	Unable to determine
QRS duration	0.10 sec
Identification	Controlled atrial fibrillation at 29 beats/min; this patient was diagnosed with digitalis toxicity

Figure 4-35 answer

Ventricular rate/rhythm	68 to 150 beats/min, irregular
Atrial rate/rhythm	Unable to determine
PR interval	Unable to determine
QRS duration	0.08 sec
Identification	Atrial flutter with a ventricular response of 68 to 150 beats/min

Figure 4-36 answer

Ventricular rate/rhythm	111 beats/min, regular except for event
Atrial rate/rhythm	111 beats/min, regular except for event
PR interval	0.18 sec
QRS duration	0.08 sec
Identification	Sinus tachycardia at 111 beats/min with a nonconducted PAC

Figure 4-37 answer

Ventricular rate/rhythm	186 beats/min, regular
Atrial rate/rhythm	Unable to determine
PR interval	Unable to determine
QRS duration	0.06 sec
Identification	AVNRT at 186 beats/min with ST-segment depression

Figure 4-38 answer

Ventricular rate/rhythm	55 to 94 beats/min, irregular
Atrial rate/rhythm	Unable to determine
PR interval	Unable to determine
QRS duration	0.10 sec
Identification	Controlled atrial fibrillation at 55 to 94 beats/min

Figure 4-39 answer

Ventricular rate/rhythm	88 beats/min, regular
Atrial rate/rhythm	Unable to determine
PR interval	Unable to determine
QRS duration	0.06 sec
Identification	Atrial flutter at 88 beats/min with ST-segment depression

Figure 4-40 answer

Ventricular rate/rhythm	83 beats/min (sinus beats), regular except for events
Atrial rate/rhythm	83 beats/min (sinus beats)/ regular except for events
PR interval	0.16 sec
QRS duration	0.04 to 0.08 sec
Identification	Sinus rhythm at 83 beats/min with frequent PACs (atrial bigeminy), ST-segment depression, inverted T waves (beats 3, 5, 7, and 9 are PACs)

Figure 4-41 answer

Ventricular rate/rhythm	64 to 83 beats/min, irregular
Atrial rate/rhythm	Unable to determine
PR interval	Unable to determine
QRS duration	0.08 sec
Identification	Atrial flutter at 64 to 83 beats/min

Figure 4-42 answer

Ventricular rate/rhythm	115 to 215 beats/min, irregular
Atrial rate/rhythm	Unable to determine, irregular
PR interval	Varies
QRS duration	0.04 to 0.06 sec
Identification	Multifocal atrial tachycardia at 115 to 215 beats/min with ST-segment depression

Figure 4-43 answer

Ventricular rate/rhythm	96 to 214 beats/min, irregular
Atrial rate/rhythm	96 to 214 beats/min, irregular
PR interval	0.16 sec (sinus beats)
QRS duration	0.08 sec
Identification	Sinus rhythm at 96 beats/min with a PAC precipitating a run of PSVT at 214 beats/min, back to a sinus rhythm at 96 beats/min

Figure 4-44 answer

Ventricular rate/rhythm	93 beats/min (sinus beats), regular except for the event
Atrial rate/rhythm	93 beats/min (sinus beats), regular except for the event
PR interval	0.16 sec (sinus beats)
QRS duration	0.04 sec (sinus beats)
Identification	Sinus rhythm at 93 beats/min with a PAC (PAC is the seventh beat from the left)

Junctional Rhythms

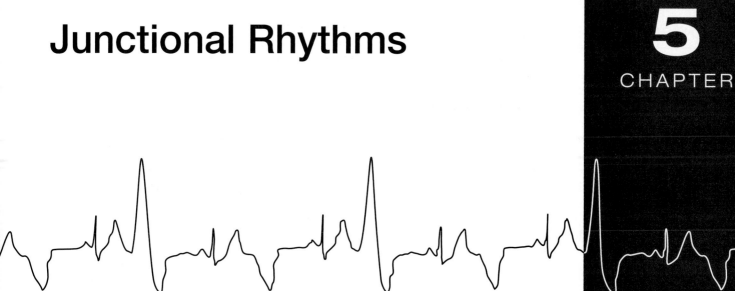

OBJECTIVES

On completion of this chapter, you will be able to:

1. Describe the ECG characteristics, possible causes, signs and symptoms, and initial emergency care for premature junctional complexes (PJCs).
2. Describe the ECG characteristics and possible causes for junctional escape beats.
3. Explain the difference between premature junctional complexes and junctional escape beats.
4. Describe the ECG characteristics, possible causes, signs and symptoms, and initial emergency care for a junctional escape rhythm.
5. Describe the ECG characteristics, possible causes, signs and symptoms, and initial emergency care for an accelerated junctional rhythm.
6. Describe the ECG characteristics, possible causes, signs and symptoms, and initial emergency care for junctional tachycardia.

INTRODUCTION

The AV node is a group of specialized cells located in the lower part of the right atrium, above the base of the tricuspid valve. The AV node's main job is to delay an electrical impulse. This allows the atria to contract and complete filling of the ventricles with blood before the next ventricular contraction.

After passing through the AV node, the electrical impulse enters the **bundle of His**. The bundle of His is located in the upper part of the interventricular septum. It connects the AV node with the two bundle branches. The bundle of His has pacemaker cells that are capable of discharging at a rhythmic rate of 40 to 60 beats/min. The AV node and the nonbranching portion of the bundle of His are called the **AV junction** (Figure 5-1). The bundle of His conducts the electrical impulse to the right and left bundle branches.

Remember that the SA node is normally the heart's pacemaker. The AV junction may assume responsibility for pacing the heart if:

- The SA node fails to discharge (such as sinus arrest)
- An impulse from the SA node is generated but blocked as it exits the SA node (such as SA block)
- The rate of discharge of the SA node is slower than that of the AV junction (such as a sinus bradycardia or the slower phase of a sinus arrhythmia)
- An impulse from the SA node is generated and is conducted through the atria but is not conducted to the ventricles (such as an AV block)

Rhythms that begin in the AV junction used to be called nodal rhythms until electrophysiologic studies proved the AV node does not contain pacemaker cells. The cells nearest the bundle of His are actually responsible for secondary pacing function. Rhythms originating from the AV junction are now called **junctional dysrhythmias**.

If the AV junction paces the heart, the electrical impulse must travel in a backward (**retrograde**) direction to activate the atria. If a P wave is seen, it will be inverted in leads II, III, and aVF because the impulse is traveling away from the positive electrode (Figure 5-2). If the atria depolarize before the ventricles, an inverted P wave will be seen *before* the QRS complex (Figure 5-3) and the PR interval will usually measure 0.12 second or less. The PR interval is shorter than usual because an impulse that begins in the AV junction does not have to travel as far to stimulate the ventricles. If the atria and ventricles depolarize at the same time, a P wave will not be visible because it will be hidden in the QRS complex. When the atria are depolarized after the ventricles, the P wave typically distorts the end of the QRS complex and an inverted P wave will appear *after* the QRS.

ECG Pearl

P waves are usually positive (upright) in lead I. Inverted P waves may be seen in some, all, or none of the chest leads.

PREMATURE JUNCTIONAL COMPLEXES (PJCs)

How Do I Recognize It?

[OBJECTIVE 1]

A **premature junctional complex** (PJC) occurs when an irritable site (focus) within the AV junction fires before the next SA node impulse is due to fire. This interrupts the sinus rhythm. Because the impulse is conducted through the ventricles in the usual manner, the QRS complex will usually measure 0.10 second or less. PJCs are sometimes called premature junctional extrasystoles. A noncompensatory

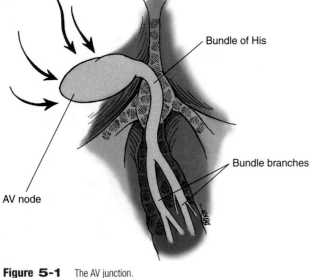

Figure 5-1   The AV junction.

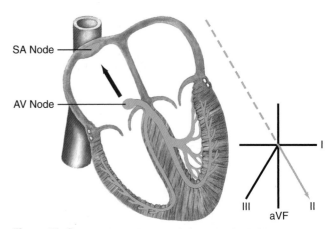

Figure 5-2   If the AV junction paces the heart, the electrical impulse must travel in a backward (retrograde) direction to activate the atria. If a P wave is seen, it will be inverted in leads II, III, and aVF because the impulse is traveling away from the positive electrode.

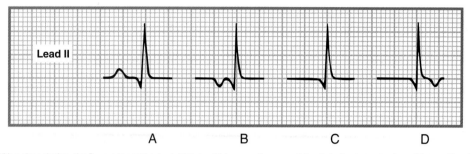

Figure 5-3   **A,** With a sinus rhythm, the P wave is positive (upright) in lead II because the wave of depolarization is moving toward the positive electrode. The P wave associated with a junctional beat (in lead II) may be: **B,** inverted (retrograde) and appear before the QRS; **C,** be hidden by the QRS, or **D,** appear after the QRS.

(incomplete) pause often follows a PJC. This pause represents the delay during which the SA node resets its rhythm for the next beat. PJCs may occur in patterns—couplets, bigeminy, trigeminy, and quadrigeminy.

You can usually tell the difference between a PAC and a PJC by the P wave. A PAC typically has an upright P wave before the QRS complex in leads II, III, and aVF. A P wave may or may not be present with a PJC. If a P wave is present, it is inverted (retrograde) and may precede or follow the QRS. PJCs can be misdiagnosed when the P wave of a PAC is buried in the preceding T wave.

Junctional complexes may come early (before the next expected sinus beat) or late (after the next expected sinus beat). If the complex is *early* it is called a premature junctional complex. If the complex is *late* it is called a junctional escape beat. To determine if a complex is early or late, we need to see at least two sinus beats in a row to establish the regularity of the underlying rhythm.

Let's look at Figure 5-4. Looking at the overall rhythm, it appears to be irregular. All QRS complexes appear to be narrow, so we assume that all impulses started from above the ventricles. Using a pen or pencil, mark an "S" (for SA node) above each normal looking P wave. Mark a "J" (for junctional) above those P waves that are inverted or absent. When you are finished, you should have a "J" marked over the P waves in beats 2, 5, 8, and 11. The rest of the P waves should be marked with an "S." Now take your calipers or a piece of paper and mark the third and fourth complexes in Figure 5-4. We already determined that these complexes came from the SA node. These beats reflect the underlying rhythm. Calculate the atrial and ventricular rate between these beats. It is 136 beats/min (1500 ÷ 11 small boxes). We now know that the underlying rhythm is a sinus tachycardia at 136 beats/min. Now move your calipers or paper to the right. If beat 5 occurred on time (when the next sinus beat was expected), it will line up with your calipers (or paper). The fifth complex is early. It occurred *before* the next expected sinus beat. Therefore this complex is a PJC. The other beats that have an inverted P wave before the QRS are also PJCs.

A PJC is not an entire rhythm—it is a single beat. When identifying a rhythm, be sure to specify the underlying rhythm and the origin of the ectopic beat(s). In this rhythm strip, we found that the underlying rhythm was a sinus tachycardia at 136 beats/min. All of the ectopic beats were early and came from the AV junction. Therefore we would identify this rhythm strip as "sinus tachycardia at 136 beats/min with frequent PJCs." The ECG characteristics of PJCs are shown in Table 5-1.

What Causes It?

PJCs are less common than either PACs or PVCs. Causes of PJCs include:

- Congestive heart failure
- Acute coronary syndromes
- Mental and physical fatigue
- Valvular heart disease
- Digitalis toxicity
- Electrolyte imbalance
- Rheumatic heart disease
- Stimulants: caffeine, tobacco, cocaine

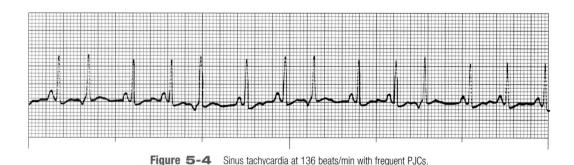

Figure 5-4   Sinus tachycardia at 136 beats/min with frequent PJCs.

TABLE **5-1**	Characteristics of Premature Junctional Complexes (PJCs)
Rate	Usually within normal range, but depends on underlying rhythm
Rhythm	Regular with *premature* beats
P waves	May occur before, during, or after the QRS; if visible, the P wave is inverted in leads II, III, and aVF
PR interval	If a P wave occurs before the QRS, the PR interval will usually be 0.12 sec or less; if no P wave occurs before the QRS, there will be no PR interval
QRS duration	Usually 0.10 sec or less unless it is aberrantly conducted or an intraventricular conduction delay exists

What Do I Do About It?

PJCs do not normally require treatment because most individuals who have PJCs are asymptomatic. However, PJCs may lead to symptoms of palpitations or the feeling of skipped beats. Light-headedness, dizziness, and other signs of decreased cardiac output can occur if PJCs are frequent. If PJCs occur because of ingestion of stimulants or digitalis toxicity, these substances should be withheld.

ECG Pearl

Keep in mind that inverted P waves are normal in lead V₁. To determine if a beat or rhythm came from the AV junction using this lead, look for a short PR interval. Use lead II, III, or aVF to confirm your findings.

JUNCTIONAL ESCAPE BEATS/ RHYTHM

How Do I Recognize It?

[OBJECTIVES 2, 3, 4]

A junctional escape beat begins in the AV junction and appears *late* (after the next expected sinus beat). Junctional escape beats frequently occur during episodes of sinus arrest or follow pauses of nonconducted PACs. Take a look at

Figure 5-5. Looking at the rhythm strip, you can see two normal looking beats on the left and two more on the far right. In the center of the strip is an odd-looking beat that appears in the middle of a very long pause between beats 2 and 4. Looking more closely at beats 1, 2, 4, and 5 you can see an upright P wave before each QRS complex. These beats came from the SA node. When you calculate the atrial and ventricular rates between these beats you will find that it is 71 beats/min (1500 ÷ 21 small boxes). With this information we know that the underlying rhythm is a sinus rhythm. Using your calipers or a piece of paper, mark the first and second complexes. When you move the calipers or paper to the right, you can see that beat No. 3 came *late*—after the next expected sinus beat.

Now let's try to figure out where beat No. 3 came from and why. If you put your finger over beat No. 3, can you explain what happened? The long pause between beats 2 and 4 is an episode of sinus arrest. Remember that if the SA node fails to initiate an impulse, an escape pacemaker site (the AV junction or ventricles) should assume responsibility for pacing the heart. Look closely at beat No. 3. The QRS complex is narrow, the ST-segment is depressed, and there is no P wave before the QRS complex. If you compare the ST-segment of beat 3 with the others in the rhythm strip, you can see that the ST-segment in beat 3 is shaped differently. It appears that there is an inverted P wave in the ST-segment of this beat. The narrow-QRS complex and absence of a positive P wave before the QRS complex tells us the beat came from the AV junction. Because the beat is *late*, it is a junctional escape beat. (If beat 3 had been *early*, we would call it a PJC). So what happened here? The SA node fired in beats 1 and 2. When the sinus did not fire again when it should have, the AV junction kicked in and fired. Thus a junctional escape beat is *protective*—preventing cardiac standstill. There is a noncompensatory pause after the junctional escape beat during which the SA node resets. This is followed by two sinus beats.

The ST-segments of the beats in this rhythm strip are depressed. The PR interval of the sinus beats is prolonged; measuring 0.24 second. Complete identification of the events that occurred in this rhythm strip would include the following description, "Sinus rhythm at 71 beats/min with a prolonged PR interval (0.24 sec), an episode of sinus arrest, a junctional escape beat, and ST-segment depression." The ECG characteristics of junctional escape beats are shown in Table 5-2.

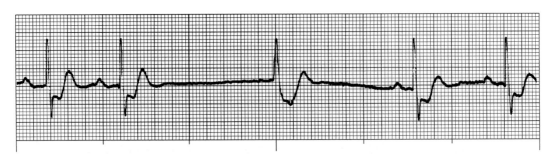

Figure 5-5   Sinus rhythm at 71 beats/min with a prolonged PR interval (0.24 sec), an episode of sinus arrest, a junctional escape beat, and ST-segment depression.

TABLE 5-2	Characteristics of Junctional Escape Beats
Rate	Usually within normal range, but depends on underlying rhythm
Rhythm	Regular with *late* beats
P waves	May occur before, during, or after the QRS; if visible, the P wave is inverted in leads II, III, and aVF
PR interval	If a P wave occurs before the QRS, the PR interval will usually be 0.12 sec or less; if no P wave occurs before the QRS, there will be no PR interval
QRS duration	Usually 0.10 sec or less unless it is aberrantly conducted or an intraventricular conduction delay exists

ECG Pearl

Junctional escape beats and rhythms occur when the SA node fails to pace the heart or AV conduction fails.

A junctional *rhythm* is several sequential junctional escape *beats*. The terms junctional rhythm and junctional escape rhythm are used interchangeably. Remember that the intrinsic rate of the AV junction is 40 to 60 beats/min. Because a junctional rhythm starts from above the ventricles, the QRS complex is usually narrow and its rhythm is very regular. If the AV junction paces the heart at a rate slower than 40 beats/min, the resulting rhythm is called a **junctional bradycardia**. This may seem confusing because the AV junction's normal pacing rate (40-60 beats/min) *is* bradycardic. However, the term junctional bradycardia refers to a rate slower than normal for the AV junction.

Figure 5-6 is a continuous rhythm strip. In A, you can see inverted (retrograde) P waves before the QRS complexes. In B, note the change in the location of the P waves. In the first beat, the retrograde P wave is seen before the QRS. In the second beat, no P wave is seen. In the remaining beats, the P wave is seen after the QRS complexes. The ECG characteristics of a junctional rhythm are shown in Table 5-3.

What Causes It?

Junctional escape beats frequently occur during episodes of sinus arrest or following pauses of nonconducted PACs. Junctional escape beats may also be observed in healthy individuals during sinus bradycardia. Causes of a junctional rhythm include:

- Acute coronary syndromes (particularly inferior wall MI)
- Hypoxia
- Rheumatic heart disease
- Valvular disease
- SA node disease
- Increased parasympathetic tone
- Immediately after cardiac surgery
- Effects of medications including digitalis, quinidine, beta-blockers, and calcium channel blockers

What Do I Do About It?

The patient may be asymptomatic with a junctional escape rhythm or may experience signs and symptoms that may be associated with the slow heart rate and decreased cardiac output. Treatment depends on the cause of the dysrhythmia and the patient's presenting signs and symptoms. Signs and symptoms may include weakness, chest pain or pressure, syncope, an altered level of consciousness, and hypotension.

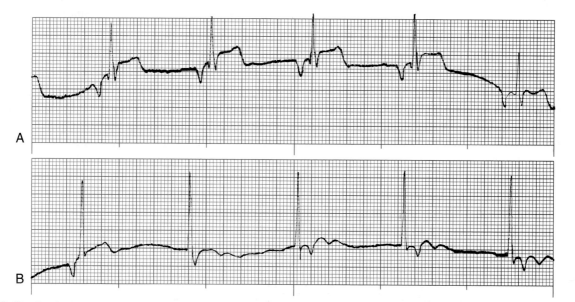

Figure 5-6 Junctional escape rhythm. Continuous strips. **A,** Note the inverted (retrograde) P waves before the QRS complexes. **B,** Note the change in the location of the P waves. In the first beat, the retrograde P wave is seen before the QRS. In the second beat, no P wave is seen. In the remaining beats, the P wave is seen after the QRS complexes.

TABLE 5-3	Characteristics of Junctional Escape Rhythm
Rate	40-60 beats/min
Rhythm	Very regular
P waves	May occur before, during, or after the QRS; if visible, the P wave is inverted in leads II, III, and aVF
PR interval	If a P wave occurs before the QRS, the PR interval will usually be 0.12 sec or less; if no P wave occurs before the QRS, there will be no PR interval
QRS duration	Usually 0.10 sec or less unless it is aberrantly conducted or an intraventricular conduction delay exists

TABLE 5-4	Characteristics of Accelerated Junctional Rhythm
Rate	61-100 beats/min
Rhythm	Very regular
P waves	May occur before, during, or after the QRS; if visible, the P wave is inverted in leads II, III, and aVF
PR interval	If a P wave occurs before the QRS, the PR interval will usually be 0.12 sec or less; if no P wave occurs before the QRS, there will be no PR interval
QRS duration	Usually 0.10 sec or less unless it is aberrantly conducted or an intraventricular conduction delay exists

If the dysrhythmia is caused by digitalis toxicity, this medication should be withheld. If the patient's signs and symptoms are related to the slow heart rate, atropine and/or transcutaneous pacing should be considered. Other medications that may be used in the treatment of symptomatic bradycardia include dopamine and epinephrine intravenous infusions.

ACCELERATED JUNCTIONAL RHYTHM

How Do I Recognize It?

[OBJECTIVE 5]

If the AV junction speeds up and fires at a rate of 61 to 100 beats/min, the resulting rhythm is called an **accelerated junctional rhythm**. This rhythm is caused by enhanced automaticity of the bundle of His. The only ECG difference between a junctional rhythm and an accelerated junctional rhythm is the increase in the ventricular rate. An example of an accelerated junctional rhythm is shown in Figure 5-7. The ECG characteristics of this rhythm are shown in Table 5-4.

What Causes It?

Causes of this dysrhythmia include digitalis toxicity, acute myocardial infarction, cardiac surgery, rheumatic fever, COPD, and hypokalemia.

What Do I Do About It?

The patient is usually asymptomatic because the ventricular rate is 61 to 100 beats/min; however, the patient should be monitored closely. If the rhythm is caused by digitalis toxicity, this medication should be withheld.

ECG Pearl

Junctional Dysrhythmias at a Glance
- Junctional rhythm—40-60 beats/min
- Accelerated junctional rhythm—61-100 beats/min
- Junctional tachycardia—101-180 beats/min

JUNCTIONAL TACHYCARDIA

How Do I Recognize It?

[OBJECTIVE 6]

Junctional tachycardia is an ectopic rhythm that begins in the pacemaker cells found in the bundle of His. When three or more sequential PJCs occur at a rate of more than 100 beats/min, a junctional tachycardia exists. Nonparoxysmal (gradual onset) junctional tachycardia usually starts as an accelerated junctional rhythm but the heart rate gradually increases to more than 100 beats/min. The usual ventricular rate for nonparoxysmal junctional tachycardia is 101 to 140 beats/min. Paroxysmal junctional tachycardia

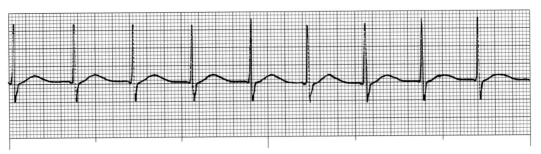

Figure 5-7 Accelerated junctional rhythm at 93 beats/min.

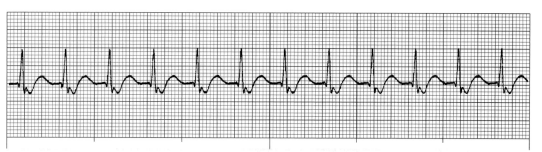

Figure 5-8   Junctional tachycardia at 120 beats/min.

starts and ends suddenly and is often precipitated by a PJC. The ventricular rate for paroxysmal junctional tachycardia is generally faster, 140 beats/min or more. When the ventricular rate is greater than 150 beats/min, it is difficult to distinguish junctional tachycardia from AV nodal reentrant tachycardia and AV reentrant tachycardia. An example of junctional tachycardia is shown in Figure 5-8. The ECG characteristics of this rhythm are shown in Table 5-5.

What Causes It?

Junctional tachycardia is an uncommon rhythm. It is probably caused by enhanced automaticity. It may occur because of an acute coronary syndrome, congestive heart failure, theophylline administration, or digitalis toxicity.

What Do I Do About It?

With sustained ventricular rates of 150 beats/min or more, the patient may complain of a "racing heart" and severe anxiety. Because of the fast ventricular rate, the ventricles may be unable to fill completely, resulting in decreased cardiac output. The more rapid the rate, the greater the incidence of symptoms due to increased myocardial oxygen demand. Junctional tachycardia associated with an acute coronary syndrome may:

- Increase myocardial ischemia
- Increase the frequency and severity of chest pain
- Extend the size of a myocardial infarction
- Cause congestive heart failure, hypotension, or cardiogenic shock
- Predispose the patient to ventricular dysrhythmias

Treatment depends on the severity of the patient's signs and symptoms. If the patient tolerates the rhythm,

TABLE 5-5	Characteristics of Junctional Tachycardia
Rate	101-180 beats/min
Rhythm	Very regular
P waves	May occur before, during, or after the QRS; if visible, the P wave is inverted in leads II, III, and aVF
PR interval	If a P wave occurs before the QRS, the PR interval will usually be 0.12 sec or less; if no P wave occurs before the QRS, there will be no PR interval
QRS duration	Usually 0.10 sec or less unless it is aberrantly conducted or an intraventricular conduction delay exists

observation is often all that is needed. If the patient is symptomatic as a result of the rapid rate, initial treatment should include oxygen and IV access. Since it is often difficult to distinguish junctional tachycardia from other narrow-QRS tachycardias, vagal maneuvers and, if necessary, IV adenosine may be used to help determine the origin of the rhythm. A beta-blocker or calcium channel blocker may be ordered (if no contraindications exist). In adults, junctional tachycardia is often a symptom of digitalis toxicity. If the rhythm is the result of digitalis toxicity, the drug should be withheld. In some cases, an antibody called Digibind may be indicated in the treatment of digitalis toxicity, depending on the patient's clinical condition. If the rhythm is the result of theophylline administration, the infusion should be slowed or stopped. A summary of junctional rhythm characteristics can be found in Table 5-6.

TABLE **5-6**	Junctional Rhythms—Summary of Characteristics

	PJCs	Junctional Escape Beat	Junctional Escape Rhythm	Accelerated Junctional Rhythm	Junctional Tachycardia
Rate	Usually within normal range, but depends on underlying rhythm	Usually within normal range, but depends on underlying rhythm	40-60 beats/min	61-100 beats/min	101-180 beats/min
Rhythm	Regular with *premature* beats	Regular with *late* beats	Regular	Regular	Regular
P Waves (leads II, III, aVF)	May occur before, during, or after the QRS; if visible, the P wave is inverted in leads II, III, and aVF	May occur before, during, or after the QRS; if visible, the P wave is inverted in leads II, III, and aVF	May occur before, during, or after the QRS; if visible, the P wave is inverted in leads II, III, and aVF	May occur before, during, or after the QRS; if visible, the P wave is inverted in leads II, III, and aVF	May occur before, during, or after the QRS; if visible, the P wave is inverted in leads II, III, and aVF
PR Interval	If a P wave occurs before the QRS, the PR interval will usually be 0.12 sec or less; if no P wave occurs before the QRS, there will be no PR interval	If a P wave occurs before the QRS, the PR interval will usually be 0.12 sec or less; if no P wave occurs before the QRS, there will be no PR interval	If a P wave occurs before the QRS, the PR interval will usually be 0.12 sec or less; if no P wave occurs before the QRS, there will be no PR interval	If a P wave occurs before the QRS, the PR interval will usually be 0.12 sec or less; if no P wave occurs before the QRS, there will be no PR interval	If a P wave occurs before the QRS, the PR interval will usually be 0.12 sec or less; if no P wave occurs before the QRS, there will be no PR interval
QRS	Usually 0.10 sec or less unless it is aberrantly conducted or an intraventricular conduction delay exists	Usually 0.10 sec or less unless it is aberrantly conducted or an intraventricular conduction delay exists	Usually 0.10 sec or less unless it is aberrantly conducted or an intraventricular conduction delay exists	Usually 0.10 sec or less unless it is aberrantly conducted or an intraventricular conduction delay exists	Usually 0.10 sec or less unless it is aberrantly conducted or an intraventricular conduction delay exists

STOP & REVIEW

True/False

Indicate whether the sentence or statement is true or false.

_____ **1.** PJCs are more common than PACs or PVCs.

_____ **2.** A PJC produces a positive (upright) P wave in leads II, III, and aVF that comes before, during, or after the QRS complex.

_____ **3.** Atropine is the drug of choice when treating a symptomatic patient with a junctional rhythm at a rate of 40 beats/min.

Completion

Complete each sentence or statement.

4. If the AV junction paces the heart, the electrical impulse must travel in a backward direction to activate the atria. This is called _____ conduction.

5. A beat originating from the AV junction that appears later than the next expected sinus beat is called a _____ _____ _____.

Matching

_____ **6.** Location of the P wave on the ECG if atrial depolarization precedes ventricular depolarization

_____ **7.** A beat originating from the AV junction that appears earlier than the next expected sinus beat

_____ **8.** Normal rate for the AV junction

_____ **9.** Primary waveform used to differentiate PJCs from PACs

_____ **10.** Medication used to increase heart rate

_____ **11.** Location of the P wave on the ECG if atrial and ventricular depolarization occur simultaneously

_____ **12.** Toxicity/excess of this medication is a common cause of junctional dysrhythmias

_____ **13.** Name given to a dysrhythmia that originates in the AV junction with a ventricular rate between 61 to 100 beats/min

_____ **14.** Impulse originating from a source other than the SA node

_____ **15.** Location of the P wave on the ECG if atrial depolarization occurs after ventricular depolarization

a. Digitalis

b. Atropine

c. Inverted P wave occurs after the QRS complex in leads II, III, and aVF

d. P wave

e. Hidden within the QRS complex (not visible)

f. Accelerated junctional rhythm

g. 40 to 60 beats/min

h. Inverted P wave appears before the QRS complex in leads II, III, and aVF

i. Ectopic

j. Premature junctional complex

Short Answer

16. Indicate the ventricular rates for each of the following junctional dysrhythmias.
   1. Junctional bradycardia   _____
   2. Junctional tachycardia   _____
   3. Accelerated junctional rhythm   _____
   4. Junctional rhythm   _____

17. List four (4) reasons why the AV junction may assume responsibility for pacing the heart.

1.

2.

3.

4.

JUNCTIONAL RHYTHMS—*PRACTICE RHYTHM STRIPS*

For each of the following rhythm strips, determine the atrial and ventricular rate and rhythm, measure the PR interval and QRS duration, and then identify the rhythm. All strips were recorded in lead II unless otherwise noted. Note: These rhythm strips include sinus, atrial, and junctional rhythms.

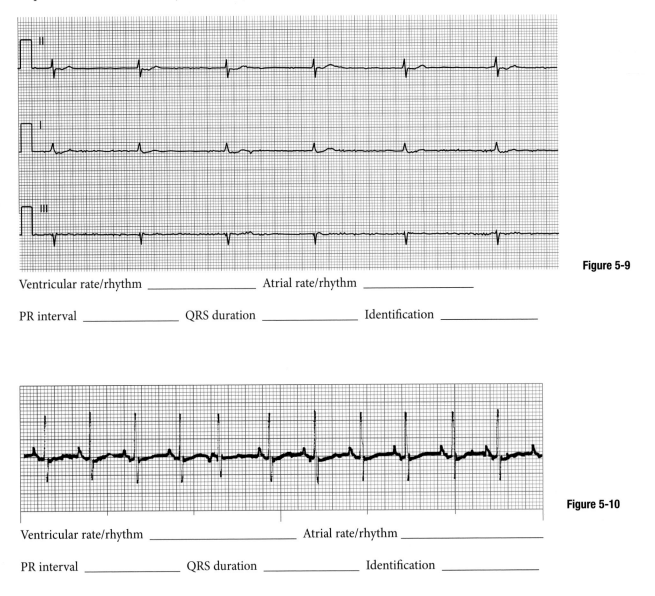

Figure 5-9

Ventricular rate/rhythm _____ Atrial rate/rhythm _____

PR interval _____ QRS duration _____ Identification _____

Figure 5-10

Ventricular rate/rhythm _____ Atrial rate/rhythm _____

PR interval _____ QRS duration _____ Identification _____

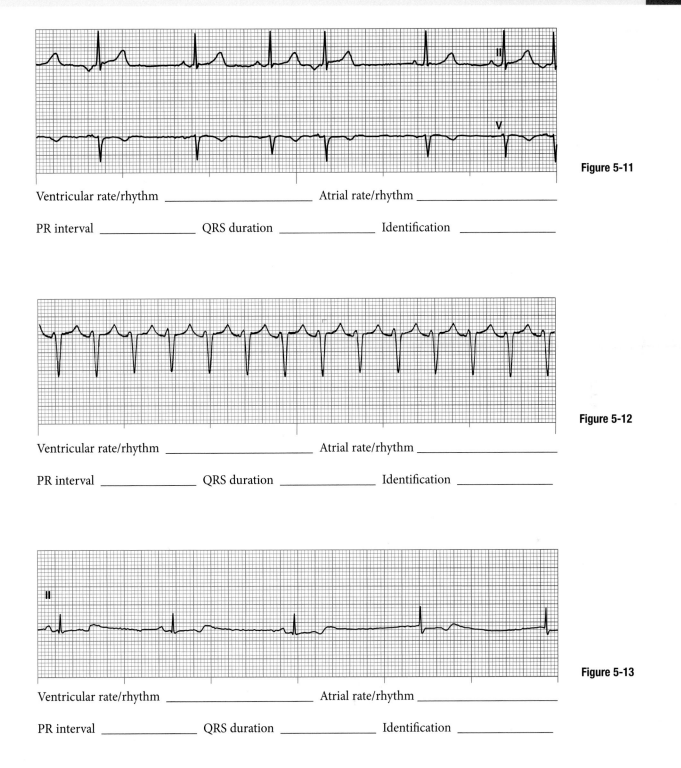

Figure 5-11

Ventricular rate/rhythm _____ Atrial rate/rhythm _____

PR interval _____ QRS duration _____ Identification _____

Figure 5-12

Ventricular rate/rhythm _____ Atrial rate/rhythm _____

PR interval _____ QRS duration _____ Identification _____

Figure 5-13

Ventricular rate/rhythm _____ Atrial rate/rhythm _____

PR interval _____ QRS duration _____ Identification _____

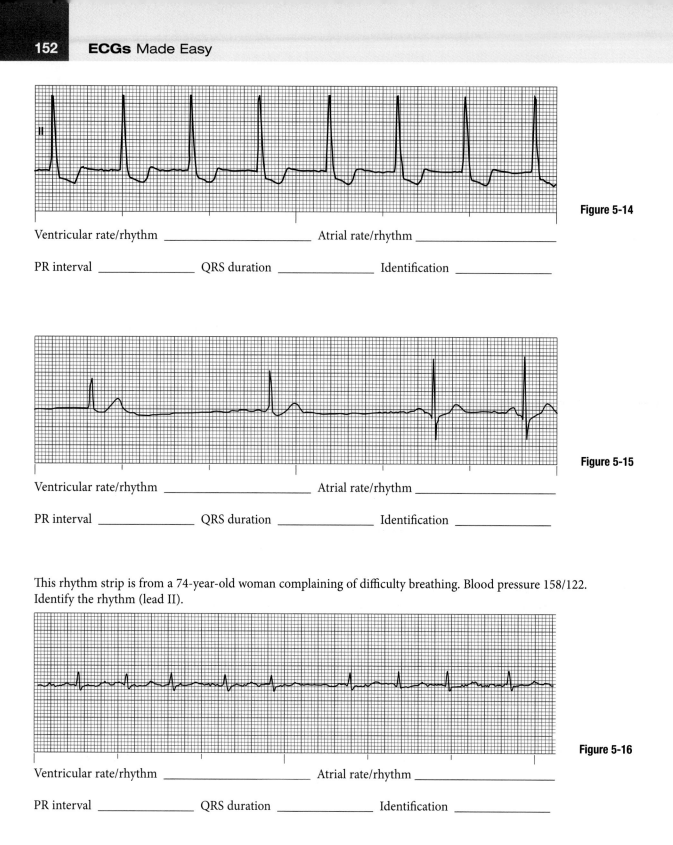

Figure 5-14

Ventricular rate/rhythm _____ Atrial rate/rhythm _____

PR interval _____ QRS duration _____ Identification _____

Figure 5-15

Ventricular rate/rhythm _____ Atrial rate/rhythm _____

PR interval _____ QRS duration _____ Identification _____

This rhythm strip is from a 74-year-old woman complaining of difficulty breathing. Blood pressure 158/122. Identify the rhythm (lead II).

Figure 5-16

Ventricular rate/rhythm _____ Atrial rate/rhythm _____

PR interval _____ QRS duration _____ Identification _____

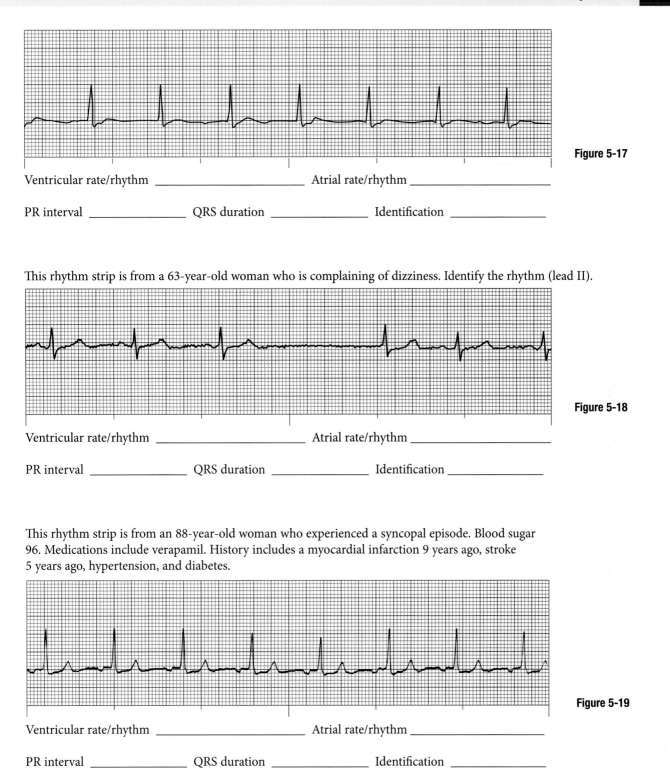

Figure 5-17

Ventricular rate/rhythm _____   Atrial rate/rhythm _____

PR interval _____   QRS duration _____   Identification _____

This rhythm strip is from a 63-year-old woman who is complaining of dizziness. Identify the rhythm (lead II).

Figure 5-18

Ventricular rate/rhythm _____   Atrial rate/rhythm _____

PR interval _____   QRS duration _____   Identification _____

This rhythm strip is from an 88-year-old woman who experienced a syncopal episode. Blood sugar 96. Medications include verapamil. History includes a myocardial infarction 9 years ago, stroke 5 years ago, hypertension, and diabetes.

Figure 5-19

Ventricular rate/rhythm _____   Atrial rate/rhythm _____

PR interval _____   QRS duration _____   Identification _____

This rhythm strip is from a 51-year-old man found unresponsive. He has a history of esophageal varices and gastrointestinal bleeding. Blood pressure 182/100. Identify the rhythm (lead I).

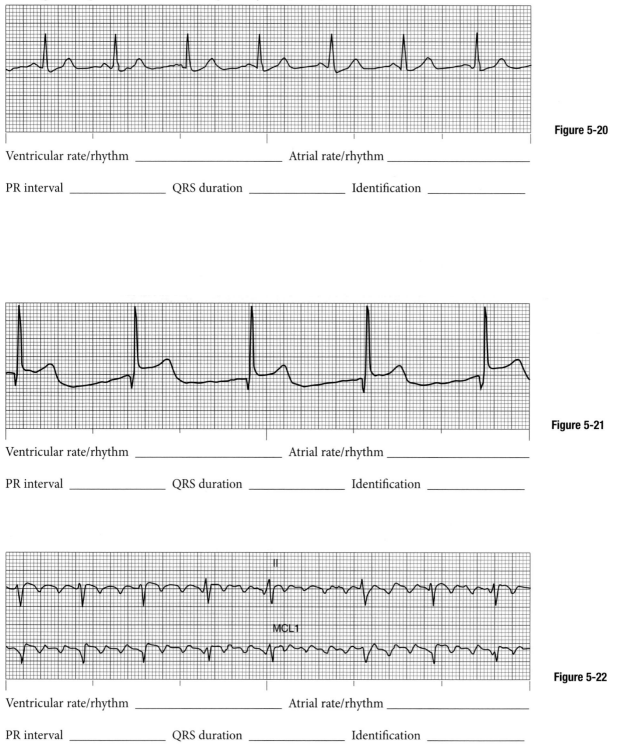

Figure 5-20

Ventricular rate/rhythm _____ Atrial rate/rhythm _____

PR interval _____ QRS duration _____ Identification _____

Figure 5-21

Ventricular rate/rhythm _____ Atrial rate/rhythm _____

PR interval _____ QRS duration _____ Identification _____

Figure 5-22

Ventricular rate/rhythm _____ Atrial rate/rhythm _____

PR interval _____ QRS duration _____ Identification _____

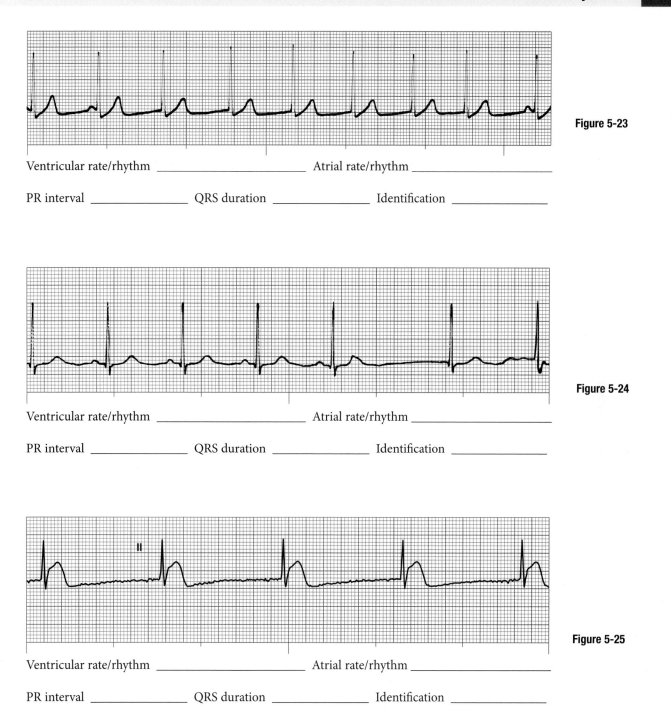

Figure 5-23

Ventricular rate/rhythm _____ Atrial rate/rhythm _____

PR interval _____ QRS duration _____ Identification _____

Figure 5-24

Ventricular rate/rhythm _____ Atrial rate/rhythm _____

PR interval _____ QRS duration _____ Identification _____

Figure 5-25

Ventricular rate/rhythm _____ Atrial rate/rhythm _____

PR interval _____ QRS duration _____ Identification _____

True/False

1. F

2. F

3. T

Completion

4. If the AV junction paces the heart, the electrical impulse must travel in a backward direction to activate the atria. This is called *retrograde* conduction.

5. A beat originating from the AV junction that appears later than the next expected sinus beat is called a *junctional escape beat.*

Matching

6. h

7. j

8. g

9. d

10. b

11. e

12. a

13. f

14. i

15. c

Short Answer

16.

1. Junctional bradycardia	Less than 40 beats/min
2. Junctional tachycardia	101 to 180 beats/min
3. Accelerated junctional rhythm	61 to 100 beats/min
4. Junctional rhythm	40 to 60 beats/min

17.

The AV junction may assume responsibility for pacing the heart if:

1. The SA node fails to discharge (such as sinus arrest)

2. An impulse from the SA node is generated but blocked as it exits the SA node (such as SA block)

3. The rate of discharge of the SA node is slower than that of the AV junction (such as a sinus bradycardia or the slower phase of a sinus arrhythmia)

4. An impulse from the SA node is generated and is conducted through the atria but is not conducted to the ventricles (such as an AV block)

Answer for Figure 5-9

Ventricular rate/rhythm	45 beats/min, regular
Atrial rate/rhythm	None
PR interval	None
QRS duration	0.06 sec
Identification	Junctional rhythm at 45 beats/min

Answer for Figure 5-10

Ventricular rate/rhythm	115 beats/min (sinus beats), regular except for the event
Atrial rate/rhythm	115 beats/min (sinus beats), regular except for the event
PR interval	0.16 sec (sinus beats)
QRS duration	0.06 sec (sinus beats)
Identification	Sinus tachycardia at 115 beats/min with a PJC (fifth beat is the PJC)

Answer for Figure 5-11

Ventricular rate/rhythm	63 beats/min (sinus beats), regular except for events (every third beat is a PJC)
Atrial rate/rhythm	63 beats/min (sinus beats), regular except for events (every third beat is a PJC)
PR interval	0.12 to 0.16 sec (sinus beats)
QRS duration	0.06 sec (sinus beats)
Identification	Sinus rhythm at 63 beats/min with PJCs (junctional trigeminy)

Answer for Figure 5-12

Ventricular rate/rhythm	138 beats/min, regular
Atrial rate/rhythm	Unable to determine
PR interval	Unable to determine
QRS	0.10 sec
Identification	Narrow-QRS tachycardia, probably junctional tachycardia, at 138 beats/min

Answer for Figure 5-13

Ventricular rate/rhythm	33 beats/min (sinus beats); 32 beats/min (junctional beats)
Atrial rate/rhythm	33 beats/min (sinus beats); unable to determine (junctional beats)
PR interval	0.20 sec (sinus beats)
QRS duration	0.04 to 0.06 sec
Identification	Sinus bradycardia at 33 beats/min to junctional bradycardia at 32 beats/min

Answer for Figure 5-14

Ventricular rate/rhythm	75 beats/min, regular
Atrial rate/rhythm	None
PR interval	None
QRS duration	0.08 sec
Identification	Accelerated junctional rhythm at 75 beats/min; ST-segment depression

Answer for Figure 5-15

Ventricular rate/rhythm	30 beats/min (junctional beats) to 56 beats/min (sinus beats), irregular
Atrial rate/rhythm	None (junctional beats) to 56 beats/min (sinus beats)
PR interval	None (junctional beats) to 0.18 sec (sinus beats)
QRS duration	0.04 sec (junctional beats) to 0.08 sec (sinus beats)
Identification	Junctional bradycardia at 30 beats/min to sinus bradycardia at 56 beats/min

Answer for Figure 5-16

Ventricular rate/rhythm	65 to 103 beats/min, irregular
Atrial rate/rhythm	Unable to determine
PR interval	Unable to determine
QRS duration	0.06 to 0.08 sec
Identification	Atrial fibrillation at 65 to 103 beats/min

Answer for Figure 5-17

Ventricular rate/rhythm	75 beats/min, regular
Atrial rate/rhythm	None
PR interval	None
QRS duration	0.06 sec
Identification	Accelerated junctional rhythm at 75 beats/min

Answer for Figure 5-18

Ventricular rate/rhythm	64 beats/min (sinus beats), regular except for the event
Atrial rate/rhythm	64 beats/min (sinus beats), regular except for the event
PR interval	0.16 to 0.18 sec
QRS duration	0.08 sec
Identification	Sinus rhythm at 64 beats/min with an episode of sinus arrest and a junctional escape beat

Answer for Figure 5-19

Ventricular rate/rhythm	75 beats/min, regular
Atrial rate/rhythm	75 beats/min, regular
PR interval	0.16 sec
QRS duration	0.08 sec
Identification	Accelerated junctional rhythm at 75 beats/min

Answer for Figure 5-20

Ventricular rate/rhythm	75 beats/min/regular
Atrial rate/rhythm	75 beats/min, regular
PR interval	0.12 sec
QRS duration	0.08 sec
Identification	Sinus rhythm at 75 beats/min

Answer for Figure 5-21

Ventricular rate/rhythm	45 beats/min, regular
Atrial rate/rhythm	None
PR interval	None
QRS duration	0.08 sec
Identification	Junctional rhythm at 45 beats/min; ST-segment elevation

Answer for Figure 5-22

Ventricular rate/rhythm	58 to 79 beats/min, irregular
Atrial rate/rhythm	Unable to determine
PR interval	Unable to determine
QRS duration	Unable to determine
Identification	Atrial flutter at 58 to 79 beats/min

Answer for Figure 5-23

Ventricular rate/rhythm	79 beats/min, regular (junctional beats)
Atrial rate/rhythm	Not measurable in junctional beats
PR interval	Not measurable in junctional beats
QRS duration	0.06 sec
Identification	Sinus rhythm changing to an accelerated junctional rhythm at 79 beats/min, back to a sinus rhythm

Answer for Figure 5-24

Ventricular rate/rhythm	70 beats/min, regular except for the event
Atrial rate/rhythm	70 beats/min, regular except for the event
PR interval	0.16 sec
QRS duration	0.08 sec
Identification	Sinus rhythm at 70 beats/min with a nonconducted PAC (note distortion of the T wave of the beat preceding the pause) and a junctional escape beat

Answer for Figure 5-25

Ventricular rate/rhythm	44 beats/min, regular
Atrial rate/rhythm	44 beats/min, regular
PR interval	0.14 sec
QRS duration	0.08 sec
Identification	Junctional rhythm at 44 beats/min; ST-segment elevation

Ventricular Rhythms

OBJECTIVES

On completion of this chapter, you will be able to:

1. Describe the ECG characteristics, possible causes, signs and symptoms, and initial emergency care for premature ventricular complexes (PVCs).
2. Explain the terms bigeminy, trigeminy, quadrigeminy, and "run" when used to describe premature complexes.
3. Explain the difference between premature ventricular complexes and ventricular escape beats.
4. Describe the ECG characteristics of ventricular escape beats.
5. Describe the ECG characteristics, possible causes, signs and symptoms, and initial emergency care for a ventricular escape (idioventricular) rhythm (IVR).
6. Explain the term pulseless electrical activity.
7. Describe the ECG characteristics, possible causes, signs and symptoms, and initial emergency care for an accelerated idioventricular rhythm (AIVR).
8. Explain the terms sustained and nonsustained ventricular tachycardia and monomorphic and polymorphic ventricular tachycardia.
9. Describe the ECG characteristics, possible causes, signs and symptoms, and initial emergency care for monomorphic ventricular tachycardia (VT).
10. Describe the ECG characteristics, possible causes, signs and symptoms, and initial emergency care for polymorphic VT.
11. Describe the ECG characteristics, possible causes, signs and symptoms, and initial emergency care for torsades de pointes (TdP).
12. Discuss long QT syndrome (LQTS).
13. Describe the ECG characteristics, possible causes, signs and symptoms, and initial emergency care for ventricular fibrillation (VF).
14. State the purpose, indications, and procedure for defibrillation.
15. Describe the ECG characteristics, possible causes, signs and symptoms, and initial emergency care for asystole.
16. Explain the term P wave asystole.

INTRODUCTION

The ventricles are the heart's least efficient pacemaker. If the ventricles function as the heart's pacemaker, they normally generate impulses at a rate of 20 to 40 beats/min. The ventricles may assume responsibility for pacing the heart if:

- The SA node fails to discharge
- An impulse from the SA node is generated but blocked as it exits the SA node
- The rate of discharge of the SA node is slower than that of the ventricles
- An irritable site in either ventricle produces an early beat or rapid rhythm

The shape of the QRS complex is influenced by the site of origin of the electrical impulse. Normally an electrical impulse that begins in the SA node, atria, or AV junction results in depolarization of the right and left ventricles at about the same time. The resulting QRS complex is usually narrow, measuring less than 0.10 second in duration.

If an area of either ventricle becomes ischemic or injured, it can become irritable. This irritability affects the manner in which impulses are conducted. Ventricular beats and rhythms can start in any part of the ventricles and may occur because of reentry, enhanced automaticity, or triggered activity. When an ectopic site within a ventricle assumes responsibility for pacing the heart, the electrical impulse bypasses the normal intraventricular conduction pathway. This results in stimulation of the ventricles at slightly different times. As a result, ventricular beats and rhythms usually have QRS complexes that are abnormally shaped and longer than normal (greater than 0.12 sec). If the atria are depolarized after the ventricles, retrograde P waves may be seen.

Because ventricular depolarization is abnormal, ventricular repolarization is also abnormal. This results in changes in ST-segments and T waves. T waves are usually in a direction opposite that of the QRS complex. In other words, if the major QRS deflection is negative, the ST-segment is usually elevated and the T wave positive (upright). If the major QRS deflection is positive, the ST-segment is usually depressed and the T wave is usually negative (inverted). P waves are usually not seen with ventricular dysrhythmias but if they are visible, they have no consistent relationship to the QRS complex (AV dissociation).

PREMATURE VENTRICULAR COMPLEXES (PVCs)

How Do I Recognize It?

[OBJECTIVE 1]

A premature ventricular complex (PVC) arises from an irritable site within either ventricle. PVCs are also called premature ventricular extrasystoles or ventricular premature beats. PVCs may be caused by enhanced automaticity or reentry. By definition, a PVC is *premature*, occurring earlier than the next expected sinus beat. The QRS of a PVC is typically equal to or greater than 0.12 second because the PVC causes the ventricles to fire prematurely and in an abnormal manner (Figure 6-1). The T wave is usually in the opposite direction of the QRS complex. A full **compensatory pause** often follows a PVC (Figure 6-2). This occurs because the SA node is not affected by the PVC. It discharges at its regular rate and rhythm, including the period during and after the PVC.

ECG Pearl

To determine whether or not the pause following a premature complex is compensatory or noncompensatory, measure the distance between three normal beats. Compare the distance between three beats, one of which includes the premature complex. The pause is compensatory (also called full or complete) if the normal beat following the premature complex occurs when expected (i.e., when the distance is the same).

ECG Pearl

"A full compensatory pause does not reliably differentiate ventricular ectopy from atrial ectopy because atrial ectopy may produce a similar compensatory pattern if it does not reset the SA node. In addition, when PVCs are retrogradely conducted to the atria, as in slow sinus rates, they can reset the SA node and a full compensatory pause may not be present."[1]

A **fusion beat** (Figure 6-3) is a result of an electrical impulse from a supraventricular site (such as the SA node) discharging at the same time as an ectopic site in the ventricles. Because fusion beats are a result of both supraventricular and ventricular depolarization, these beats do not resemble normally conducted beats, nor do they resemble true ventricular beats.

PVCs: Patterns

PVCs may occur in patterns:
- Pairs (couplets): Two sequential PVCs
- "Runs" or "bursts": Three or more PVCs in a row
  - Three or more PVCs in a row at a rate of more than 100 beats/min is a run of ventricular tachycardia.
- Bigeminal PVCs (ventricular bigeminy): Every other beat is a PVC
- Trigeminal PVCs (ventricular trigeminy): Every third beat is a PVC
- Quadrigeminal PVCs (ventricular quadrigeminy): Every fourth beat is a PVC.

Types of PVCs
Uniform and Multiformed PVCs
[OBJECTIVE 2]

Premature ventricular beats that look alike in the same lead and begin from the same anatomic site (focus) are called **uniform** PVCs (Figure 6-4). PVCs that look different

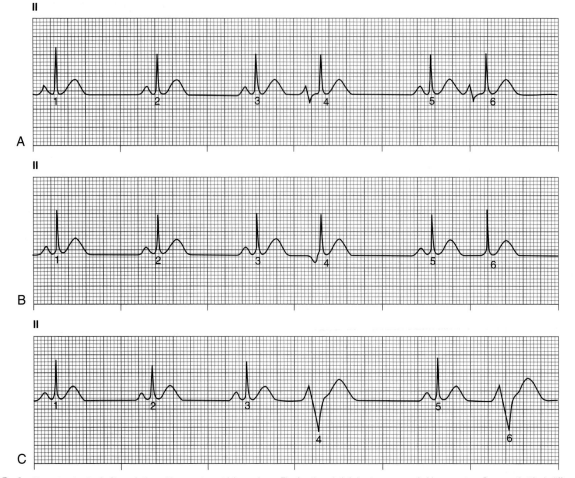

Figure 6-1   Premature beats. **A,** Sinus rhythm with premature atrial complexes. The fourth and sixth beats are preceded by premature P waves that look different from the normally conducted sinus beats. Note that the QRS complex that follows each of these PACs is narrow and identical in appearance to that of the sinus-conducted beats. **B,** Sinus rhythm with premature junctional complexes. The fourth and sixth beats are PJCs. Beat No. 4 is preceded by an inverted P wave with a short PR interval. There is no identifiable atrial activity associated with beat No. 6. **C,** Sinus rhythm with premature ventricular complexes. The fourth and sixth beats are very different in appearance from the normally conducted sinus beats. Beats 4 and 6 are PVCs. They are not preceded by P waves.

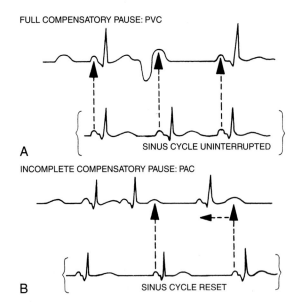

Figure 6-2   A premature ventricular complex (PVC) is often followed by a full compensatory pause. A premature atrial complex (PAC) is often followed by a non-compensatory (incomplete) pause.

from one another in the same lead are called **multiform** PVCs (Figure 6-5). The terms unifocal and multifocal are sometimes used to describe PVCs that are similar or different in appearance. Uniform PVCs are unifocal, but multiform PVCs are not necessarily multifocal.[2] A PVC is not an entire rhythm—it is a single beat. Therefore it is important to identify the underlying rhythm and the ectopic beat(s) (i.e., "sinus tachycardia at 138 beats/min with frequent PVCs").

ECG Pearl

Multiform PVCs often, but do not always, arise from different anatomic sites.

Interpolated PVCs

A PVC may occur without interfering with the normal cardiac cycle. An **interpolated** PVC does not have a full compensatory pause (Figure 6-6). It is "squeezed" between two regular complexes and does not disturb the underlying rhythm. The

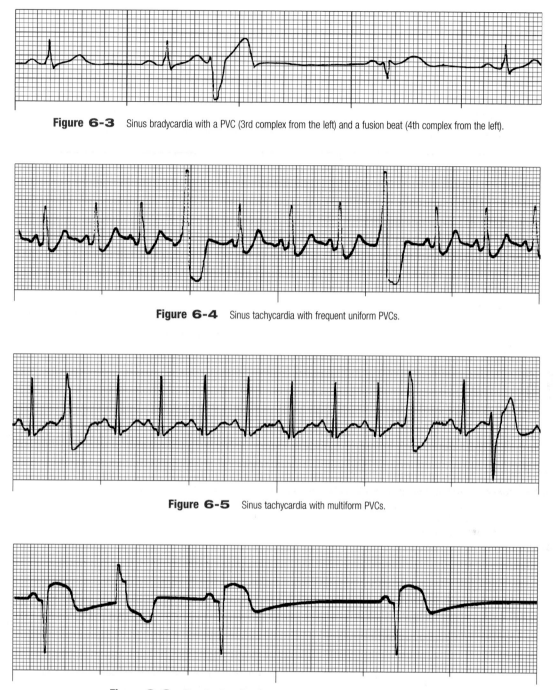

Figure 6-3   Sinus bradycardia with a PVC (3rd complex from the left) and a fusion beat (4th complex from the left).

Figure 6-4   Sinus tachycardia with frequent uniform PVCs.

Figure 6-5   Sinus tachycardia with multiform PVCs.

Figure 6-6   Sinus bradycardia with an interpolated PVC and ST-segment elevation.

PR interval of the cardiac cycle following the PVC may be longer than normal. If an interpolated PVC produces a palpable pulse, frequent interpolated PVCs may cause signs and symptoms because of an increased heart rate.

R-on-T PVCs

R-on-T PVCs occur when the R wave of a PVC falls on the T wave of the preceding beat (Figure 6-7). Because the T wave is vulnerable (relative refractory period) to any electrical stimulation, it is possible that a PVC occurring during this period of the cardiac cycle will precipitate VT or VF; however, VT and VF most commonly occur without a preceding R-on-T PVC, and most R-on-T PVCs do not precipitate a sustained ventricular tachydysrhythmia.[2]

Paired PVCs (Couplets)

Two PVCs in a row are called a **couplet** or **paired PVC** (Figure 6-8). Couplets are also referred to as *two in a row* or *back-to-back* PVCs. The appearance of couplets indicates the ventricular ectopic site is very irritable. Three or more PVCs in a row at a rate of more than 100 beats/min is considered a "salvo," "run," or "burst" of ventricular tachycardia. The general characteristics of PVCs are shown in Table 6-1.

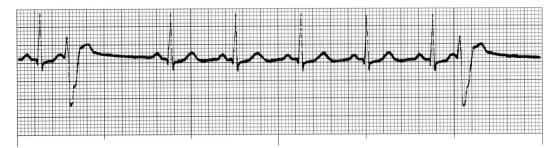

Figure 6-7   Sinus rhythm with two R-on-T PVCs.

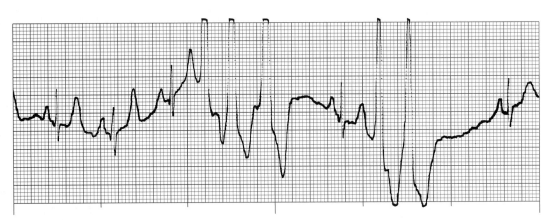

Figure 6-8   Sinus rhythm with a run of VT and one episode of couplets.

TABLE 6-1	Characteristics of Premature Ventricular Complexes (PVCs)
Rate	Usually within normal range, but depends on underlying rhythm
Rhythm	Essentially regular with *premature* beats; if the PVC is an interpolated PVC, the rhythm will be regular
P waves	Usually absent or, with retrograde conduction to the atria, may appear after the QRS (usually upright in the ST-segment or T wave)
PR interval	None with the PVC because the ectopic originates in the ventricles
QRS duration	Usually 0.12 sec or greater, wide and bizarre; T wave usually in opposite direction of the QRS complex

Box 6-1	Common Causes of PVCs

Normal variant
Hypoxia
Stress, anxiety
Exercise
Digitalis toxicity
Acid-base imbalance
Myocardial ischemia
Electrolyte imbalance
Congestive heart failure
Increased sympathetic tone
Acute coronary syndromes
Stimulants (caffeine, tobacco)
Medications (sympathomimetics, tricyclic antidepressants, phenothiazines)

What Causes It?

PVCs are the most common dysrhythmia in healthy individuals and in those with organic heart disease. PVCs can occur in healthy persons with apparently normal hearts and for no apparent cause. The frequency with which PVCs occur increases with age. PVCs can occur at rest or may be associated with exercise. Common causes of PVCs are shown in Box 6-1.

What Do I Do About It?

Patients often describe premature beats as "flip-flops." PVCs may or may not produce palpable pulses. Patients experiencing PVCs may be asymptomatic or complain of palpitations, a "racing heart," skipped beats, or chest or neck discomfort. These symptoms may be caused by the greater than normal contractile force of the postectopic beats or the feeling that the heart has stopped during the long pause after the premature complexes.[3] If the PVCs are frequent, signs of decreased cardiac output may be present.

Routine use of medications to treat PVCs is no longer recommended. Treatment of PVCs depends on the cause, patient's signs and symptoms, and on the clinical situation. Most patients experiencing PVCs do not require treatment with antiarrhythmic medications. Treatment of PVCs focuses on treatment of the underlying cause. In the setting of an acute coronary syndrome, treatment is directed at:

- Ensuring adequate oxygenation
- Relieving pain
- Rapidly identifying and correcting hypoxia, heart failure, and electrolyte or acid-base abnormalities

VENTRICULAR ESCAPE BEATS/ RHYTHM

How Do I Recognize It?

[OBJECTIVES 3,4,5]

Remember that premature beats are *early* and escape beats are *late*. In order to determine if a complex is early or late, we need to see at least two sinus beats in a row to establish the regularity of the underlying rhythm. Although ventricular escape beats share some of the same physical characteristics as PVCs (wide QRS complexes, T waves deflected in a direction opposite the QRS), they differ in some very important areas.

A PVC appears *early*, before the next expected sinus beat. PVCs often reflect irritability in some area of the ventricles. When PVCs cause *serious* symptoms, medications are sometimes used to reduce the frequency with which they occur or eliminate them completely.

A **ventricular escape beat** occurs after a pause in which a supraventricular pacemaker failed to fire. Thus the escape beat is *late*, appearing after the next expected sinus beat. A ventricular escape beat is a *protective* mechanism. It protects the heart from more extreme slowing or even asystole. Because it is protective, you would not want to administer any medication that would "wipe out" the escape beat.

Take a look at Figure 6-9. When looking at this rhythm strip, one of the first things you notice is the beat with wide QRS complex. Although it looks interesting, let us first examine the rhythm systemically. The rhythm is essentially regular except for the single wide-QRS beat. There are upright P waves before beats 1, 2, 3, 5, and 6. When you calculate the atrial and ventricular rate, you find that the rate is 63 beats/min. Now we know that the underlying rhythm is a sinus rhythm at 63 beats/min. Next, let us examine the wide-QRS beat more closely and see what happened here. Look to the left of the wide-QRS beat and see if anything looks amiss. When you look closely at the T wave of beat 3, it has an extra "hump." If you take a moment to plot P waves across the strip, you will find that this extra hump is actually an early P wave that was not conducted. This is a nonconducted PAC. When plotting the P waves, you should have noticed that the wide-QRS beat occurred *late*—after the next expected sinus beat. This is an escape beat. Because the QRS associated with it is *wide*, it is a *ventricular* escape beat. (A *junctional* escape beat is also late, but it usually has a *narrow* QRS). Notice that the T wave of this beat is deflected in a direction opposite its QRS complex. When you look at the PR intervals and ST-segment, you will find that the PR interval is longer than normal (about 0.24 sec). For now, we will simply say that it is prolonged. We will explore the reasons for this and give it a name in the next chapter. ST-segment depression is also present. Our identification of this rhythm would include a description like, "Sinus rhythm at 63 beats/min with a prolonged PR interval, nonconducted PAC, ventricular escape beat, and ST-segment depression." My goodness!! That was one complicated rhythm strip! The ECG characteristics of ventricular escape beats are shown in Table 6-2.

A ventricular escape or **idioventricular rhythm (IVR)** exists when three or more ventricular escape beats occur in a row at a rate of 20 to 40 beats/min. This rate is the intrinsic

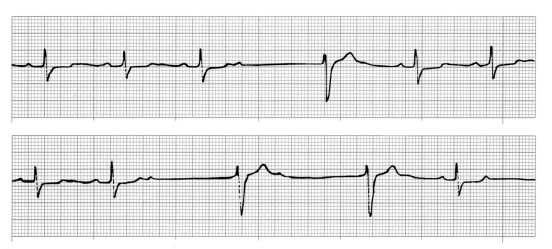

Figure 6-9   Sinus rhythm with a prolonged PR interval, ST-segment depression. Note the ventricular escape beats following nonconducted premature atrial complexes.

TABLE 6-2	Characteristics of Ventricular Escape Beats
Rate	Usually within normal range, but depends on underlying rhythm
Rhythm	Essentially regular with *late* beats; the ventricular escape beat occurs *after* the next expected sinus beat
P waves	Usually absent or, with retrograde conduction to the atria, may appear after the QRS (usually upright in the ST-segment or T wave)
PR interval	None with the ventricular escape beat because the ectopic beat originates in the ventricles
QRS duration	0.12 sec or greater, wide and bizarre, T wave frequently in opposite direction of the QRS complex

TABLE 6-3	Characteristics of Idioventricular Rhythm (IVR)
Rate	Ventricular rate 20-40 beats/min
Rhythm	Ventricular rhythm is essentially regular
P waves	Usually absent or, with retrograde conduction to the atria, may appear after the QRS (usually upright in the ST-segment or T wave)
PR interval	None
QRS duration	0.12 sec or greater, T wave frequently in opposite direction of the QRS complex

firing rate of the ventricles. The QRS complexes seen in IVR are wide and bizarre because the impulses begin in the ventricles, bypassing the normal conduction pathway. When the ventricular rate slows to a rate of less than 20 beats/min, some refer to the rhythm as an *agonal rhythm* or "dying heart." An example of IVR is shown in Figure 6-10. The characteristics of this rhythm are described in Table 6-3.

What Causes It?

IVR may occur when:
- The SA node and the AV junction fail to initiate an electrical impulse
- The rate of discharge of the SA node or AV junction becomes less than the intrinsic rate of the ventricles
- Impulses generated by a supraventricular pacemaker site are blocked

IVR may also occur because of myocardial infarction, digitalis toxicity, or metabolic imbalances.

What Do I Do About It?

[OBJECTIVE 6]
Because the ventricular rate associated with IVR is slow (20 to 40 beats/min) with a loss of atrial kick, the patient may experience serious signs and symptoms because of decreased cardiac output. If the patient has a pulse and is

symptomatic because of the slow rate, transcutaneous pacing may be attempted. Medications such as lidocaine should be avoided in the management of this rhythm because lidocaine may abolish ventricular activity, possibly causing asystole in a patient with IVR. If the patient is not breathing and has no pulse despite the appearance of organized electrical activity on the cardiac monitor, a clinical situation called **pulseless electrical activity** (PEA) exists. Management of PEA should include CPR, giving oxygen, possible placement of an advanced airway, starting an IV, and an aggressive search for the underlying cause of the situation.

ACCELERATED IDIOVENTRICULAR RHYTHM (AIVR)

How Do I Recognize It?

[OBJECTIVE 7]
An **accelerated idioventricular rhythm (AIVR)** exists when three or more ventricular beats occur in a row at a rate of 41 to 100 beats/min (Figure 6-11). Some cardiologists consider the ventricular rate range of AIVR to be 41 to 120 beats/min.

AIVR is usually considered a benign escape rhythm that appears when the sinus rate slows and disappears when the sinus rate speeds up. Episodes of AIVR usually last a few seconds to a minute. Because AIVR usually begins and ends gradually, it is also called *nonparoxysmal VT.* Fusion beats are often seen at the onset and end of the rhythm. The ECG characteristics of AIVR are shown in Table 6-4.

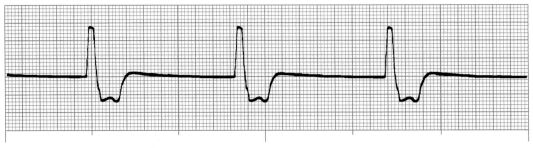

Figure 6-10   Idioventricular rhythm (IVR) at 35 beats/min.

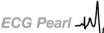

ECG Pearl

The memory aids "PATCH-4-MD" and "The 5 Hs and 5 Ts" may be used to recall possible treatable causes of cardiac emergencies.

PATCH-4-MD
Pulmonary embolism
Acidosis
Tension pneumothorax
Cardiac tamponade
Hypovolemia
Hypoxia
Heat/cold (hypothermia/hyperthermia)
Hypokalemia/hyperkalemia (and other electrolytes)
Myocardial infarction
Drug overdose/accidents

Five Hs and Five Ts	
Hypovolemia	Tamponade, cardiac
Hypoxia	Tension pneumothorax
Hypothermia	Thrombosis: lungs (massive pulmonary embolism)
Hypokalemia/Hyperkalemia	Thrombosis: heart (acute coronary syndromes)
Hydrogen ion (acidosis)	Tablets/toxins: drug overdose

What Causes It?

AIVR is usually considered a benign escape rhythm. It is often seen during the first 12 hours of myocardial infarction. It is particularly common after successful reperfusion therapy. AIVR has been observed in patients with:

- Digitalis toxicity
- Cocaine toxicity
- Subarachnoid hemorrhage
- Acute myocarditis
- Hypertensive heart disease
- Dilated cardiomyopathy

What Do I Do About It?

AIVR generally requires no treatment because the rhythm is protective and often transient, spontaneously resolving on its own. However possible dizziness, lightheadedness, or other signs of hemodynamic compromise may occur because of the loss of atrial kick. Atropine may be ordered in an attempt to block the vagus nerve and stimulate the SA node to over-drive the ventricular rhythm. *Atrial* (not ventricular) pacing may be attempted to suppress AIVR.

ECG Pearl

Electrical shocks are delivered to the heart of a patient in ventricular fibrillation (VF) or pulseless ventricular tachycardia (VT). What should you do if a shock terminates VF or pulseless VT and AIVR is now present on the monitor? A quick assessment reveals the patient has a pulse and is breathing on his own about 4 to 6 times per minute. As you direct a co-worker to assist the patient's respirations, the patient's pulse and blood pressure are assessed. The patient's BP is 94/53. The monitor shows AIVR at a rate of 100 beats/min. Should anything be done about the patient's rhythm?

Confusion about what treatment should be instituted is common because the patient was previously pulseless and now has a pulse, although the rhythm on the monitor is ventricular in origin. AIVR can be mistaken for VT if the ventricular rate is not counted and the patient assessed. Keep in mind that most patients do not develop serious signs and symptoms related to a tachycardia until the rate exceeds 150 beats/min. Although medications are often used to suppress VT that causes serious signs and symptoms, they are not generally used to suppress AIVR. In our patient scenario, a patient who was pulseless now has a pulse and is attempting to breathe on his own. These are positive signs. In a case such as this, "watchful waiting" is a reasonable course of action. Remember, AIVR is usually a transient rhythm. Close monitoring of the patient's vital signs and cardiac rhythm is essential.

TABLE 6-4	Characteristics of Accelerated Idioventricular Rhythm (AIVR)
Rate	Ventricular rate 41-100 beats/min (some experts consider the ventricular rate range to be 41-120 beats/min)
Rhythm	Ventricular rhythm is essentially regular
P waves	Usually absent or, with retrograde conduction to the atria, may appear after the QRS (usually upright in the ST-segment or T wave)
PR interval	None
QRS duration	Greater than 0.12 sec, T wave frequently in opposite direction of the QRS complex

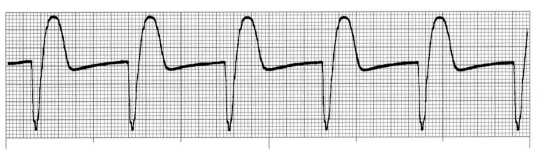

Figure 6-11 Accelerated idioventricular rhythm (AIVR) at 56 beats/min.

VENTRICULAR TACHYCARDIA (VT)

How Do I Recognize It?

[OBJECTIVES 8, 9, 10]

Ventricular tachycardia (VT) exists when three or more PVCs occur in a row at a rate greater than 100 beats/min. If VT occurs as a short run lasting less than 30 seconds, it is called *nonsustained VT* (Figure 6-12). When VT persists for more than 30 seconds it is called *sustained VT* (Figure 6-13).

Monomorphic VT

VT, like PVCs, may originate from an ectopic focus in either ventricle. When the QRS complexes of VT are of the same shape and amplitude, the rhythm is called **monomorphic VT** (Figure 6-14). Monomorphic VT with a ventricular rate greater than 200 beats/min is called ventricular flutter by some cardiologists. The ECG characteristics of monomorphic VT are shown in Table 6-5.

Polymorphic VT

[OBJECTIVES 11, 12]

When the QRS complexes of VT vary in shape and amplitude from beat to beat, the rhythm is called **polymorphic VT** (Figure 6-15). In polymorphic VT, the QRS complexes appear to twist from upright to negative or negative to upright and back.

Polymorphic VT is divided into two classifications based on its association with a normal or prolonged QT interval:

1. Normal QT
2. Long QT syndrome (LQTS)
   a. Acquired (iatrogenic)
   b. Congenital (idiopathic)

Polymorphic VT that occurs in the presence of a long QT interval is called **torsades de pointes (TdP)**. *Torsades de pointes* is French for "twisting of the points," which describes the QRS that changes in shape, amplitude, and width and appears to "twist" around the isoelectric line, resembling a spindle. Polymorphic VT that occurs in the presence

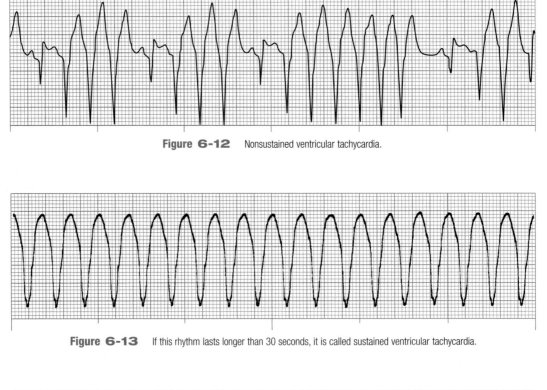

Figure 6-12   Nonsustained ventricular tachycardia.

Figure 6-13   If this rhythm lasts longer than 30 seconds, it is called sustained ventricular tachycardia.

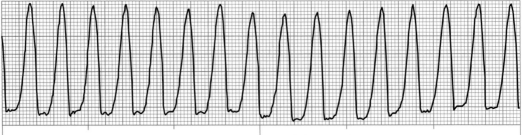
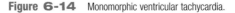

Figure 6-14   Monomorphic ventricular tachycardia.

TABLE 6-5	Characteristics of Monomorphic Ventricular Tachycardia
Rate	Ventricular rate 101-250 beats/min (some experts consider the rate 121-250 beats/min)
Rhythm	Ventricular rhythm is essentially regular
P waves	May be present or absent; if present, they have no set relationship to the QRS complexes appearing between the QRS's at a rate different from that of the VT
PR interval	None
QRS duration	0.12 sec or greater; often difficult to differentiate between the QRS and T wave

TABLE 6-6	Characteristics of Polymorphic Ventricular Tachycardia
Rate	Ventricular rate 150-300 beats/min, typically 200-250 beats/min
Rhythm	Ventricular rhythm may be regular or irregular
P waves	None
PR interval	None
QRS duration	0.12 sec or greater; gradual alteration in amplitude and direction of the QRS complexes; a typical cycle consists of 5-20 QRS complexes

of a normal QT interval is simply referred to as *polymorphic VT*. The ECG characteristics of polymorphic VT are shown in Table 6-6.

Long QT syndrome (LQTS) is an abnormality of the heart's electrical system. The mechanical function of the heart is entirely normal. The electrical problem is caused by defects in sodium and potassium channels that affect repolarization. These electrical defects prolong the QT interval, predisposing affected persons to TdP.

LQTS may be acquired or inherited. The acquired form of LQTS is more common and usually caused by medications that prolong the QT interval. Inherited LQTS is caused by mutations of genes that encode the sodium and potassium channels.

- Symptoms most commonly begin in preteen to teenage years, but may present from a few days of age to middle age.
- About one third of individuals who have LQTS never exhibit symptoms. A lack of symptoms does not exclude an individual or family from having LQTS.
- The usual symptoms of LQTS include syncope or sudden death. These events usually occur during

physical activity or emotional stress, but they can also occur during sleep. The syncopal episodes are often misdiagnosed as the common faint (vasovagal event) or a seizure. Actual seizures are uncommon in LQTS, but epilepsy is one of the common errors in diagnosis.

Cases in which LQTS should be considered include:
- Recurrent syncope during physical exertion or emotional stress
- Sudden and unexplained loss of consciousness during childhood and teenage years
- Family history of unexplained syncope
- Family history of sudden, unexpected death
- Any young person who has an unexplained cardiac arrest
- Epilepsy in children

Common triggers of LQTS include swimming, running, being startled (an alarm clock, a loud horn, a ringing phone), anger, crying, test taking, and other stressful situations. The diagnosis of LQTS is commonly suspected or made from the ECG. Children and young adults should have an ECG as part of their evaluation for an unexplained loss of consciousness episode. Beta-blockers, potassium supplements, pacemakers, and implantable defibrillators have been used for treatment of LQTS.

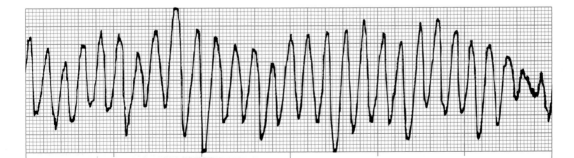

Figure 6-15 Polymorphic ventricular tachycardia. This rhythm strip is from a 77-year-old man 3 days post myocardial infarction (MI). His chief complaint at the onset of this episode was chest pain. He had a past medical history of a previous MI and an abdominal aortic aneurysm repair. The patient was given lidocaine and defibrillated several times without success. Lab work revealed a serum potassium (K+) level of 2.0. IV K+ was administered and the patient converted to a sinus rhythm with the next defibrillation.

What Causes It?

Sustained monomorphic VT is often associated with underlying heart disease, particularly myocardial ischemia. It rarely occurs in patients without underlying heart disease. Common causes of VT include:

- Acute coronary syndromes
- Cardiomyopathy
- Tricyclic antidepressant overdose
- Digitalis toxicity
- Valvular heart disease
- Cocaine abuse
- Mitral valve prolapse
- Acid-base imbalance
- Trauma (e.g., myocardial contusion, invasive cardiac procedures)
- Electrolyte imbalance (e.g., hypokalemia, hyperkalemia, hypomagnesemia)

What Do I Do About It?

Signs and symptoms associated with VT vary. VT may occur with or without pulses. Sustained VT does not always produce signs of hemodynamic instability. In fact, the patient who has sustained monomorphic VT may be stable for long periods. However, when the ventricular rate is very fast, or when myocardial ischemia is present, monomorphic VT can degenerate to polymorphic VT or ventricular fibrillation.

Syncope or near-syncope may occur because of an abrupt onset of VT. The patient's only warning symptom may be a brief period of lightheadedness. During VT, the severity of the patient's symptoms depend on how rapid the ventricular rate is, how long the tachycardia has been present, and the presence and extent of underlying heart disease. Signs and symptoms of hemodynamic instability related to VT may include the following:

- Altered mental status
- Shock
- Chest pain
- Hypotension
- Shortness of breath
- Pulmonary congestion

Treatment is based on the patient's signs and symptoms and the type of VT. If the rhythm is monomorphic VT (and the patient's symptoms are due to the tachycardia):

- Stable but symptomatic patients are treated with oxygen, IV access, and ventricular antiarrhythmics (such as amiodarone) to suppress the rhythm
- Unstable patients (usually a sustained heart rate of 150 beats/min or more) are treated with oxygen, IV access, and sedation (if awake and time permits) followed by synchronized cardioversion. CPR and defibrillation are used to treat the pulseless patient in VT. In all cases, an aggressive search must be made for the cause of the VT.

If the rhythm is polymorphic VT, it is important to determine if the patient's QT interval just before the tachycardia is normal or prolonged. If the QT interval is normal and the patient is symptomatic due to the tachycardia, treat ischemia if present, correct electrolyte abnormalities, and proceed with electrical therapy or antiarrhythmic medications if necessary. If the QT interval is prolonged and the patient is symptomatic due to the tachycardia, discontinue any medications the patient may be taking that prolong the QT interval, correct electrolyte abnormalities, and proceed with electrical therapy or antiarrhythmic medications if necessary.

ECG Pearl

A supraventricular tachycardia with an intraventricular conduction delay may be difficult to distinguish from VT. Keep in mind that VT is considered a potentially life-threatening dysrhythmia. If you are unsure whether a regular, wide-QRS tachycardia is VT or SVT with an intraventricular conduction delay, treat the rhythm as VT until proven otherwise. Obtaining a 12-lead ECG may help differentiate VT from SVT, but do not delay treatment if the patient is symptomatic.

VENTRICULAR FIBRILLATION (VF)

How Do I Recognize It?

[OBJECTIVE 13]

Ventricular fibrillation (VF) is a chaotic rhythm that begins in the ventricles. In VF, there is no organized depolarization of the ventricles. The ventricular muscle quivers. As a result, there is no effective myocardial contraction and no pulse. The resulting rhythm looks chaotic with deflections that vary in shape and amplitude. No normal-looking waveforms are visible. VF with waves that are 3 or more millimeters high is called "coarse" VF (Figure 6-16). VF with low amplitude waves (less than 3 mm) is called "fine" VF (Figure 6-17). Table 6-7 lists the ECG characteristics of VF. Figure 6-18 illustrates a comparison of ventricular dysrhythmias.

ECG Pearl

Because artifact can mimic VF, *always* check the patient's pulse before beginning treatment.

What Causes It?

Factors that increase the susceptibility of the myocardium to fibrillate include the following:

- Increased sympathetic nervous system activity
- Vagal stimulation
- Electrolyte imbalance
- Antiarrhythmics and other medications
- Environmental factors (e.g., electrocution)
- Hypertrophy
- Acute coronary syndromes
- Heart failure
- Arrhythmias

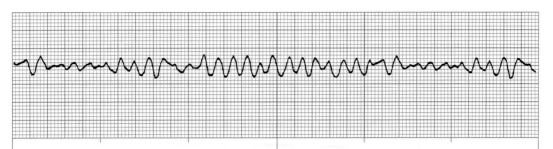

Figure 6-16 Coarse ventricular fibrillation.

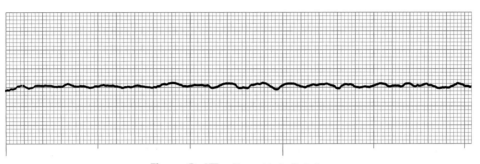

Figure 6-17 Fine ventricular fibrillation.

What Do I Do About It?

The patient in VF is unresponsive, apneic, and pulseless. Since no drugs used in cardiac arrest have been shown to improve survival to hospital discharge, the priorities of care in cardiac arrest due to pulseless VT or VF are CPR and defibrillation. When a cardiac arrest is witnessed and the patient's heart rhythm is VF, the patient's survival rate decreases 7% to 10% for every minute that passes between collapse and defibrillation if no CPR is provided.[4] The decrease in survival rates is less rapid (averaging 3% to 4% per minute from collapse to defibrillation) when bystander CPR is provided.[5] CPR and defibrillation may be followed by medications per current resuscitation guidelines.

TABLE 6-7	Characteristics of Ventricular Fibrillation (VF)
Rate	Cannot be determined because there are no discernible waves or complexes to measure
Rhythm	Rapid and chaotic with no pattern or regularity
P waves	Not discernible
PR interval	Not discernible
QRS duration	Not discernible

ECG Pearl

Cardiac Arrest Rhythms
- Ventricular tachycardia
- Ventricular fibrillation
- Asystole
- Pulseless electrical activity

VT and VF are "shockable" rhythms. This means that delivering a shock to the heart by means of a defibrillator may result in termination of the rhythm. Asystole and PEA are nonshockable rhythms.

Defibrillation

[OBJECTIVE 14]

Defibrillation is indicated in the treatment of pulseless VT and ventricular fibrillation. Defibrillation is the therapeutic delivery of an unsynchronized electrical current (the delivery of energy has no relationship to the cardiac cycle) through the myocardium over a very brief period to terminate a cardiac dysrhythmia. The shock attempts to deliver a uniform electrical current of sufficient intensity to simultaneously depolarize ventricular cells, including fibrillating cells, causing momentary asystole. This provides an opportunity for the heart's natural pacemakers to resume normal activity. The pacemaker with the highest degree of automaticity should then assume responsibility for pacing the heart. The steps for performing defibrillation are shown in Skill 6-1.

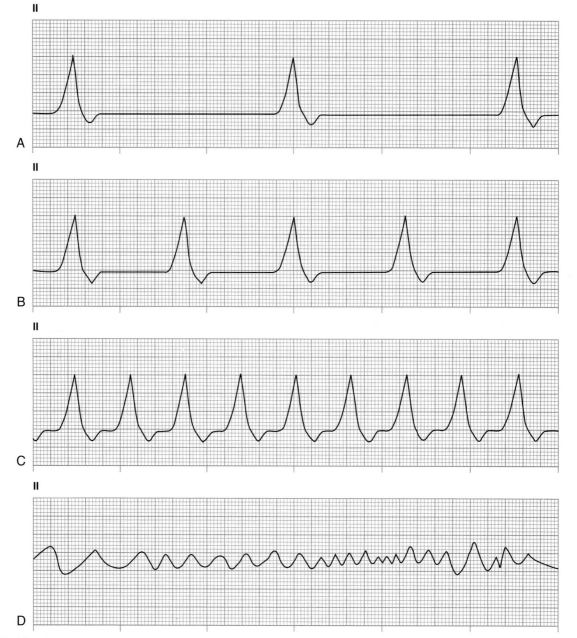

Figure 6-18   Comparison of ventricular arrhythmias. **A,** Idioventricular rhythm at 38 beats/min. **B,** Accelerated idioventricular rhythm at 75 beats/min. **C,** Monomorphic ventricular tachycardia at 150 beats/min. **D,** Coarse ventricular fibrillation.

ASYSTOLE (CARDIAC STANDSTILL)

How Do I Recognize It?

[OBJECTIVES 15, 16]

Asystole is a total absence of ventricular electrical activity (Figure 6-19). There is no ventricular rate or rhythm, no pulse, and no cardiac output. Some atrial electrical activity may be evident. If atrial electrical activity is present, the rhythm is called "P wave" asystole or ventricular standstill

(Figure 6-20). The ECG characteristics of asystole are shown in Table 6-8.

What Causes It?

The causes of asystole are the same as those for pulseless electrical activity. In addition, ventricular asystole may occur temporarily following termination of a tachycardia with medications, defibrillation, or synchronized cardioversion (Figure 6-21).

SKILL 6-1 Defibrillation

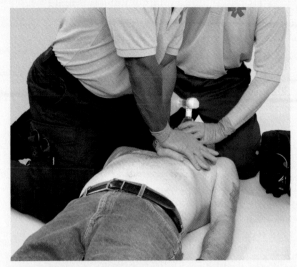

Step 1 Take appropriate standard precautions and verify that the procedure is indicated. Identify the rhythm on the cardiac monitor.

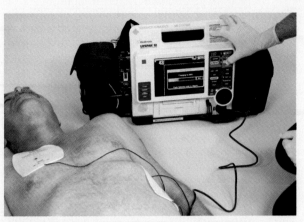

Step 3 Charge the defibrillator. Because oxygen flow over the patient's chest during electrical therapy increases the risk of spark/fire, make sure oxygen is not flowing over the patient's chest.

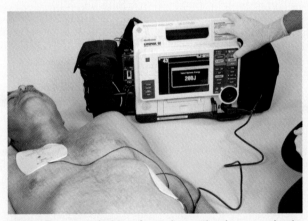

Step 2 Remove clothing from the patient's upper body. Using gloves, remove nitroglycerin paste/patches from the patient's chest if present and quickly wipe away any medication residue. Do not apply alcohol, tincture of benzoin, or antiperspirant to the skin.

If using multipurpose adhesive electrodes, place them in proper position on the patient's bare chest. If excessive hair is present in the areas where the paddles/electrodes will be placed, quickly check to see if you have two pairs of adhesive electrodes available. If so, quickly apply and then immediately remove the first set of electrodes. This will remove some of the chest hair, allowing better contact when you apply the second set. If using standard paddles, you must use defibrillation gel or defibrillation gel pads between the paddle electrode surface and the patient's skin. Place pregelled defibrillator pads on the patient's chest (or apply defibrillator gel to the electrode surface of the paddles).

Once the pads are in place, recheck the ECG rhythm and then select the appropriate energy level.

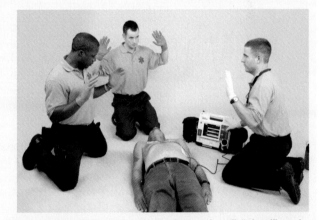

Step 4 If the ECG rhythm is unchanged, call "clear!" and look around you. Make sure everyone is clear of the patient, bed, and any equipment connected to the patient. If CPR is in progress, all team members with the exception of the person performing chest compressions should immediately clear the patient. Once the defibrillator is charged, the chest compressor should clear the patient and a shock should be delivered immediately to the patient.

If the area is clear, press the shock control. If using standard paddles, depress the shock control on both paddles at the same time. Release the shock controls after the shock has been delivered. Recheck the rhythm on the monitor.

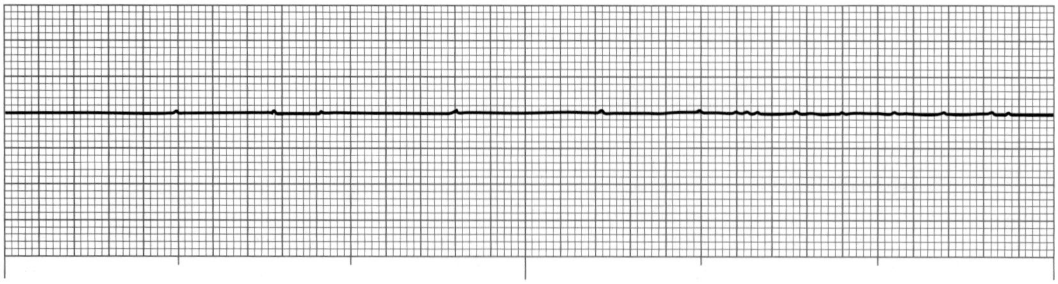

Figure 6-19 Asystole.

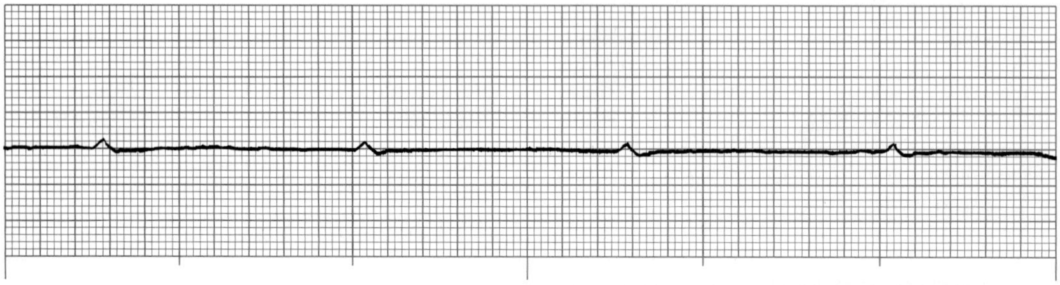

Figure 6-20 "P wave" asystole (also known as ventricular standstill).

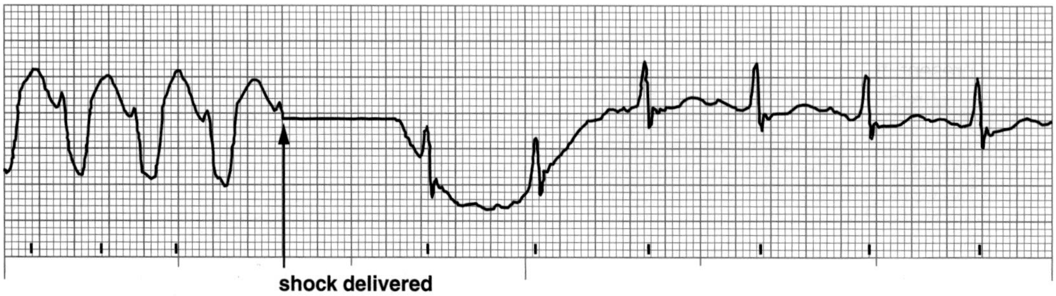

shock delivered

Figure 6-21 This rhythm strip is from a 62-year-old man complaining of palpitations. The patient's initial rhythm was monomorphic ventricular tachycardia. A synchronized shock was delivered, resulting in a sinus rhythm with a prolonged PR interval. Note the short period of asystole after the shock was delivered.

ECG Pearl

Do the following when a "flat line" is observed on an ECG:

- Make sure the power to the monitor is on
- Check the lead/cable connections
- Make sure the correct lead is selected
- Turn up the gain (ECG size) on the monitor

If the rhythm appears to be asystole, confirm the rhythm in second lead because it is possible (although rare) that coarse VF may be present in some leads.

What Do I Do About It?

Treatment of asystole includes the following:
- Confirmation of the absence of a pulse
- Immediate CPR
- Confirmation of the rhythm in two leads
- Possible insertion of an advanced airway

TABLE 6-8	Characteristics of Asystole
Rate	Ventricular usually not discernible but atrial activity may be seen ("P wave" asystole)
Rhythm	Ventricular not discernible, atrial may be discernible
P waves	Usually not discernible
PR interval	Not measurable
QRS duration	Absent

- IV access
- Consideration of the possible causes of the rhythm
- Medications per current resuscitation guidelines
- Consider termination of efforts

A summary of all ventricular rhythm characteristics can be found in Table 6-9.

TABLE 6-9 Ventricular Rhythms—Summary of Characteristics

	PVCs	Ventricular Escape Beat	Idioventricular Rhythm (IVR)	Accelerated Idioventricular Rhythm (AIVR)
Rate	Usually within normal range, but depends on underlying rhythm	Usually within normal range, but depends on underlying rhythm	20-40 beats/min	41-100 beats/min (some experts consider the rate 41-120 beats/min)
Rhythm	Regular with *early* beats	Regular with *late* beats	Essentially regular	Essentially regular
P Waves (lead II)	Usually absent or, with retrograde conduction to the atria, may appear after the QRS (usually upright in ST-segment or T wave)	Usually absent or, with retrograde conduction to the atria, may appear after the QRS (usually upright in ST-segment or T wave)	Usually absent or, with retrograde conduction to the atria, may appear after the QRS (usually upright in ST-segment or T wave)	Usually absent or, with retrograde conduction to the atria, may appear after the QRS (usually upright in ST-segment or T wave)
PR Interval	None	None	None	None
QRS	Usually 0.12 sec or greater	0.12 sec or greater	0.12 sec or greater	0.12 sec or greater

	Monomorphic Ventricular Tachycardia	Polymorphic VT	Ventricular Fibrillation	Asystole
Rate	101-250 beats/min (some experts consider the rate 121-250 beats/min)	150-300 beats/min	Not discernible	None
Rhythm	Usually regular	Irregular	Chaotic	None
P Waves (lead II)	May be present or absent. If present, they have no set relationship to the QRS complexes appearing between the QRSs at a rate different from that of the VT.	Independent or none	Absent	Atrial activity may be observed ("P wave" asystole)
PR Interval	None	None	None	None
QRS	0.12 sec or greater	0.12 sec or greater	Not discernible	Absent

REFERENCES

1. Crawford MV, Spence MI: Electrical complications in coronary artery disease: Arrhythmias in common sense approach to coronary care, ed 6, St Louis, 1995, Mosby, p 220.
2. Goldberger AL: Clinical electrocardiography: A simplified approach, ed 7, St Louis, 2006, Mosby.
3. Kinney MR, Packa DR, editors: Andreoli's comprehensive cardiac care, ed 8, St Louis, 1996, Mosby.
4. Larsen MP, Eisenberg MS, Cummins RO et al: Predicting survival from out-of-hospital cardiac arrest: A graphic model. Ann Emerg Med 1993;22(11):1652-1658.
5. 2005 American Heart Association Guidelines for Cardiopulmonary Resuscitation and Emergency Cardiovascular Care, Part 5: Electrical Therapies: Automated External Defibrillators, Defibrillation, Cardioversion, and Pacing. Circulation. 2005;112(suppl IV):IV-36.

STOP & REVIEW

True/False

Decide whether each statement is true or false. In the space provided, write T for true or F for false.

_____ **1.** Torsades de pointes (TdP) is a type of monomorphic ventricular tachycardia.

_____ **2.** Transcutaneous pacing is the treatment of choice for pulseless ventricular tachycardia or ventricular fibrillation.

Matching

Match each item with the correct statement below.

_____ **3.** Absence of electrical activity on the cardiac monitor

_____ **4.** The result of an electrical impulse from a supra-ventricular site discharging at the same time as an ectopic site in the ventricles

_____ **5.** Two sequential PVCs

_____ **6.** Premature ventricular beats that look alike in the same lead and begin from the same anatomic site

_____ **7.** Chaotic rhythm associated with no breathing or pulse

_____ **8.** Pattern in which every other beat is an ectopic beat

_____ **9.** Essentially regular ventricular rhythm with a ventricular rate of 20 to 40 beats/min

_____ **10.** Name given a PVC falling on the T wave of the preceding beat

_____ **11.** Clinical situation in which organized electrical activity (other than VT) is observed on the cardiac monitor, but there is an absence of mechanical contraction of the myocardial fibers

_____ **12.** Essentially regular ventricular rhythm with a ventricular rate of 41 to 100 beats/min

a. Accelerated idioventricular rhythm

b. Uniform premature ventricular complexes

c. R-on-T phenomenon

d. Pair or couplet

e. Pulseless electrical activity

f. Idioventricular rhythm

g. Asystole

h. Ventricular fibrillation

i. Bigeminy

j. Fusion beat

Short Answer

13. Explain the difference between a PVC and a ventricular escape beat.

14. List four (4) common causes of premature ventricular complexes.
1.

2.

3.

4.

15. How do coarse and fine ventricular fibrillation differ?

16. What is the name given to polymorphic VT that occurs in the presence of a long QT interval?

17. List three (3) potential sites of origin of ectopic beats.
1.

2.

3.

18. List three (3) reasons why the ventricles may assume responsibility for pacing the heart.
1.

2.

3.

19. List five (5) possible causes of asystole or pulseless electrical activity.
1.

2.

3.

4.

5.

20. How would you differentiate a junctional escape rhythm at 40 beats/min from a ventricular escape rhythm at the same rate?

VENTRICULAR RHYTHMS—*PRACTICE RHYTHM STRIPS*

For each of the following rhythm strips, determine the atrial and ventricular rate and rhythm, measure the PR interval and strips include sinus, atrial, junctional, and ventricular rhythms. All strips were recorded in lead II unless otherwise noted. Note: These rhythm strips include sinus, atrial, junctional, and ventricular rhythms.

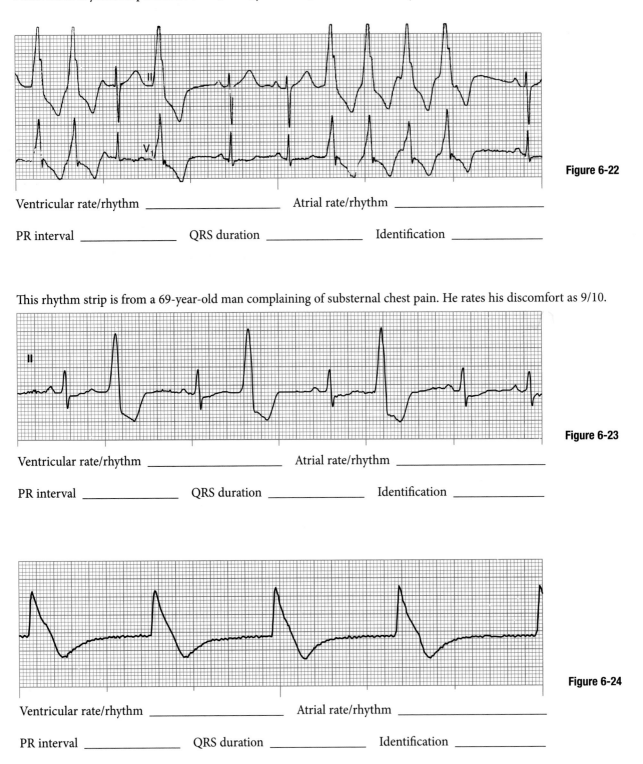

Figure 6-22

Ventricular rate/rhythm _____   Atrial rate/rhythm _____

PR interval _____   QRS duration _____   Identification _____

This rhythm strip is from a 69-year-old man complaining of substernal chest pain. He rates his discomfort as 9/10.

Figure 6-23

Ventricular rate/rhythm _____   Atrial rate/rhythm _____

PR interval _____   QRS duration _____   Identification _____

Figure 6-24

Ventricular rate/rhythm _____   Atrial rate/rhythm _____

PR interval _____   QRS duration _____   Identification _____

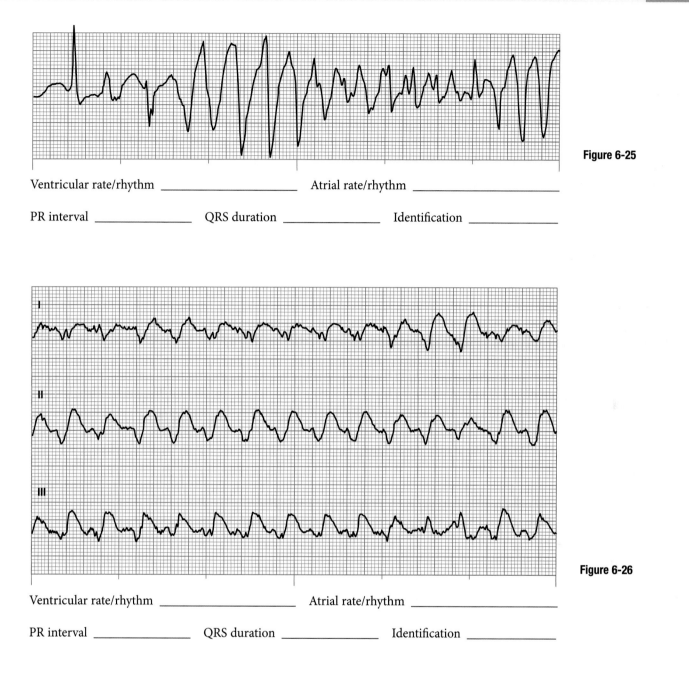

Figure 6-25

Ventricular rate/rhythm _____   Atrial rate/rhythm _____

PR interval _____   QRS duration _____   Identification _____

Figure 6-26

Ventricular rate/rhythm _____   Atrial rate/rhythm _____

PR interval _____   QRS duration _____   Identification _____

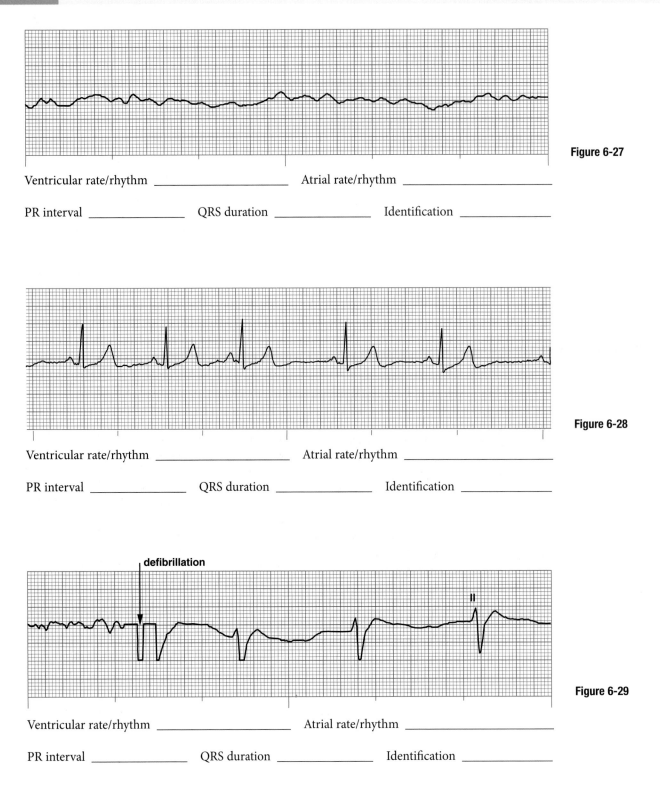

Figure 6-27

Ventricular rate/rhythm _____   Atrial rate/rhythm _____

PR interval _____   QRS duration _____   Identification _____

Figure 6-28

Ventricular rate/rhythm _____   Atrial rate/rhythm _____

PR interval _____   QRS duration _____   Identification _____

defibrillation

Figure 6-29

Ventricular rate/rhythm _____   Atrial rate/rhythm _____

PR interval _____   QRS duration _____   Identification _____

This rhythm strip is from a 32-year-old woman complaining of dizziness and shortness of breath. Identify the rhythm (lead II).

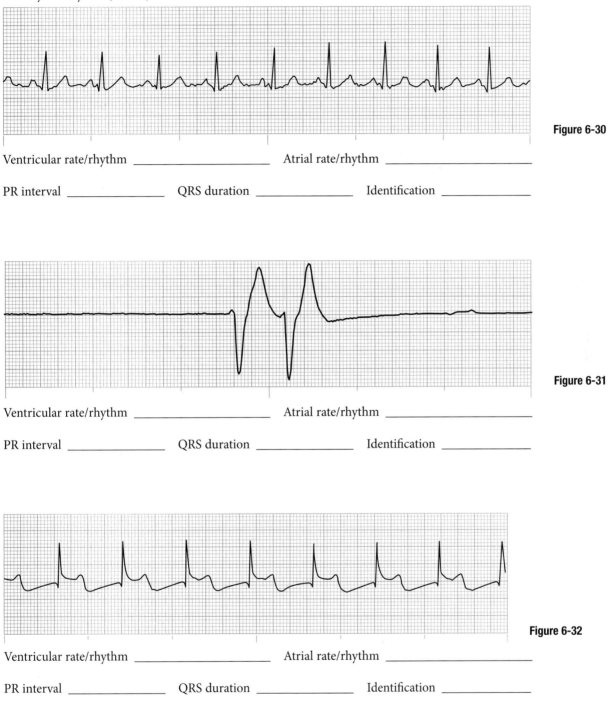

Figure 6-30

Ventricular rate/rhythm _____ Atrial rate/rhythm _____

PR interval _____ QRS duration _____ Identification _____

Figure 6-31

Ventricular rate/rhythm _____ Atrial rate/rhythm _____

PR interval _____ QRS duration _____ Identification _____

Figure 6-32

Ventricular rate/rhythm _____ Atrial rate/rhythm _____

PR interval _____ QRS duration _____ Identification _____

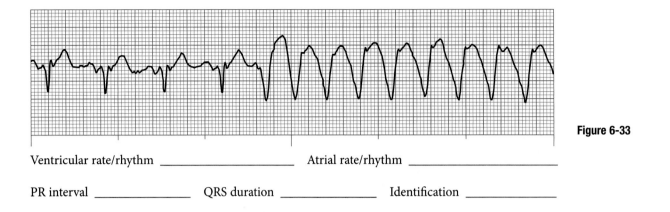

Figure 6-33

Ventricular rate/rhythm _____   Atrial rate/rhythm _____

PR interval _____   QRS duration _____   Identification _____

This rhythm strip is from a 79-year-old man complaining of palpitations. His initial blood pressure was 112/84.
His second blood pressure, 8 minutes after the first, was 78/P.
Identify the rhythm (lead II).

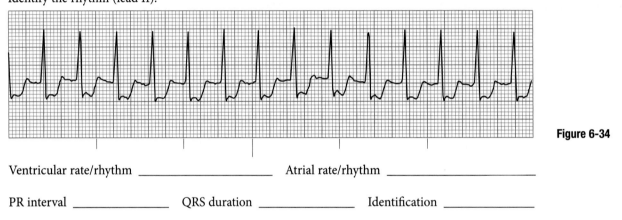

Figure 6-34

Ventricular rate/rhythm _____   Atrial rate/rhythm _____

PR interval _____   QRS duration _____   Identification _____

This rhythm strip is from a 19-year-old male who walked into the Emergency Department after ingesting a number of unknown medications (per patient) in a suicide attempt. He became unresponsive 5 minutes after his arrival. Initial rhythms before the onset of this dysrhythmia were monomorphic VT and then complete AV block. After a brief episode of the above rhythm, the patient again converted to a complete AV block. Drug screen was negative. A transvenous pacemaker was inserted and the patient admitted to CCU.

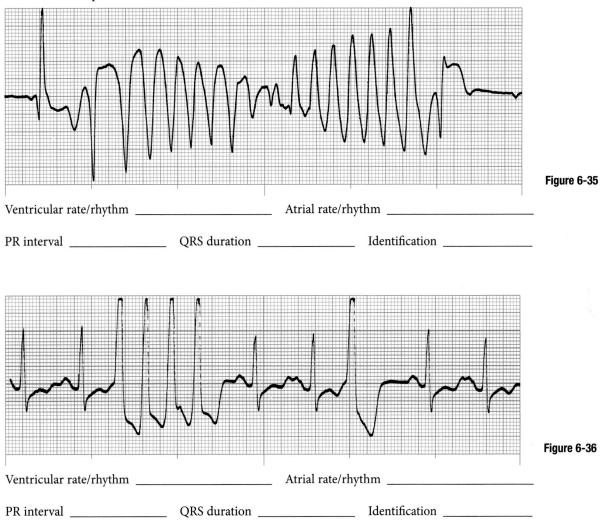

Figure 6-35

Ventricular rate/rhythm _____   Atrial rate/rhythm _____

PR interval _____   QRS duration _____   Identification _____

Figure 6-36

Ventricular rate/rhythm _____   Atrial rate/rhythm _____

PR interval _____   QRS duration _____   Identification _____

This rhythm strip is from a 63-year-old man who collapsed on the kitchen floor. He is unresponsive, apneic, and pulseless. His past medical history includes a coronary artery bypass graft 8 years ago and pacemaker implantation 5 years ago. Identify the rhythm (lead II).

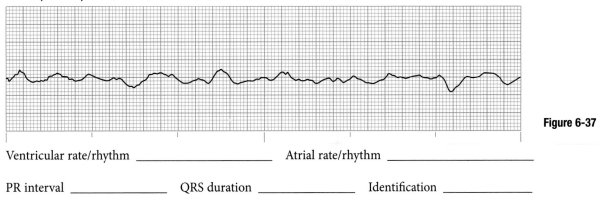

Figure 6-37

Ventricular rate/rhythm _____   Atrial rate/rhythm _____

PR interval _____   QRS duration _____   Identification _____

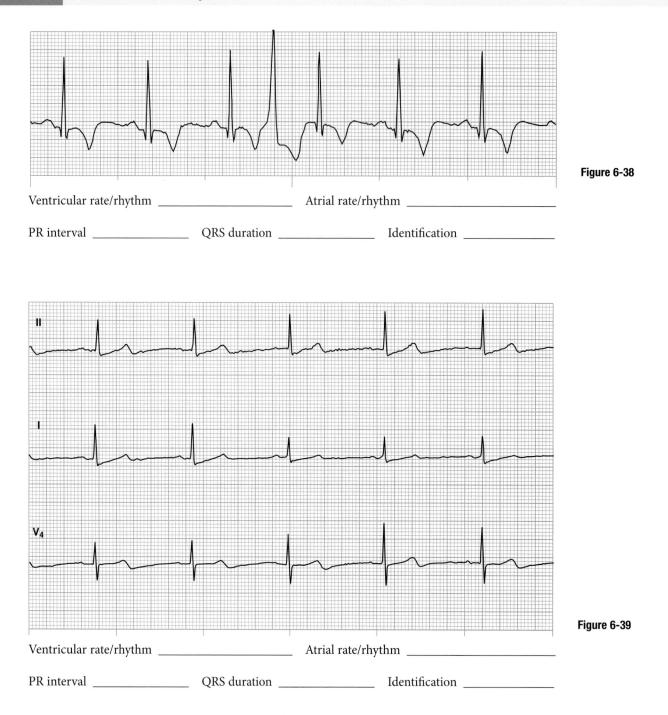

Figure 6-38

Ventricular rate/rhythm _____   Atrial rate/rhythm _____

PR interval _____   QRS duration _____   Identification _____

Figure 6-39

Ventricular rate/rhythm _____   Atrial rate/rhythm _____

PR interval _____   QRS duration _____   Identification _____

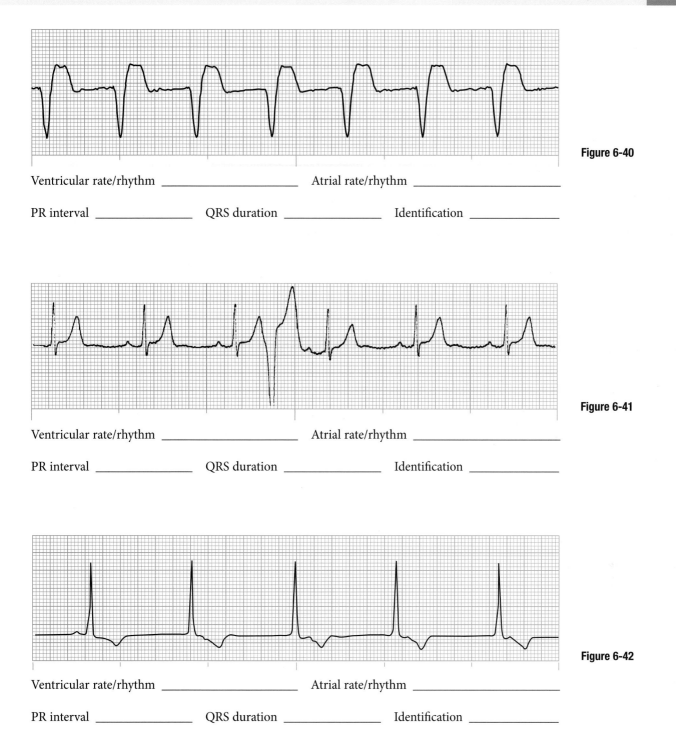

Figure 6-40

Ventricular rate/rhythm _____   Atrial rate/rhythm _____

PR interval _____   QRS duration _____   Identification _____

Figure 6-41

Ventricular rate/rhythm _____   Atrial rate/rhythm _____

PR interval _____   QRS duration _____   Identification _____

Figure 6-42

Ventricular rate/rhythm _____   Atrial rate/rhythm _____

PR interval _____   QRS duration _____   Identification _____

This rhythm strip is from a 37-year-old man who presented to the Emergency Department with seizures. He had a history of a 3-day methamphetamine binge. The rhythm converted with diltiazem (Cardizem).

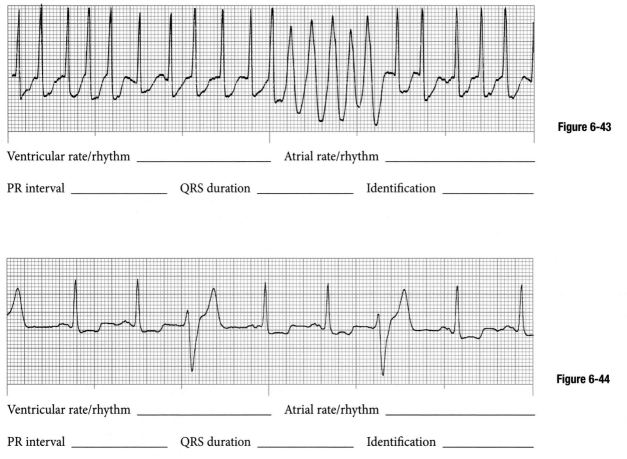

Figure 6-43

Ventricular rate/rhythm _____   Atrial rate/rhythm _____

PR interval _____   QRS duration _____   Identification _____

Figure 6-44

Ventricular rate/rhythm _____   Atrial rate/rhythm _____

PR interval _____   QRS duration _____   Identification _____

STOP & REVIEW ANSWERS

True/False

1. F

2. F

Matching

3. g

4. j

5. d

6. b

7. h

8. i

9. f

10. c

11. e

12. a

Short Answer

13. A PVC is premature and occurs before the next expected sinus beat. A ventricular escape beat is late, occurring after the next expected sinus beat.

14. Common causes of PVCs include normal variant, hypoxia, stress/anxiety, exercise, digitalis toxicity, acid-base imbalance, myocardial ischemia, electrolyte imbalance (hypokalemia, hypocalcemia, hypercalcemia, hypomagnesemia), congestive heart failure, increased sympathetic tone, acute myocardial infarction, stimulants (alcohol, caffeine, tobacco), and medications (sympathomimetics, cyclic antidepressants, phenothiazines).

15. Coarse ventricular fibrillation (VF) is 3 mm or more in amplitude. Fine VF is less than 3 mm in amplitude.

16. Polymorphic VT that occurs in the presence of a long QT interval is called "torsades de pointes."

17. Three potential sites of origin of ectopic beats are: (1) the atria (PACs); (2) the AV junction (PJCs); and (3) the ventricles (PVCs).

18. The ventricles may assume responsibility for pacing the heart if:
- SA node fails to discharge
- Impulse from the SA node is generated but blocked as it exits the SA node
- Rate of discharge of the SA node is slower than that of the ventricles
- Irritable site in either ventricle produces an early beat or rapid rhythm

19. Possible causes of asystole or pulseless electrical activity include the following

PATCH-4-MD
- **P**ulmonary embolism
- **A**cidosis
- **T**ension pneumothorax
- **C**ardiac tamponade
- **H**ypovolemia (common cause of PEA)
- **H**ypoxia
- **H**eat/cold (hypothermia/hyperthermia)
- **H**ypokalemia/hyperkalemia (and other electrolytes)
- **M**yocardial infarction
- **D**rug overdose/accidents

Five Hs and Five Ts

Hypovolemia	**T**amponade, cardiac
Hypoxia	**T**ension pneumothorax
Hypothermia	**T**hrombosis: lungs (massive
Hypokalemia/	pulmonary embolism)
Hyperkalemia	**T**hrombosis: heart (acute coronary
Hydrogen ion	syndromes)
(acidosis)	**T**ablets/toxins: drug overdose

20. The junctional escape rhythm will have a narrow QRS complex; the ventricular escape rhythm will have a wide QRS complex.

Figure 6-22 answers

Ventricular rate/rhythm	94 beats/min (sinus beats), irregular
Atrial rate/rhythm	94 beats/min (sinus beats), irregular
PR interval	0.16 sec (sinus beats)
QRS duration	0.08 sec (sinus beats)
Identification	Sinus rhythm at 94 beats/min with an episode of couplets and a run of VT

Figure 6-23 answers

Ventricular rate/rhythm	86 beats/min, irregular
Atrial rate/rhythm	86 beats/min, irregular
PR interval	0.18 sec (sinus beats)
QRS duration	0.10 sec (sinus beats)
Identification	Sinus rhythm at 86 beats/min with uniform PVCs

Figure 6-24 answers

Ventricular rate/rhythm	42 beats/min, regular
Atrial rate/rhythm	None
PR interval	None
QRS duration	0.24 sec
Identification	Accelerated idioventricular rhythm (AIVR) at 42 beats/min

Figure 6-25 answers

Ventricular rate/rhythm	250 to 333 beats/min, irregular
Atrial rate/rhythm	Unable to determine
PR interval	Unable to determine
QRS duration	0.16 sec
Identification	Polymorphic VT at 250 to 333 beats/min

Figure 6-26 answers

Ventricular rate/rhythm	150 beats/min, essentially regular
Atrial rate/rhythm	Unable to determine
PR interval	Unable to determine
QRS duration	0.12 to 0.16 sec
Identification	Monomorphic VT at 150 beats/min

Figure 6-27 answers

Ventricular rate/rhythm	None
Atrial rate/rhythm	None
PR interval	None
QRS duration	None
Identification	Coarse ventricular fibrillation

Figure 6-28 answers

Ventricular rate/rhythm	60 beats/min (sinus beats), regular except for the event
Atrial rate/rhythm	60 beats/min (sinus beats), regular except for the event
PR interval	0.16 sec
QRS duration	0.08 sec
Identification	Sinus rhythm at 60 beats/min with a PAC

Figure 6-29 answers

Ventricular rate/rhythm	None to 40 beats/min, irregular to regular
Atrial rate/rhythm	None
PR interval	None
QRS duration	None to 0.16 sec
Identification	Ventricular fibrillation – shock (defibrillation) – idioventricular rhythm at 40 beats/min

Figure 6-30 answers

Ventricular rate/rhythm	94 beats/min, regular
Atrial rate/rhythm	94 beats/min/regular
PR interval	0.16 sec
QRS duration	0.06 sec
Identification	Sinus rhythm at 94 beats/min

Figure 6-31 answers

Ventricular rate/rhythm	Two ventricular complexes to none
Atrial rate/rhythm	None
PR interval	None
QRS duration	0.14 sec to none
Identification	Agonal rhythm/asystole

Figure 6-32 answers

Ventricular rate/rhythm	79 beats/min, regular
Atrial rate/rhythm	None
PR interval	None
QRS duration	0.08 sec
Identification	Accelerated junctional rhythm at 79 beats/min with ST-segment elevation

Figure 6-33 answers

Ventricular rate/rhythm	94 beats/min (sinus beats) to 150 beats/min (VT), regular (sinus beats), regular (VT)
Atrial rate/rhythm	94 beats/min (sinus beats), regular (sinus beats) to unable to determine (VT)
PR interval	0.16 sec (sinus beats)
QRS duration	0.10 sec (sinus beats) to 0.14 sec (VT)
Identification	Sinus rhythm at 94 beats/min to monomorphic VT at 150 beats/min

Figure 6-34 answers

Ventricular rate/rhythm	147 beats/min, regular
Atrial rate/rhythm	Unable to determine
PR interval	Unable to determine
QRS duration	0.06 to 0.08 sec
Identification	Narrow-QRS tachycardia (SVT) at 147 beats/min with ST-segment depression

Figure 6-35 answers

Ventricular rate/rhythm	230 to 300 beats/min, irregular
Atrial rate/rhythm	Unable to determine
PR interval	Unable to determine
QRS duration	Varies
Identification	Polymorphic VT at 230 to 300 beats/min

Figure 6-36 answers

Ventricular rate/rhythm	88 beats/min (sinus beats), regular except for the events
Atrial rate/rhythm	88 beats/min (sinus beats), regular except for the events
PR interval	0.20 sec (sinus beats)
QRS duration	0.08 sec (sinus beats)
Identification	Sinus rhythm at 88 beats/min with a PVC and run of VT, ST-segment depression, inverted T waves

Figure 6-37 answers

Ventricular rate/rhythm	None
Atrial rate/rhythm	None
PR interval	None
QRS duration	None
Identification	Coarse ventricular fibrillation

Figure 6-38 answers

Ventricular rate/rhythm	62 beats/min, essentially regular
Atrial rate/rhythm	62 beats/min, essentially regular
PR interval	0.20 sec
QRS duration	0.10 sec
Identification	Sinus rhythm at 62 beats/min with an interpolated PVC; inverted T waves

Figure 6-39 answers

Ventricular rate/rhythm	52 beats/min, regular
Atrial rate/rhythm	52 beats/min/regular
PR interval	0.16 to 0.20 sec
QRS duration	0.06 sec
Identification	Sinus bradycardia at 52 beats/min

Figure 6-40 answers

Ventricular rate/rhythm	71 beats/min, regular
Atrial rate/rhythm	Unable to determine
PR interval	Unable to determine
QRS duration	0.12 sec
Identification	Accelerated idioventricular rhythm (AIVR) at 71 beats/min; ST-segment elevation

Figure 6-41 answers

Ventricular rate/rhythm	60 beats/min, regular
Atrial rate/rhythm	60 beats/min, regular
PR interval	0.20 sec (sinus beats)
QRS duration	0.08 sec (sinus beats)
Identification	Sinus rhythm at 60 beats/min with R-on-T interpolated PVC; tall T waves

Figure 6-42 answers

Ventricular rate/rhythm	52 beats/min, regular
Atrial rate/rhythm	None
PR interval	None
QRS duration	0.06 sec
Identification	Sinus beat to junctional escape rhythm at 52 beats/min with inverted T waves

Figure 6-43 answers

Ventricular rate/rhythm	150 to 250 beats/min, irregular
Atrial rate/rhythm	None
PR interval	None
QRS duration	0.06 sec (atrial beats)
Identification	Atrial fib with a rapid ventricular response of 150 to 250 beats/min and a run of VT

Figure 6-44 answers

Ventricular rate/rhythm	83 beats/min (sinus beats), regular except for events (PVCs)
Atrial rate/rhythm	83 beats/min (sinus beats), regular except for events (PVCs)
PR interval	0.16 sec (sinus beats)
QRS duration	0.08 sec (sinus beats)
Identification	Sinus rhythm at 83 beats/min with ventricular trigeminy, ST-segment depression, inverted T waves

Atrioventricular (AV) Blocks

OBJECTIVES

On completion of this chapter, you will be able to:

1. Describe the ECG characteristics, possible causes, signs and symptoms, and emergency management for first-degree AV block.
2. Describe the ECG characteristics, possible causes, signs and symptoms, and emergency management for second-degree AV block, type I.
3. Describe the ECG characteristics, possible causes, signs and symptoms, and emergency management for second-degree AV block, type II.
4. Describe the ECG characteristics, possible causes, signs and symptoms, and emergency management for second-degree AV block, 2:1 conduction.
5. Describe the ECG characteristics, possible causes, signs and symptoms, and emergency management for third-degree AV block.

INTRODUCTION

The **AV junction** is an area of specialized conduction tissue that provides the electrical links between the atrium and ventricle. If a delay or interruption in impulse conduction occurs within the AV node, bundle of His, or His-Purkinje system, the resulting dysrhythmia is called an atrioventricular (AV) block. AV blocks have been traditionally classified in two ways: according to the *degree* of block and/or according to the *site* of the block.

Remember that the PR interval reflects depolarization of the right and left atria (P wave) and the spread of the impulse through the AV node, bundle of His, right and left bundle branches, and the Purkinje fibers (reflected by the PR-segment). The PR interval is the key to differentiating the *type* of AV block. The key to differentiating the *level* (location) of the block is the width of the QRS complex and, in second- and third-degree AV blocks, the rate of the escape rhythm.

ECG Pearl

Depolarization and repolarization are slow in the AV node making this area vulnerable to blocks in conduction (AV blocks).

In first-degree AV block, impulses from the SA node to the ventricles are *delayed* (not blocked). First-degree AV block usually occurs at the AV node (Figure 7-1). With second-degree AV blocks, there is an *intermittent* disturbance in conduction of impulses between the atria and ventricles. The site of block in second-degree AV block type I is typically at the AV node. The site of block in second-degree AV block type II is the bundle of His or, more commonly, the bundle branches. In third-degree AV block, there is a *complete* block in conduction of impulses between the atria and ventricles. The site of block in a third-degree AV block may be the AV node or, more commonly, the bundle of His or bundle branches (Table 7-1).

Second and third-degree AV blocks may become serious enough to require the use of a natural escape pacemaker. Should such a pacemaker become a necessity, AV blocks that occur at the level of the AV node have a tremendous advantage. If required, there is usually a reliable junctional pacemaker available that can fire at 40 to 60 beats/min. However, when the location of an AV block is below the AV junction, the only available pacemaker may be a slow ventricular one, firing at 20 to 40 beats/min. Not only are ventricular pacemakers slow, they are prone to long pauses, making them less than reliable. Therefore, AV blocks at the level of the AV node usually have a more effective and reliable escape pacemaker than do AV blocks at the bundle of His or below.

ECG Pearl

The clinical significance of an AV block depends on:

- The degree (severity) of the block
- The rate of the escape pacemaker (junctional vs. ventricular)
- The patient's response to that ventricular rate

TABLE 7-1	Classification of AV Blocks

CLASSIFICATION BY DEGREE

Name of Block	Type of Block
First-degree AV block	Incomplete
Second-degree AV block type I	Incomplete
Second-degree AV block type II	Incomplete
Third-degree AV block	Complete

CLASSIFICATION BY SITE/LOCATION

Site	Name of Block
AV node	First-degree AV block
	Second-degree AV block type I
	Third-degree AV block
Infranodal (Subnodal)	
Bundle of His	Second-degree AV block type II (uncommon)
	Third-degree AV block
Bundle branches	Second-degree AV block type II (more common)
	Third-degree AV block

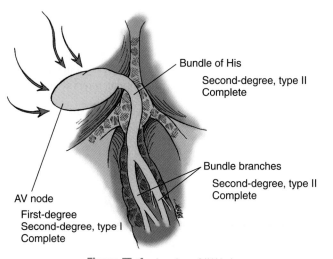

Bundle of His
Second-degree, type II
Complete

Bundle branches
Second-degree, type II
Complete

AV node
First-degree
Second-degree, type I
Complete

Figure 7-1 Locations of AV block.

FIRST-DEGREE AV BLOCK

How Do I Recognize It?

[OBJECTIVE 1]

A PR interval of normal duration (0.12-0.20 sec) indicates the electrical impulse was conducted normally through the atria, AV node, bundle of His, bundle branches, and Purkinje fibers. When a PR interval is prolonged, it is usually between 0.21 and 0.48 second. Occasionally, a PR interval greater than 0.8 second may be seen.[1] However, PR intervals as long as 1 second or more have been reported.[2]

In first-degree AV block, all components of the ECG tracing are usually within normal limits except the PR interval. This is because electrical impulses travel normally from the SA node through the atria, but there is a delay in impulse conduction, usually at the level of the AV node. In first-degree AV block, each P wave is followed by a QRS complex (1:1 relationship). Despite its name, in first-degree AV block, the sinus impulse is not blocked (all sinus beats are conducted); impulses are *delayed* for the same period before they are conducted to the ventricles. This delay in AV conduction results in a PR interval that is longer than normal (more than 0.20 second in duration) and constant.

Let's look at the rhythm shown in Figure 7-2. The ventricular rhythm is regular at a rate of 60 beats/min. Each QRS complex is preceded by an upright P wave. The atrial rhythm is also regular at a rate of 60 beats/min. We now know that the underlying rhythm is a sinus rhythm at 60 beats/min. The QRS duration is within normal limits. However the PR interval is longer than normal measuring 0.32 second, but constant before each QRS. The 1:1 relationship of P wave to QRS complex and a longer than normal PR interval fits the criteria of a first-degree AV block.

First-degree AV block is not a dysrhythmia itself. It is a condition describing the consistent prolonged PR interval viewed on the ECG rhythm strip. Our identification of the rhythm strip in Figure 7-2 must include a description of the underlying rhythm, the ventricular rate, and then describe anything that appears amiss. In this case, we will identify the rhythm as "Sinus rhythm at 60 beats/min with a first-degree AV block." The characteristics of first-degree AV block are shown in Table 7-2

What Causes It?

First-degree AV block may be a normal finding in individuals with no history of cardiac disease, especially in athletes. In some people, mild prolongation of the PR interval may be a normal variant, especially with sinus bradycardia during rest or sleep. First-degree AV block may also occur because of:

- Ischemia or injury to the AV node or junction
- Medications
- Rheumatic heart disease
- Hyperkalemia
- Acute myocardial infarction (MI)
- Increased vagal tone

ECG Pearl

Examples of medications that may cause first-degree AV block include:
- Quinidine
- Procainamide
- Beta-blockers
- Calcium channel blockers
- Digitalis
- Amiodarone

What Do I Do About It?

The patient with a first-degree AV block is often asymptomatic; however, marked first-degree AV block can lead to symptoms even in the absence of higher degrees of AV block.[3] First-degree AV block that occurs with acute MI should be monitored closely.

SECOND-DEGREE AV BLOCKS

Overview

When some, but not all, atrial impulses are blocked from reaching the ventricles, second-degree AV blocks result. Because the SA node is generating impulses in a normal manner, each P wave will occur at a regular interval across the

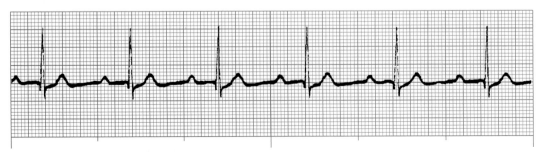

Figure 7-2   Sinus rhythm at 60 beats/min with a first-degree AV block.

TABLE 7-2	Characteristics of First-Degree AV Block
Rate	Usually within normal range, but depends on underlying rhythm
Rhythm	Regular
P waves	Normal in size and shape, one positive (upright) P wave before each QRS in leads II, III, and aVF
P-R interval	Prolonged (greater than 0.20 sec) but constant
QRS duration	Usually 0.10 sec or less unless an intraventricular conduction delay exists

rhythm strip (all P waves will plot through on time), although not every P wave will be followed by a QRS complex. This suggests that the atria are being depolarized normally, but not every impulse is being conducted to the ventricles. As a result, more P waves than QRS complexes are seen on the ECG.

Second-degree AV block is classified as type I or type II, depending on the location of the block. In second-degree AV block types I and II, the ventricular rhythm (R-R interval) is irregular. Second-degree AV block type I occurs above the bundle of His. Second-degree AV block type II occurs within or below the bundle of His.

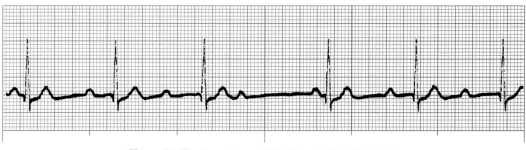

ECG Pearl

AV blocks that occur in the AV node usually produce a narrow QRS complex (just as a junctional rhythm does) and an AV block in the bundle branches usually produces a wide QRS complex (just as a ventricular rhythm does). While this rule is not absolute, it is another useful clue in determining the site of an AV block.[4]

Second-Degree AV Block Type I (Wenckebach, Mobitz Type I)

How Do I Recognize It?

[OBJECTIVE 2]

The conduction delay in second-degree AV block type I usually occurs at the level of the AV node. Let us look at the example of this type of AV block in Figure 7-3. You can quickly see that the ventricular rhythm is irregular. Since it is irregular,

calculate the rate between the shortest and longest R-R intervals. The rate range is about 43 to 60 beats/min. Now let us look at the atrial rhythm and calculate the atrial rate. Look to the left of each QRS and label each P wave in the rhythm strip. Place your calipers or a piece of paper on two P waves and begin moving from the left side of the strip to the right to see if the P waves occur on time. You will find that there is an "extra" P wave after beat No. 3. The extra P wave occurs on time, but there is no QRS after it. The remainder of the P waves occur on time. The atrial rate is about 68 beats/min.

Although we are discussing AV blocks in this chapter, how do you know that the extra P wave with no QRS after it isn't a nonconducted PAC? Well, the difference is in the timing of the P waves. If you have not been plotting P waves when analyzing a rhythm strip until now, it is *very* important that you do so when identifying AV blocks. In second and third-degree AV blocks there are more P waves than QRS complexes—and the P waves occur *on time*. This happens because the problem in second- and third-degree AV blocks is not in the SA node. The problem occurs somewhere in the conduction system *below* the SA node. So, the sinus fires regularly—as it is supposed to. The P wave that occurs after beat No. 3 is not a nonconducted PAC because all of the P waves are on time. By definition, the P wave of a nonconducted *premature* atrial complex is early.

The QRS complexes in Figure 7-3 are within normal limits. Now, look closely at the PR intervals. In second-degree AV block type I, impulses generated by the SA node take longer and longer to conduct through the AV node. This appears on the ECG as lengthening PR intervals. In order to determine if the PR intervals remain the same or lengthen, we need to see two PQRST cycles in a row that do not contain extra waveforms. Beats 1, 2, and 3 allow us to do this because there is one P wave before each QRS. When you compare the PR intervals of these beats, the PR interval of beat 1 is short. The PR interval of beat 2 is longer than beat 1 and the PR interval of beat 3 is longer than the first two beats. Thus, we can see that the PR intervals are getting progressively longer.

The lengthening PR intervals eventually result in a P wave that falls during the refractory period of the ventricles. Because the ventricles are refractory, the sinus impulse is blocked. The blocked sinus impulse appears on the ECG as a P wave with no QRS after it (dropped beat). Thus the atria are depolarized (represented by the P wave), but the AV junction fails to

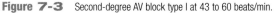

Figure 7-3   Second-degree AV block type I at 43 to 60 beats/min.

conduct the impulse from the atria to the ventricles (reflected on the ECG by the absence of a QRS complex). Because QRS complexes are periodically dropped, the ventricular rhythm is irregular. The cycle then begins again. The repetition of this cyclic pattern is called "grouped beating." In second-degree AV block type I, any P to QRS ratio may be seen. For example, 3 P waves to 2 QRS complexes (3:2), 4:3, 5:4, etc. Our identification of this rhythm strip is "Second-degree AV block type I at 43 to 60 beats/min." ECG characteristics of second-degree AV block type I are shown in Table 7-3.

ECG Pearl

Second-degree AV block type I is also known as Mobitz type I or Wenckebach. The Wenckebach pattern is the progressive lengthening of the PR interval followed by a P wave with no QRS complex.

What Causes It?

Second-degree AV block type I is usually caused by a conduction delay within the AV node. Remember that the right coronary artery supplies the AV node in 90% of the population. Thus, right coronary artery occlusions are associated with AV block occurring in the AV node.

If the right coronary artery is blocked, ischemia may develop in the AV node. As a result of this ischemia, there can be a disturbance in the balance between the parasympathetic and sympathetic divisions of the autonomic nervous system, resulting in an increase in parasympathetic tone. Once parasympathetic tone increases, conduction through the AV node is slowed. This slowing may manifest itself as a prolonged PR interval or dropped beats. An increase in parasympathetic tone is the cause of most AV blocks complicating right coronary artery occlusions (inferior wall infarctions and right ventricular infarction).

What Do I Do About It?

The patient with this type of AV block is usually asymptomatic because the ventricular rate often remains nearly normal, and cardiac output is not significantly affected. If the patient is symptomatic and the rhythm is a result of medications, these substances should be withheld. If the heart rate is slow and serious signs and symptoms occur because of the slow rate, atropine and/or temporary pacing should be considered. When associated with an acute inferior wall MI, this dysrhythmia is usually transient. It usually resolves within 48 to 72 hours as the effects of parasympathetic stimulation disappear. When this rhythm occurs in conjunction with acute MI, the patient should be observed for increasing AV block.

ECG Pearl

Two types of second-degree AV blocks based on jugular pulse tracings were first described by an early 20th century European physician named Wenckebach. In 1924, a German electrocardiographer named Mobitz identified the same dysrhythmias previously identified by Wenckebach. Mobitz termed the rhythms type I (later called Mobitz I) and type II (later known as Mobitz II).

Second-Degree AV Block, Type II (Mobitz Type II)

How Do I Recognize It?

[OBJECTIVE 3]

Second-degree AV block type II is also called Mobitz type II AV block. The conduction delay in second-degree AV block type II occurs below the AV node, either at the bundle of His or, more commonly, at the level of the bundle branches. This type of block is more serious than second-degree AV block type I and frequently progresses to third-degree AV block.

Look at Figure 7-4. You can see right away that the ventricular rhythm is irregular. Calculate the ventricular rate. Be sure to provide a rate range (slowest to fastest) since the ventricular rhythm is irregular. The ventricular rate ranges from about 20 to 60 beats/min. You can quickly see that there are more P waves than QRS complexes in this rhythm strip. Use your calipers or paper to plot the P waves and see whether or not they occur on time. They do indeed occur regularly, although not every P wave is followed by a QRS complex. Now calculate the atrial rate. It is about 60 beats/min. In second-degree AV block type II, each P wave occurs at a regular interval across the rhythm strip (all P waves will plot through on time) because the SA node is generating impulses in a normal manner. Impulses generated by the SA node are conducted to the ventricles at the same rate (appearing on the ECG as a constant PR interval) until an impulse is suddenly blocked—appearing on the ECG as a P wave with no QRS after it (dropped beat). Because QRS complexes are periodically dropped, the ventricular rhythm is irregular.

Look at the QRS complexes in Figure 7-4. They are wider than normal, measuring about 0.16 second. Remember that in second-degree AV block type I, the QRS is usually narrow because the block occurs at the level of the AV node. In second-degree AV block type II, the site of the block is lower

TABLE 7-3	Characteristics of Second-Degree AV Block Type I
Rate	Atrial rate is greater than the ventricular rate
Rhythm	Atrial regular (Ps plot through on time); ventricular irregular
P waves	Normal in size and shape; some P waves are not followed by a QRS complex (more Ps than QRSs)
PR interval	Lengthens with each cycle (although lengthening may be very slight), until a P wave appears without a QRS complex; the PRI *after* the nonconducted beat is shorter than the interval preceding the nonconducted beat
QRS duration	Usually 0.10 sec or less but is periodically dropped

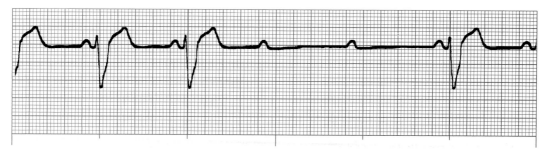

Figure 7-4 Second-degree AV block type II at 20 to 60 beats/min, ST-segment elevation.

in the conduction system; in the bundle of His (uncommon) or bundle branches (more common). If the block occurs in the bundle of His, the QRS will remain narrow. If the block occurs below the bundle of His, the QRS will be wide (more than 0.10 sec in duration).

ECG Pearl

When AV block occurs in the setting of a left coronary artery occlusion (septal and anterior infarctions), the block is usually located in the bundle branches and most likely due to serious tissue injury or tissue death.

Now look closely at the PR intervals in the first two PQRST cycles in Figure 7-4 and compare them. Are they the same or different? Remember that in second-degree AV block type I, we found that the PR intervals lengthened until a P wave appeared with no QRS after it. In this rhythm strip, the PR intervals are the same and then a P wave suddenly appears with no QRS after it. When the PR intervals measure the same, we say that the PR interval is *constant*. This is an important difference between second-degree AV block type I and second-degree AV block type II. In second-degree AV block type II, the PR interval is usually within normal limits or slightly prolonged, but it is constant for the conducted beats. Examination of the ST-segments in this rhythm strip reveals ST-segment elevation. Our identification of the rhythm in Figure 7-4 is "Second-degree AV block type II at a rate of 20 to 60 beats/min with ST-segment elevation." The ECG characteristics of second-degree AV block type II are shown in Table 7-4.

What Causes It?

The bundle branches receive their primary blood supply from the left coronary artery. Thus disease of the left coronary artery or an anterior MI is usually associated with blocks that occur within the bundle branches. Second-degree AV block type II may also occur because of acute myocarditis or other types of organic heart disease.

What Do I Do About It?

The patient's response to this rhythm is usually related to the ventricular rate. If the ventricular rate is within normal limits, the patient may be asymptomatic. More commonly, the ventricular rate is significantly slowed and serious signs and

TABLE 7-4	Characteristics of Second-Degree AV Block Type II
Rate	Atrial rate is greater than the ventricular rate; ventricular rate is often slow
Rhythm	Atrial regular (Ps plot through on time), ventricular irregular
P waves	Normal in size and shape; some P waves are not followed by a QRS complex (more Ps than QRSs)
PR interval	Within normal limits or slightly prolonged but constant for the conducted beats; there may be some shortening of the PR interval that follows a nonconducted P wave
QRS duration	Usually greater than 0.10 sec, periodically absent after P waves

symptoms result because of the slow rate and decreased cardiac output.

Second-degree AV block type II may rapidly progress to third-degree AV block without warning. Preparations should be made for pacing when this rhythm is recognized. The use of atropine should be avoided. In this situation, atropine will usually not improve the block but will increase the rate of discharge of the SA node. This may trigger a situation in which even fewer impulses are conducted through to the ventricles and the ventricular rate is further slowed. Second-degree AV block type II is usually an indication for a permanent pacemaker.

ECG Pearl

Locating the probable site of an AV block plays a critical part in developing an effective treatment plan for AV block. Remember, when AV block is associated with an inferior wall MI and produces a narrow QRS complex, it is probably located in the AV node. However, when an anterior wall MI produces AV block it usually occurs in the bundle branches (infranodal) and displays a wide QRS complex. Infranodal AV blocks may quickly progress to a near-asystole state. Therefore, standby pacing is indicated when infranodal AV block complicates anterior wall MI. The rationale behind this strategy is this: If an AV block is known to be unstable and unlikely to respond to atropine, then applying the pacemaker on standby—even when the AV block is presently stable—is the best defense.[4]

Second-Degree AV Block, 2:1 Conduction (2:1 AV Block)

How Do I Recognize It?

[OBJECTIVE 4]

Second-degree AV block with 2:1conduction may be due to a block within the AV node (type I) or more distal block within the His-Purkinje system (type II). Before we discuss more about 2:1 AV block, let us review a couple of very important points regarding second-degree AV blocks. So far you have learned how important it is to plot P waves to make sure they occur on time. You have also learned that there are differences in the PR interval patterns in second-degree AV block type I and type II. In order to compare PR intervals, we must see two PQRST cycles in a row. If there are more P waves than QRSs and the P waves occur on time, you now know that you have some type of AV block. If you then look at the PR intervals, you can begin to differentiate what type of AV block it is.

For example, if the PR intervals get progressively longer and then a P wave appears with no QRS after it, you know that the rhythm is a second-degree AV block type I. If the PR intervals remain the same (constant) before the conducted beats, you know that the rhythm is a second-degree AV block type II. The QRS complex in a second-degree AV block type I is usually narrow. It is usually wide in a second-degree AV block type II.

In 2:1 AV block, two P waves occur for every one QRS complex (2:1 conduction). Since there are no two PQRST cycles in a row from which to compare PR intervals, the decision as to what to term the rhythm is based on the width of the QRS complex. A 2:1 AV block associated with a narrow QRS complex (0.10 sec or less) usually represents a form of second-degree AV block, type I (Figure 7-5). A

2:1 AV block associated with wide QRS complexes (greater than 0.10 sec) is usually associated with a delay in conduction below the bundle of His. Thus, it is usually a type II block (Figure 7-6).

The terms *high-grade* or *advanced* second-degree AV block may be used to describe two or more consecutive P waves that are not conducted. For example, in 3:1 block, every third P wave is conducted; in 4:1 block, every fourth P wave is conducted. In cases of advanced AV block, it may be difficult to determine the type of second-degree block because the block may involve either a type I or type II mechanism. If the PR interval varies and its length is inversely related to the interval between the P wave and its preceding R wave, the rhythm is most likely a second-degree block type I.[5] If the PR interval is constant for all conducted beats, the rhythm is most likely a second-degree AV block type II.

A comparison of the types of second-degree AV blocks is shown in Figure 7-7. The ECG characteristics of 2:1 AV block are summarized in Table 7-5.

ECG Pearl

When two conducted P waves occur in a row, the PR intervals of the consecutive beats should be compared to identify either type I or type II second-degree AV block.

What Causes It? What Do I Do About It?

The causes and management of second-degree AV block with 2:1 conduction are those of type I or type II blocks previously discussed.

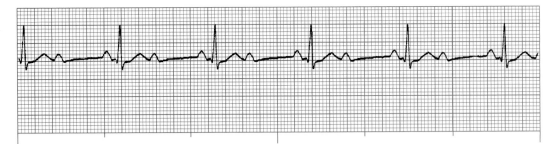

Figure 7-5   Second-degree AV block, 2:1 conduction, probably type I.

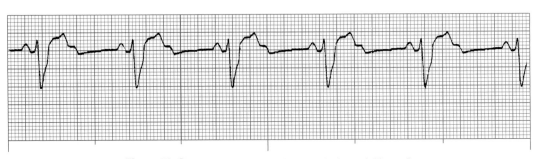

Figure 7-6   Second-degree AV block, 2:1 conduction, probably type II.

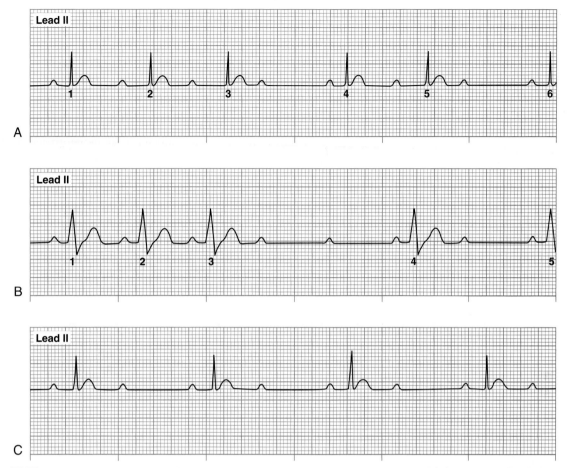

Figure 7-7 Types of second-degree AV block. **A,** Second-degree AV block type I. **B,** Second-degree AV block type II. **C,** Second-degree AV block 2:1 conduction.

ECG Pearl

A Quick Look at P Waves and AV Blocks

AV Block	P Wave Conduction
First-degree	All P waves conducted but delayed
Second-degree	Some P waves conducted, others blocked
Third-degree	No P waves conducted

TABLE 7-5	Characteristics of Second-Degree AV Block 2:1 Conduction (2:1 AV Block)
Rate	Atrial rate is twice the ventricular rate
Rhythm	Atrial regular (Ps plot through on time), ventricular regular
P waves	Normal in size and shape; every other P wave is followed by a QRS complex (more Ps than QRSs)
PR interval	Constant
QRS duration	Within normal limits, if the block occurs above the bundle of His (probably type I); wide if the block occurs below the bundle of His (probably type II); absent after every other P wave

THIRD-DEGREE AV BLOCK

How Do I Recognize It?

[OBJECTIVE 5]

Second-degree AV blocks are types of *incomplete* blocks because the AV junction conducts at least some impulses to the ventricles. In third-degree AV block, impulses generated by the SA node are blocked before reaching the ventricles so no P waves are conducted. The atria and ventricles beat independently of each other. Thus third-degree AV block is also called *complete* AV block. The block may occur at the AV node, bundle of His, or bundle branches. A secondary pacemaker (either junctional or ventricular) stimulates the ventricles; therefore, the QRS may be narrow or wide, depending on the location of the escape pacemaker and the condition of the intraventricular conduction system.

Third-degree AV block associated with an inferior MI is thought to be the result of a block above the bundle of His. It often occurs after progression from first-degree AV block or second-degree AV block type I. The resulting rhythm is usually stable because the escape pacemaker is usually junctional (narrow QRS complexes) with a ventricular rate of more than 40 beats/min (Figure 7-8).

Third-degree AV block associated with an anterior MI is usually preceded by second-degree AV block type II or an intraventricular conduction delay (right or left bundle branch block). The resulting rhythm is usually unstable because the escape pacemaker is usually ventricular (wide QRS complexes) with a ventricular rate of less than 40 beats/min (Figure 7-9). The ECG characteristics of third-degree AV block are shown in Table 7-6.

What Causes It?

When associated with an inferior MI, third-degree AV block often resolves on its own within 1 week. Third-degree AV block associated with an anterior MI may develop suddenly and without warning, usually 12 to 24 hours after the onset of acute ischemia.

What Do I Do About It?

The patient's signs and symptoms will depend on the origin of the escape pacemaker (junctional vs. ventricular) and the patient's response to a slower ventricular rate. If the QRS is narrow and the patient is symptomatic due to the slow rate, initial management consists of atropine and/or transcutaneous pacing. If the QRS is wide and the patient is symptomatic due to the slow rate, transcutaneous pacing should be instituted while preparations are made for insertion of a transvenous pacemaker. Third-degree AV block that occurs with an acute anterior MI is often an indication for insertion of a permanent pacemaker.

Table 7-7 will help you learn to recognize the differences between second- and third-degree AV blocks. First, determine if the ventricular rhythm is regular or irregular. Next, look at the PR intervals. Based on this information, you should be able to identify the rhythm strips in this chapter. A summary of AV block characteristics can be found in Table 7-8.

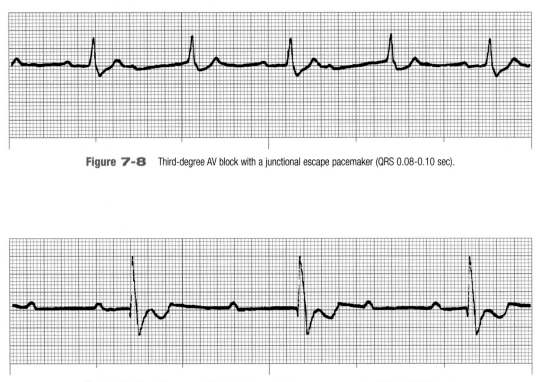

Figure 7-8   Third-degree AV block with a junctional escape pacemaker (QRS 0.08-0.10 sec).

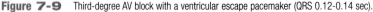

Figure 7-9   Third-degree AV block with a ventricular escape pacemaker (QRS 0.12-0.14 sec).

TABLE 7-6	Characteristics of Third-Degree AV Block
Rate	Atrial rate is greater than (and independent of) the ventricular rate; ventricular rate determined by origin of the escape rhythm
Rhythm	Atrial regular (Ps plot through on time), ventricular regular; there is no relationship between the atrial and ventricular rhythms
P waves	Normal in size and shape
PR interval	None—the atria and ventricles beat independently of each other, thus there is no true PR interval
QRS duration	Narrow or wide depending on the location of the escape pacemaker and the condition of the intraventricular conduction system; narrow = junctional pacemaker, wide = ventricular pacemaker

TABLE 7-7	AV Blocks—Quick Summary	
	Second-Degree AV Block Type I	**Second-Degree AV Block Type II**
Ventricular rhythm	Irregular	Irregular
PR interval	Progressively lengthening	Constant
QRS width	Usually narrow	Usually wide
	Second-Degree AV Block 2:1 Conduction	**Third-Degree (Complete) AV Block**
Ventricular rhythm	Regular	Regular
PR interval	Constant	None—no relationship between P waves and QRS complexes
QRS width	May be narrow or wide	May be narrow or wide

TABLE 7-8	AV Blocks—Summary of Characteristics				
	First-Degree	**Second-Degree Type I**	**Second-Degree Type II**	**Second-Degree 2:1 Conduction**	**Third-Degree (Complete)**
Rate	Usually within normal range, but depends on underlying rhythm	Atrial rate greater than ventricular rate; both often within normal limits	Atrial rate greater than ventricular rate; ventricular rate often slow	Atrial rate greater than ventricular rate	Atrial rate greater than ventricular rate; ventricular rate determined by origin of escape rhythm
Rhythm	Atrial regular, ventricular regular	Atrial regular, ventricular irregular	Atrial regular, ventricular irregular	Atrial regular, ventricular regular	Atrial regular, ventricular regular
P Waves (lead II)	Normal, one P wave precedes each QRS	Normal in size and shape; some P waves are not followed by a QRS complex (more Ps than QRSs)	Normal in size and shape; some P waves are not followed by a QRS complex (more Ps than QRSs)	Normal in size and shape; every other P wave is not followed by a QRS complex (more Ps than QRSs)	Normal in size and shape; some P waves are not followed by a QRS complex (more Ps than QRSs)
PR Interval	Greater than 0.20 sec and constant	Lengthens with each cycle until a P wave appears without a QRS	Normal or slightly prolonged but constant for conducted beats	Constant	None—the atria and ventricles beat independently of each other, thus there is no true PR interval
QRS	Usually 0.10 sec or less unless an intraventricular conduction delay exists	Usually 0.10 sec or less unless an intraventricular conduction delay exists	Usually greater than 0.10 sec, periodically absent after P waves	Within normal limits if block above bundle of His (probably type I); wide if block below bundle of His (probably type II); absent after every other P wave	Narrow or wide depending on location of escape pacemaker and condition of intraventricular conduction system

REFERENCES

1. Kahn MG: Rapid ECG interpretation, Philadelphia, 1997, WB Saunders.
2. Rusterholz AP, Marriott HJL: How long can the P-R interval be? Am J Noninvasive Cardiol 1994;8:11-13.
3. Barold SS: Indications for permanent cardiac pacing in first-degree AV block: Class I, II, or III? PACE 1996;19:747-751.
4. Phalen T, Aehlert B: The 12-lead ECG in acute coronary syndromes, St Louis 2006, Elsevier.
5. Chou T, Knilans TK: Electrocardiography in clinical practice: Adult and pediatric, Philadelphia, 1996, WB Saunders.

STOP & REVIEW

True/False

Decide whether each statement is true or false. In the space provided, write T for true or F for false.

____ 1. The site of block in second-degree AV block type II is the bundle of His or the bundle branches.

____ 2. The ventricular rhythm is regular in second-degree AV block type I.

____ 3. During a first-degree AV block, the PR intervals are completely variable because the atria and ventricles beat independently of each other.

____ 4. Second-degree AV blocks are examples of *incomplete* AV blocks.

Matching

Match each item with the correct statement below.

____ 5. A _____ escape rhythm may occur with a third-degree AV block; ventricular rate is usually 40 beats/min or less.

____ 6. Second-degree AV block type II is most commonly associated with a(n) _____ myocardial infarction.

____ 7. AV block that often progresses to a third-degree AV block without warning

____ 8. AV block characterized by regular P-P intervals, regular R-R intervals, and a PR interval with no consistent value or pattern

____ 9. PR interval pattern in second-degree AV block type II

____ 10. Second-degree AV block type I is most commonly associated with a(n) _____ myocardial infarction.

____ 11. PR interval pattern in second-degree AV block type I

____ 12. Ventricular rhythm pattern in second-degree AV block types I and II

____ 13. Normal duration of the PR interval

____ 14. AV block characterized by a PR interval greater than 0.20 second and one P wave for each QRS complex

____ 15. Location of the block in a third-degree AV block

____ 16. Ventricular rhythm pattern in second-degree AV block 2:1 conduction and third-degree AV block

____ 17. Location of the block in a second-degree AV block type II

____ 18. Common location of the block in a second-degree AV block type I

____ 19. A _____ escape rhythm may occur with a third-degree AV block, usually has a narrow QRS and a ventricular rate of 40 to 60 beats/min.

a. 0.12-0.20 sec

b. Regular

c. Bundle of His or bundle branches

d. Progressive lengthening

e. AV node

f. First-degree AV block

g. Ventricular

h. AV node, bundle of His, bundle branches

i. Inferior wall

j. Third-degree AV block

k. Junctional

l. Anterior wall

m. Irregular

n. Constant

o. Second-degree AV block type II

Short Answer

20. Indicate the ECG criteria for the following dysrhythmias.

Second-degree AV block type I	*Third-degree AV block*	*Ventricular*
Rhythm	_____	_____
PR interval	_____	_____
QRS width	_____	_____

21. Complete the following ECG criteria for second-degree AV block type I.

Rate   _____

Rhythm   _____

P waves   _____

PR interval   _____

QRS duration _____

22. Which type of AV block has the greatest potential to deteriorate to sudden, third-degree AV block?

AV BLOCKS—*PRACTICE RHYTHM STRIPS*

For each of the following rhythm strips, determine the atrial and ventricular rate and rhythm, measure the PR interval and QRS duration, and then identify the rhythm. All strips were recorded in lead II unless otherwise noted. Note: These rhythm strips also include sinus, atrial, junctional, and ventricular rhythms.

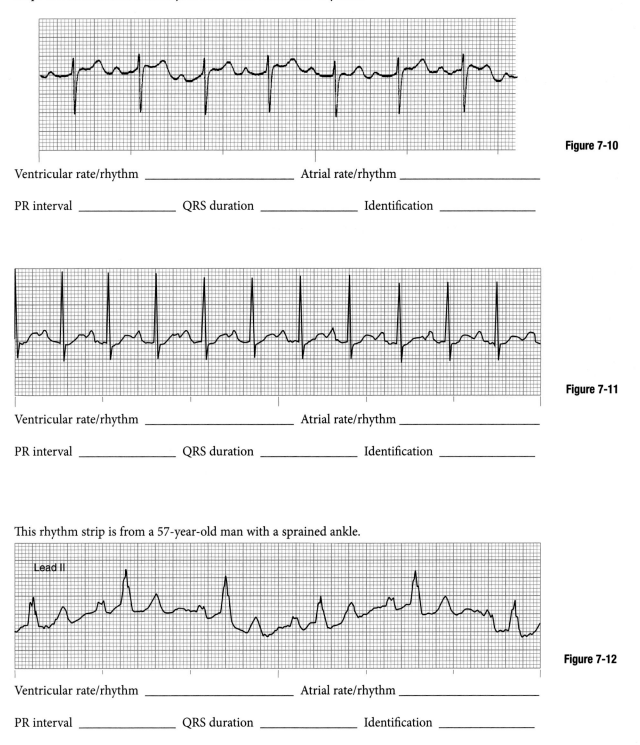

Figure 7-10

Ventricular rate/rhythm _____ Atrial rate/rhythm _____

PR interval _____ QRS duration _____ Identification _____

Figure 7-11

Ventricular rate/rhythm _____ Atrial rate/rhythm _____

PR interval _____ QRS duration _____ Identification _____

This rhythm strip is from a 57-year-old man with a sprained ankle.

Lead II

Figure 7-12

Ventricular rate/rhythm _____ Atrial rate/rhythm _____

PR interval _____ QRS duration _____ Identification _____

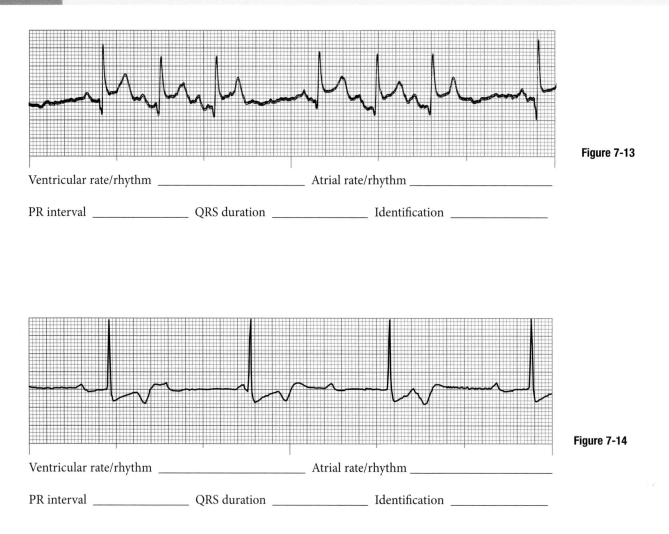

Figure 7-13

Ventricular rate/rhythm _____   Atrial rate/rhythm _____

PR interval _____   QRS duration _____   Identification _____

Figure 7-14

Ventricular rate/rhythm _____   Atrial rate/rhythm _____

PR interval _____   QRS duration _____   Identification _____

These rhythm strips are from a 77-year-old woman complaining of shortness of breath and weakness. BP 140/86.

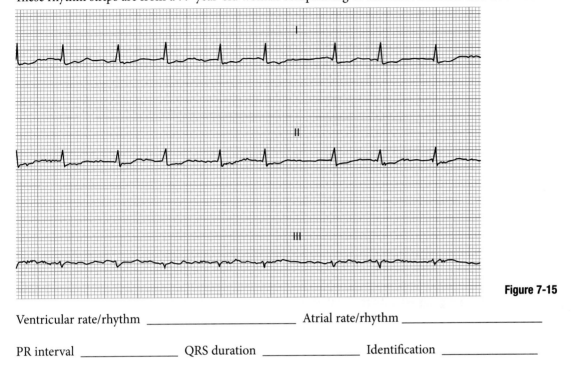

Figure 7-15

Ventricular rate/rhythm _____ Atrial rate/rhythm _____

PR interval _____ QRS duration _____ Identification _____

This rhythm strip is from a 69-year-old man complaining of shortness of breath. Lung sounds reveal bilateral crackles. Blood pressure 160/58.

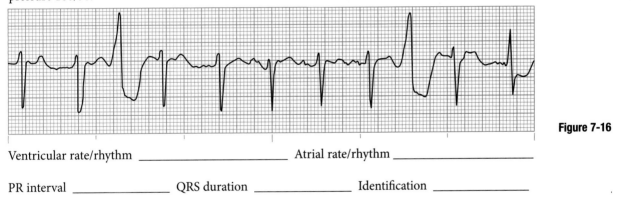

Figure 7-16

Ventricular rate/rhythm _____ Atrial rate/rhythm _____

PR interval _____ QRS duration _____ Identification _____

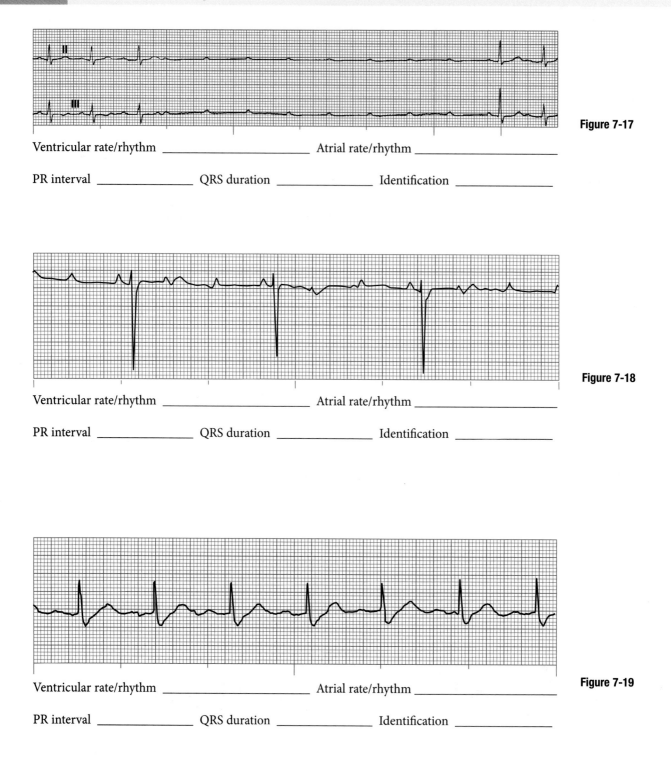

Figure 7-17

Ventricular rate/rhythm _____ Atrial rate/rhythm _____

PR interval _____ QRS duration _____ Identification _____

Figure 7-18

Ventricular rate/rhythm _____ Atrial rate/rhythm _____

PR interval _____ QRS duration _____ Identification _____

Figure 7-19

Ventricular rate/rhythm _____ Atrial rate/rhythm _____

PR interval _____ QRS duration _____ Identification _____

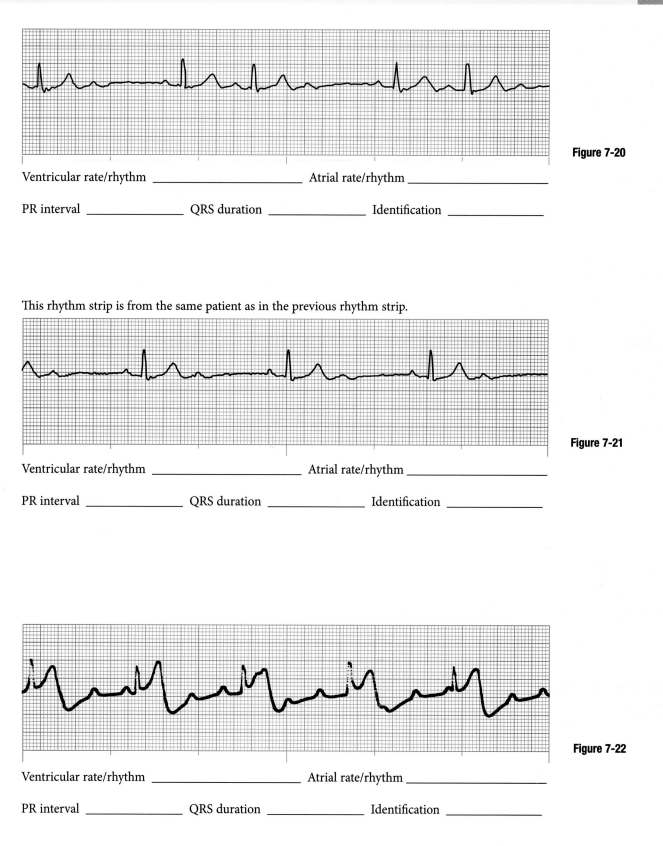

Figure 7-20

Ventricular rate/rhythm _____ Atrial rate/rhythm _____

PR interval _____ QRS duration _____ Identification _____

This rhythm strip is from the same patient as in the previous rhythm strip.

Figure 7-21

Ventricular rate/rhythm _____ Atrial rate/rhythm _____

PR interval _____ QRS duration _____ Identification _____

Figure 7-22

Ventricular rate/rhythm _____ Atrial rate/rhythm _____

PR interval _____ QRS duration _____ Identification _____

This rhythm strip is from a 77-year-old woman who stated she felt fine. She stopped at a blood pressure machine in Wal-Mart, and the machine would not read her pulse rate. She later went to her physician's office and then to the emergency department.

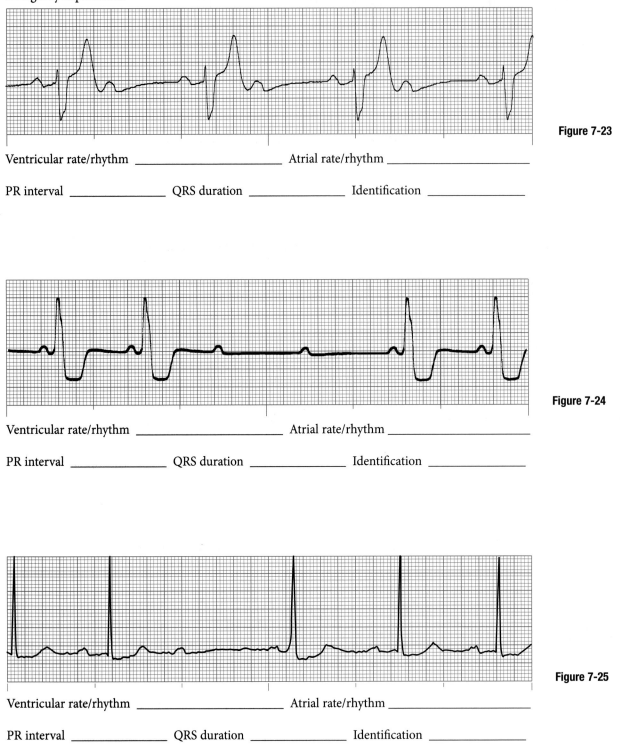

Figure 7-23

Ventricular rate/rhythm _____   Atrial rate/rhythm _____

PR interval _____   QRS duration _____   Identification _____

Figure 7-24

Ventricular rate/rhythm _____   Atrial rate/rhythm _____

PR interval _____   QRS duration _____   Identification _____

Figure 7-25

Ventricular rate/rhythm _____   Atrial rate/rhythm _____

PR interval _____   QRS duration _____   Identification _____

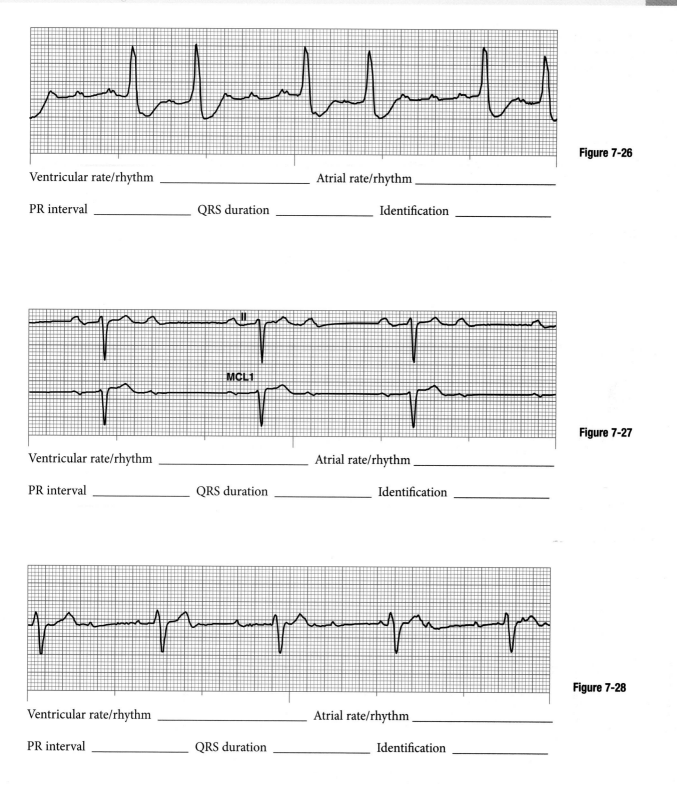

Figure 7-26

Ventricular rate/rhythm _____ Atrial rate/rhythm _____

PR interval _____ QRS duration _____ Identification _____

Figure 7-27

Ventricular rate/rhythm _____ Atrial rate/rhythm _____

PR interval _____ QRS duration _____ Identification _____

Figure 7-28

Ventricular rate/rhythm _____ Atrial rate/rhythm _____

PR interval _____ QRS duration _____ Identification _____

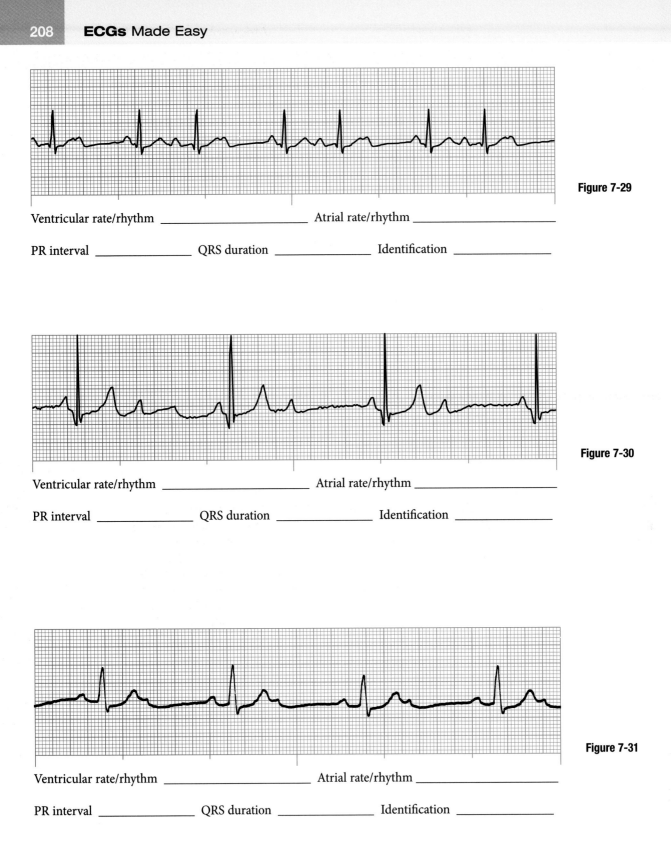

Figure 7-29

Ventricular rate/rhythm _____   Atrial rate/rhythm _____

PR interval _____   QRS duration _____   Identification _____

Figure 7-30

Ventricular rate/rhythm _____   Atrial rate/rhythm _____

PR interval _____   QRS duration _____   Identification _____

Figure 7-31

Ventricular rate/rhythm _____   Atrial rate/rhythm _____

PR interval _____   QRS duration _____   Identification _____

STOP & REVIEW ANSWERS

True/False

1. T

2. F

3. F

4. T

Matching

5. g

6. l

7. o

8. j

9. n

10. i

11. d

12. m

13. a

14. f

15. h

16. b

17. c

18. e

19. k

Short Answer

20.

	Second-degree AV block type I	*Third-degree AV block*	*Ventricular*
Rhythm		Irregular	Regular
PR interval		Progressively lengthening	None
QRS width		Usually narrow	Narrow or wide

21.

Rate	*Rhythm*	*P waves*	*PR interval*
Atrial rate is greater than the ventricular rate	Atrial regular (Ps plot through); ventricular irregular	Normal in size and shape; some P waves are not followed by a QRS complex (more Ps than QRSs)	Lengthens with each cycle (although lengthening may be very slight), until a P wave appears without a QRS complex; the PR interval after the nonconducted beat is shorter than the interval preceding the nonconducted beat QRS duration Usually 0.10 sec or less but is periodically dropped

22. Second-degree AV block type II

Figure 7-10 answer

Ventricular rate/rhythm	88 beats/min, regular
Atrial rate/rhythm	88 beats/min, regular
PR interval	0.28 sec
QRS duration	0.08 sec
Identification	Sinus rhythm at 88 beats/min with first-degree AV block; ST-segment elevation

Figure 7-11 answer

Ventricular rate/rhythm	107 beats/min, regular
Atrial rate/rhythm	107 beats/min, regular
PR interval	0.24 sec
QRS duration	0.08 sec
Identification	Sinus tachycardia at 107 beats/min with first-degree AV block

Figure 7-12 answer

Ventricular rate/rhythm	54 beats/min, regular
Atrial rate/rhythm	54 beats/min, regular
PR interval	0.28 sec
QRS duration	0.12 sec
Identification	Sinus bradycardia at 54 beats/min with first-degree AV block, notched P waves and a wide, notched QRS

Figure 7-13 answer

Ventricular rate/rhythm	50 to 94 beats/min, irregular
Atrial rate/rhythm	94 beats/min, regular
PR interval	Lengthens
QRS duration	0.10 sec
Identification	Second-degree AV block type I at 50 to 94 beats/min, ST-segment elevation

Figure 7-14 answer

Ventricular rate/rhythm	38 beats/min, regular
Atrial rate/rhythm	68 beats/min, regular
PR interval	Varies
QRS duration	0.06 sec
Identification	Third-degree AV block at 38 beats/min with ST-segment depression and inverted T waves

Figure 7-15 answer

Ventricular rate/rhythm	94 to 107 beats/min, irregular
Atrial rate/rhythm	Unable to determine
PR interval	None
QRS duration	0.06 sec
Identification	Atrial fibrillation at 94 to 107 beats/min with ST-segment depression

Figure 7-16 answer

Ventricular rate/rhythm	107 beats/min (sinus beats), regular
Atrial rate/rhythm	107 beats/min (sinus beats), regular
PR interval	0.20 sec (sinus beats)
QRS duration	0.08 sec (sinus beats)
Identification	Sinus tachycardia at 107 beats/min with uniform PVCs

Figure 7-17 answer

Ventricular rate/rhythm	Less than 20 to 94 beats/min, irregular
Atrial rate/rhythm	94 beats/min, regular
PR interval	Lengthens
QRS duration	0.08 sec
Identification	Second-degree AV block type I at less than 20 to 94 beats/min (leads II and III)

Figure 7-18 answer

Ventricular rate/rhythm	36 beats/min, regular
Atrial rate/rhythm	108 beats/min, regular
PR interval	0.16 sec
QRS duration	0.08 to 0.10 sec
Identification	High-grade second-degree AV block with 3:1 conduction at 36 beats/min

Figure 7-19 answer

Ventricular rate/rhythm	68 beats/min, regular
Atrial rate/rhythm	68 beats/min, regular
PR interval	0.28 sec
QRS	0.06 sec
Identification	Sinus rhythm with first-degree AV block at 68 beats/min, ST-segment depression

Figure 7-20 answer

Ventricular rate/rhythm	75 beats/min, regular
Atrial rate/rhythm	None
PR interval	None
QRS duration	0.08 sec
Identification	Accelerated junctional rhythm at 75 beats/min; ST-segment depression

Figure 7-21 answer

Ventricular rate/rhythm	36 beats/min, regular
Atrial rate/rhythm	72 beats/min, regular
PR interval	0.20 to 0.22 sec
QRS duration	0.06 to 0.08 sec
Identification	2:1 AV block, probably type I at 36 beats/min

Figure 7-22 answer

Ventricular rate/rhythm	50 beats/min, regular
Atrial rate/rhythm	167 beats/min, regular
PR interval	Varies
QRS duration	0.06 sec
Identification	Third-degree AV block at 50 beats/min, ST-segment elevation

Figure 7-23 answer

Ventricular rate/rhythm	30 beats/min, regular
Atrial rate/rhythm	68 beats/min, regular
PR interval	0.28 sec
QRS duration	0.16 sec
Identification	2:1 AV block, probably type II at 30 beats/min; ST-segment elevation

Figure 7-24 answer

Ventricular rate/rhythm	Less than 20 to 60 beats/min, irregular
Atrial rate/rhythm	60 beats/min, regular
PR interval	0.16 sec
QRS duration	0.12 sec
Identification	Second-degree AV block type II at less than 20 to 60 beats/min, ST-segment depression

Figure 7-25 answer

Ventricular rate/rhythm	28 to 58 beats/min, irregular
Atrial rate/rhythm	58 beats/min, regular
PR interval	Lengthens
QRS duration	0.06 to 0.08 sec
Identification	Second-degree AV block type I at 28 to 58 beats/min, ST-segment depression

Figure 7-26 answer

Ventricular rate/rhythm	48 to 83 beats/min, irregular
Atrial rate/rhythm	167 beats/min, regular
PR interval	0.24 sec
QRS duration	0.12 sec
Identification	Second-degree AV block type II at 48 to 83 beats/min; ST-segment depression

Figure 7-27 answer

Ventricular rate/rhythm	36 beats/min, regular
Atrial rate/rhythm	72 beats/min, regular
PR interval	0.32 sec
QRS duration	0.12-0.14 sec
Identification	2:1 AV block, probably type II at 36 beats/min

Figure 7-28 answer

Ventricular rate/rhythm	45 beats/min, regular
Atrial rate/rhythm	115 beats/min, regular
PR interval	Varies
QRS duration	0.16 sec
Identification	Third-degree AV block at 45 beats/min

Figure 7-29 answer

Ventricular rate/rhythm	60 to 98 beats/min, irregular
Atrial rate/rhythm	111 beats/min, regular
PR interval	Lengthens
QRS duration	0.08 sec
Identification	Second-degree AV block type I at 68 to 90 beats/min; ST-segment depression

Figure 7-30 answer

Ventricular rate/rhythm	34 beats/min, regular
Atrial rate/rhythm	68 beats/min, regular
PR interval	0.14 to 0.16 sec
QRS duration	0.10 sec
Identification	2:1 AV block, probably type I at 34 beats/min; ST-segment depression; tall T waves

Figure 7-31 answer

Ventricular rate/rhythm	40 beats/min, regular
Atrial rate/rhythm	83 beats/min, regular
PR interval	0.24 sec
QRS duration	0.12 sec
Identification	2:1 AV block, probably type II at 40 beats/min; ST-segment depression

Pacemaker Rhythms

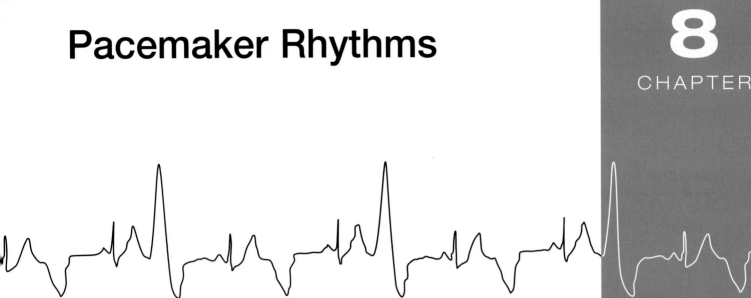

OBJECTIVES

On completion of this chapter, you will be able to:

1. Define the following terms: sensing, capture, asynchronous, synchronous, threshold.
2. Identify the components of a pacemaker system.
3. Describe a unipolar and bipolar pacing electrode.
4. Explain the differences between fixed-rate and demand pacemakers.
5. Describe the primary pacing modes.
6. Identify the cardiac chamber(s) stimulated by different pacing methods.
7. Describe the appearance of a typical pacemaker spike on the ECG.
8. Describe the appearance of the waveform on the ECG produced as a result of atrial pacing and ventricular pacing.
9. Describe the benefits of AV sequential pacing.
10. Identify the primary indications for transcutaneous pacing.
11. Describe the procedure for transcutaneous pacing.
12. List three types of pacemaker malfunction.
13. Identify possible complications of pacing.
14. Describe how to analyze pacemaker function on the ECG.

PACEMAKER TERMINOLOGY

[OBJECTIVE 1]

A wave: Atrial paced event; the atrial stimulus or the point in the intrinsic atrial depolarization (P wave) at which atrial sensing occurs; analogous to the P wave of intrinsic waveforms.

AA interval: Interval between two consecutive atrial stimuli, with or without an interceding ventricular event; analogous to the P-P interval of intrinsic waveforms.

Asynchronous pacemaker: (Fixed-rate) pacemaker that continuously discharges at a preset rate regardless of the patient's intrinsic activity.

Atrial pacing: Pacing system with a lead attached to the right atrium designed to correct abnormalities in the SA node (sick sinus syndrome).

Automatic interval: Period, expressed in milliseconds, between two consecutive paced events in the same cardiac chamber without an intervening sensed event (e.g., AA interval, VV interval); also known as the demand interval, basic interval, or pacing interval.

AV interval: In dual-chamber pacing, the length of time between an atrial sensed or atrial paced event and the delivery of a ventricular pacing stimulus; analogous to the PR interval of intrinsic waveforms; also called the artificial or electronic PR interval.

AV sequential pacemaker: Pacemaker that stimulates first the atrium, then the ventricle, mimicking normal cardiac physiology; a type of dual-chamber pacemaker.

Base rate: Rate at which the pulse generator paces when no intrinsic activity is detected; expressed in pulses per minute (ppm).

Bipolar lead: Pacing lead with two electrical poles that are external from the pulse generator; the negative pole is located at the extreme distal tip of the pacing lead; the positive pole is located several millimeters proximal to the negative electrode; the stimulating pulse is delivered through the negative electrode.

Capture: Ability of a pacing stimulus to successfully depolarize the cardiac chamber that is being paced; with one-to-one capture, each pacing stimulus results in depolarization of the appropriate chamber.

Demand (synchronous) pacemaker: Pacemaker that discharges only when the patient's heart rate drops below the preset rate for the pacemaker.

Dual-chamber pacemaker: Pacemaker that stimulates the atrium and ventricle; dual-chamber pacing is also called physiologic pacing.

Escape interval: Time measured between a sensed cardiac event and the next pacemaker output.

Fusion beat: In pacing, the ECG waveform that results when an intrinsic depolarization and a pacing stimulus occur simultaneously, and both contribute to depolarization of that cardiac chamber.

Hysteresis: Programmable feature in some demand pacemakers that allows programming of a longer escape interval between the intrinsic complex and the first paced event; the longer escape interval allows intrinsic beats an opportunity to inhibit the pacemaker.

Inhibition: Pacemaker response in which the output pulse is suppressed (inhibited) when an intrinsic event is sensed.

Interval: Period, measured in milliseconds, between any two designated cardiac events; in pacing, intervals are more useful than rate because pacemaker timing is based on intervals.

Intrinsic: Inherent; naturally occurring.

Milliampere (mA): Unit of measure of electrical current needed to elicit depolarization of the myocardium.

Output: Electrical stimulus delivered by the pulse generator, usually defined in terms of pulse amplitude (volts) and pulse width (milliseconds).

Pacemaker: Artificial pulse generator that delivers an electrical current to the heart to stimulate depolarization.

Pacemaker spike: Vertical line on the ECG that indicates the pacemaker has discharged.

Pacemaker syndrome: Adverse clinical signs and symptoms that limit a patient's everyday functioning and occur in the setting of an electrically normal pacing system; common signs and symptoms include weakness, fatigue, dizziness, near or full syncope, cough, chest pain, hypotension, dyspnea, and congestive heart failure; pacemaker syndrome is most commonly associated with a loss of AV synchrony (e.g., VVI pacing) but may also occur because of an inappropriate AV interval or inappropriate rate modulation.

Pacing interval: Period, expressed in milliseconds, between two consecutive paced events in the same cardiac chamber without an intervening sensed event (e.g., AA interval, VV interval); also known as the demand interval, basic interval, or automatic interval.

Pacing system analyzer (PSA): External testing and measuring device capable of pacing the heart during pacemaker implantation; used to determine appropriate pulse generator settings for the individual patient (e.g., pacing threshold, lead impedance, pulse amplitude).

Parameter: Value that can be measured and sometimes changed, either indirectly or directly; in pacing, parameter refers to a value that influences the function of the pacemaker (e.g., sensitivity, amplitude, mode).

Pulse generator: Power source that houses the battery and controls for regulating a pacemaker.

Rate modulation: Ability of a pacemaker to increase the pacing rate in response to physical activity or metabolic demand; some type of physiologic sensor is used by the pacemaker to determine the need for an increased pacing rate; also called rate adaptation or rate response.

R wave: In pacing, R wave refers to the entire QRS complex denoting an intrinsic ventricular event.

RV interval: Period from the intrinsic ventricular event and the ventricular-paced event that follows; the pacemaker's escape interval.

Sensing: Ability of a pacemaker to recognize and respond to intrinsic electrical activity; the pacemaker's response to sensed activity depends on its programmed mode and parameters.

Threshold: Minimum level of electrical current needed to consistently depolarize the myocardium.

Unipolar lead: Pacing lead with a single electrical pole at the distal tip of the pacing lead (negative pole) through which the stimulating pulse is delivered; in a permanent pacemaker with a unipolar lead, the positive pole is the pulse generator case.

V-A interval: In dual-chamber pacing, the interval between a sensed or ventricular-paced event and the next atrial-paced event.

V-V interval: Interval between two ventricular-paced events.

V wave: Ventricular-paced event; the ventricular stimulus or the point in the intrinsic ventricular depolarization (R wave) during which ventricular sensing occurs.

Ventricular pacing: Pacing system with a lead attached in the right ventricle.

PACEMAKER SYSTEMS

Introduction

[OBJECTIVE 2]

A **pacemaker** is an artificial pulse generator that delivers an electrical current to the heart to stimulate depolarization. Pacemaker systems are usually named according to where the electrodes are located and the route the electrical current takes to the heart. A pacemaker system consists of a **pulse generator** (power source) and pacing lead(s) (Figure 8-1). The pulse generator houses a battery and electronic circuitry. The circuitry works like a computer, converting energy from the battery into electrical pulses. A pacing lead is an insulated wire used to carry an electrical impulse from the pacemaker to the patient's heart. It also carries information about the heart's electrical activity back to the pacemaker. The exposed portion of the pacing lead is called an *electrode*, which is placed in direct contact with the heart.

Permanent Pacemakers

A permanent pacemaker is implanted in the body, usually under local anesthesia. Pacemaker wires are surrounded by plastic insulation. The pacemaker's circuitry is housed in a hermetically sealed case made of titanium that is airtight and impermeable to fluid.

The electrode of a permanent pacemaker may be unipolar or bipolar. It is placed transvenously or surgically. Once the electrode is in place, the pulse generator is usually implanted

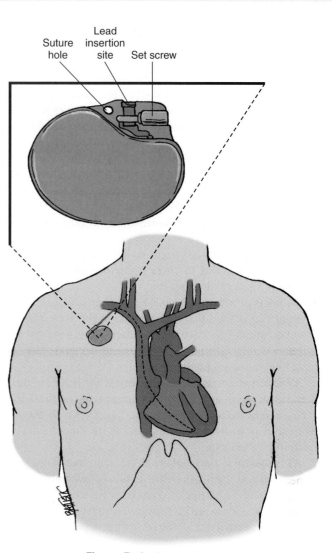

Figure 8-1 Permanent pacemaker.

into the subcutaneous tissue of the anterior chest just below the right or left clavicle. The electrode is then connected to the pulse generator. The patient's handedness, occupation, and hobbies determine whether the pacemaker is implanted on the right or left side. The nondominant side is usually chosen to minimize interference with the patient's daily activities.[1]

Lithium batteries are almost exclusively used in modern pacemakers. Battery life depends on the following:
- How much energy is required for capture
- The percentage of time the device paces
- The number of cardiac chambers paced

When the battery gets low, the entire pacemaker is replaced because the battery is sealed inside the pacemaker.

Indications

Indications for insertion of a permanent pacemaker typically include the following:[2]
- Third-degree AV block
- Symptomatic type II second-degree block

- Second-degree AV block with episodic ventricular arrhythmias
- Sick sinus syndrome
- Symptomatic bradycardias with syncope or presyncope
- Hypersensitive carotid artery syndrome
- Type I block with infra-His bundle block
- Specific subgroups of patients with triphasic and biphasic blocks at risk of developing sudden high-degree block

Temporary Pacemakers

The pulse generator of a temporary pacemaker is located externally. Temporary pacing can be accomplished through transvenous, epicardial, or transcutaneous means.

- Transvenous pacemakers stimulate the endocardium of the right atrium or ventricle (or both) by means of an electrode introduced into a central vein, such as the subclavian or cephalic vein.
- Epicardial pacing is the placement of pacing leads directly onto or through the epicardium. Epicardial leads may be used when a patient is undergoing surgery and the outer surface of the heart is easy to reach. They are frequently used in neonates, children, and adolescents because of cardiac anatomy, small body size, and/or difficulty accessing the superior vena cava.
- Transcutaneous pacing delivers pacing impulses to the heart using electrodes placed on the patient's thorax. Transcutaneous pacing is also called *temporary external pacing* or *noninvasive pacing* and is discussed later in this chapter.

Indications

Indications for emergent temporary pacing include the following:

- Hemodynamically significant bradycardia (blood pressure less than 80 mm Hg systolic, change in mental status, pulmonary edema, angina)
- Bradycardia with escape rhythms unresponsive to drug therapy
- **Overdrive pacing** of tachycardia-supraventricular or ventricular-refractory to pharmacologic therapy or electrical countershock. (During overdrive pacing, the heart is paced briefly [seconds] at a rate faster than the rate of the tachycardia. The pacemaker is then stopped to allow return of the heart's intrinsic pacemaker).

Pacemaker Electrodes

Unipolar Electrodes
[OBJECTIVE 3]

There are two types of pacemaker electrodes: unipolar and bipolar. A unipolar electrode has one pacing electrode that is located at its distal tip (Figure 8-2). The negative electrode is in contact with the heart, and the pulse generator (located outside the heart) functions as the positive electrode. The **pacemaker spikes** produced by a unipolar electrode are often large because of the distance between the positive and negative electrodes.

Bipolar Electrodes
[OBJECTIVE 3]

A bipolar pacemaker electrode contains a positive and negative electrode at the distal tip of the pacing lead wire. Most temporary transvenous pacemakers have bipolar electrodes.

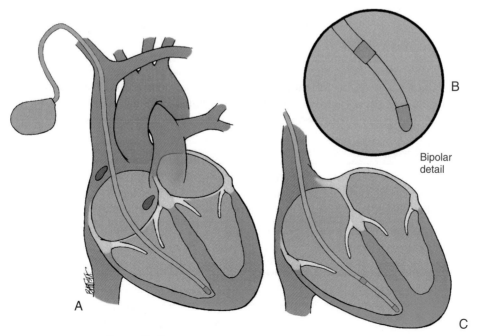

Bipolar detail

Figure 8-2 **A,** Unipolar and **(B, C)** bipolar pacemaker electrodes.

A permanent pacemaker may have either a bipolar or a unipolar electrode. The spike produced by a bipolar electrode is often small and difficult to see.

PACEMAKER MODES

Fixed-Rate (Asynchronous) Pacemakers

[OBJECTIVE 4]

A **fixed-rate pacemaker** continuously discharges at a preset rate (usually 70–80/min) regardless of the patient's heart rate. An advantage of the fixed-rate pacemaker is its simple circuitry, reducing the risk of pacemaker failure. However, this type of pacemaker does not sense the patient's own cardiac rhythm. This may result in competition between the patient's cardiac rhythm and that of the pacemaker. Ventricular tachycardia (VT) or ventricular fibrillation (VF) may be induced if the pacemaker were to fire during the T wave (vulnerable period) of a preceding patient beat. Fixed-rate pacemakers are not often used today.

Demand (Synchronous, Noncompetitive) Pacemakers

[OBJECTIVE 4]

A **demand pacemaker** discharges only when the patient's heart rate drops below the pacemaker's preset (base) rate. For example, if the demand pacemaker was preset at a rate of 70 impulses per minute, it would sense the patient's heart rate and allow electrical impulses to flow from the pacemaker through the pacing lead to stimulate the heart only when the rate fell below 70 beats/min. Demand pacemakers can be programmable or nonprogrammable. The voltage level and impulse rate are preset at the time of manufacture in nonprogrammable pacemakers.

Pacemaker Identification Codes

[OBJECTIVE 5]

Pacemaker identification codes are used to assist in identifying a pacemaker's preprogrammed pacing, sensing, and response functions (Table 8-1). The first three letters are used for

antibradycardia functions. The *first letter* of the code identifies the heart chamber (or chambers) paced (stimulated). The options available are:

O, none
A, atrium
V, ventricle
D, dual (both atrium and ventricle)

A pacemaker used to pace only a single chamber is represented by either A (atrial) or V (ventricular). A pacemaker capable of pacing in both chambers is represented by D (dual).

The *second letter* identifies the chamber of the heart where patient-initiated (intrinsic) electrical activity is sensed by the pacemaker. The letter designations for the second letter are the same as the designations for the first.

The *third letter* indicates how the pacemaker will respond when it senses patient-initiated electrical activity:

O, no sensing
T, a pacemaker stimulus is triggered in response to a sensed event
I, sensing of intrinsic impulses inhibits the pacemaker from producing a stimulus
D, dual (a combination of triggered pacing and inhibition)

Commonly encountered pacing modes are VVI, DVI, DDD, and DDDR.

The *fourth letter* is most often used in permanent pacing and identifies the availability of rate responsiveness and the number of reprogrammable functions available. A pacemaker's rate responsiveness may also be referred to as *rate modulation* or *rate adaptation*.

O, the pacemaker is not programmable or rate responsive (most commonly found on devices manufactured before mid-1970s)
P, simple programmability where the pacemaker is limited to one or two programmable parameters (such as rate or output)
M, multiprogrammability (i.e., more than two variables can be altered)
C, capability of transmitting and/or receiving data for informational or programming purposes
R, rate responsiveness, denoting the pacemaker's ability to automatically adjust its rate to meet the body's needs caused by increased physical activity

TABLE **8-1**	Pacemaker Codes			
Chamber Paced (First Letter)	Chamber Sensed (Second Letter)	Response To Sensing (Third Letter)	Programmable Functions (Fourth Letter)	Antitachycardia Functions (Fifth Letter)
O = None	O = None (fixed-rate pacemaker)	O = None (fixed-rate pacemaker)	O = None	O = None
A = Atrium	A = Atrium	T = Triggers pacing	P = Simple programmability (rate and/or output)	P = Pacing (antitachycardia)
V = Ventricle	V = Ventricle	I = Inhibits pacing	M = Multiprogrammable	S = Shock
D = Dual chamber (atrium and ventricle)	D = Dual chamber (atrium and ventricle)	D = Dual (triggers and inhibits pacing)	C = Communication	D = Dual (pacing and shock)
			R = Rate responsive	

The *fifth letter* indicates the presence of one or more active antitachycardia functions and indicates how the pacemaker will respond to tachydysrhythmias:

O, the device has no antitachycardia functions

P, the device is capable of antitachycardia pacing

S, the device is capable of delivering synchronized and unsynchronized countershocks

D, the device is capable of antitachycardia pacing, synchronized and unsynchronized countershocks

Implantable cardioverter defibrillators (ICDs) use the features designated by the fourth letter in the management of tachydysrhythmias.

When the SA node is diseased, the body loses its ability to physiologically adjust the heart rate in response to physical or emotional stressors. Rate-responsive pacemakers contain an artificial sensor (or more than one sensor) that detects physiologic changes and adjusts the heart rate accordingly. Two common types of sensors are an activity sensor and a minute ventilation sensor. When the patient's activity increases, the sensor becomes the regulator of the patient's heart rate. The sensor detects a signal indicating a need for a rate faster than the pacemaker's base rate and instructs the pacemaker to provide electrical stimuli (output) at the sensor-indicated rate. The patient's physician determines the pacemaker's base rate and the upper sensor-driven rate of the device.

Metabolic parameters and nonmetabolic markers can be used to assess the body's physiologic demands. For example, vibration sensors detect body movement, impedance sensors detect respiratory rate and minute ventilation, and special sensors on the pacing electrode can detect central venous temperature, right atrial pressure, pH, and catecholamine levels, among other parameters.

Single-Chamber Pacemakers

[OBJECTIVE 6, 7, 8]

A pacemaker that paces a single heart chamber (either the atrium or ventricle) has one lead placed in the heart. Atrial pacing is achieved by placing the pacing electrode in the right atrium. Stimulation of the atria produces a pacemaker spike on the ECG, followed by a P wave (Figure 8-3). Atrial pacing may be used when the SA node is diseased or damaged, but conduction through the AV junction and ventricles is normal. This type of pacemaker is ineffective if an AV block develops because it cannot pace the ventricles.

Ventricular pacing is accomplished by placing the pacing electrode in the right ventricle. Stimulation of the ventricles produces a pacemaker spike on the ECG followed by a wide QRS, resembling a ventricular ectopic beat (Figure 8-4). The QRS complex is wide because a paced impulse does not follow the normal conduction pathway in the heart.

A single-chamber ventricular pacemaker can pace the ventricles but cannot coordinate pacing with the patient's intrinsic atrial rate. This results in asynchronous contraction of the atrium and ventricle (AV asynchrony). Because of this loss of AV synchrony, a ventricular demand pacemaker is rarely used in a patient with an intact SA node. Conversely, a ventricular demand pacemaker may be used for the patient with chronic atrial fibrillation.

The **ventricular demand (VVI) pacemaker** is a common type of pacemaker. With this device, the pacemaker electrode is placed in the right ventricle (V); the ventricle is sensed (V) and the pacemaker is inhibited (I) when spontaneous ventricular depolarization occurs within a preset interval. When spontaneous ventricular depolarization does not occur within

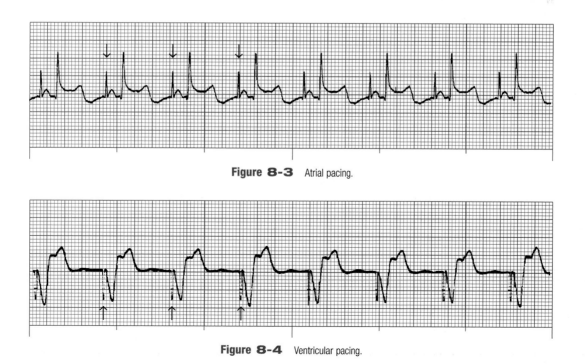

Figure 8-3 Atrial pacing.

Figure 8-4 Ventricular pacing.

this preset interval, the pacemaker fires and stimulates ventricular depolarization at a preset rate.

Because a VVI pacemaker does not sense or pace atrial activity, P waves can appear anywhere in the cardiac cycle, with no relation to the QRS complexes. A disadvantage of VVI pacing is its fixed rate, regardless of the patient's level of physical activity.

Dual-Chamber Pacemakers

[OBJECTIVE 6, 7, 8]

A pacemaker that paces both the atrium and ventricle has a two-lead system placed in the heart—one lead is placed in the right atrium, the other in the right ventricle. This type of pacemaker is called a dual-chamber pacemaker (Figure 8-5). Dual-chamber pacing is also called physiologic pacing. An **AV sequential pacemaker** is an example of a dual-chamber pacemaker. The AV sequential pacemaker stimulates the right atrium and right ventricle sequentially (stimulating first the atrium, then the ventricle), mimicking normal cardiac physiology and thus preserving the atrial contribution to ventricular filling (atrial kick) (Figure 8-6).

The dual-chamber pacemaker may also be called a DDD pacemaker, indicating that both the atrium and ventricle are paced (D), both chambers are sensed (D), and the pacemaker has both a triggered and inhibited mode of response (D). When spontaneous atrial depolarization does not occur within a preset interval, the atrial pulse generator fires and stimulates atrial depolarization at a preset rate. The pacemaker is programmed to wait—simulating the normal delay in conduction through the AV node (the PR interval). The "artificial" or "electronic" PR interval is referred to as an **AV interval**. If spontaneous ventricular depolarization does not occur within a preset interval, the pacemaker fires and stimulates ventricular depolarization at a preset rate.

The presence of a dual-chamber pacemaker does not necessarily mean that the pacemaker is in DDD mode. Dual-chamber pacemakers can be programmed to VVI mode, depending on patient need (such as the development of chronic atrial fibrillation).

TRANSCUTANEOUS PACING

Transcutaneous pacing (TCP) is the use of electrical stimulation through pacing pads positioned on a patient's torso to stimulate contraction of the heart. Although TCP is a type of electrical therapy, the current delivered is considerably less than that used for cardioversion or defibrillation. The energy levels selected for cardioversion or defibrillation are indicated in joules. The stimulating current selected for TCP is measured in **milliamperes** (mA). The range of output current of a transcutaneous pacemaker varies depending on the manufacturer. For example, the range of output current for one brand of transcutaneous pacemaker is 0 to 140 mA. The range for another brand is 0 to 200 mA. Most transcutaneous pacemakers have a heart rate selection that ranges from 30 to 180 beats/min. You must be familiar with your equipment before you need to use it.

TCP requires attaching two pacing electrodes to the skin surface of the patient's outer chest wall. The pacing pads used during TCP function as a bipolar pacing system. The electrical signal exits from the negative terminal on the machine (and subsequently the negative electrode) and passes through the chest wall to the heart. Small or medium pediatric electrodes should be used for a child weighing less than 15 kg. Adult electrodes should be used for a child weighing more than 15 kg.

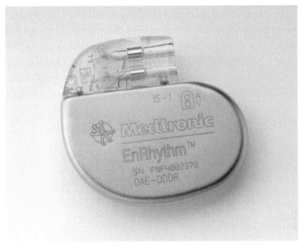

Figure 8-5 An example of a dual-chamber pacemaker.

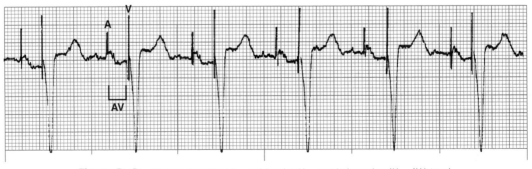

Figure 8-6 AV sequential pacing. A = atrial pacing, V = ventricular pacing, AV = AV interval.

Indications

[OBJECTIVE 10, 11]

TCP is effective, quick, safe, and the least invasive pacing technique currently available. TCP is indicated for significant bradycardias unresponsive to atropine therapy or when atropine is not immediately available or indicated. It may also be used as a bridge until transvenous pacing can be accomplished or the cause of the bradycardia is reversed (as in cases of drug overdose or hyperkalemia). The steps to perform TCP are shown in Skill 8-1.

The primary limitation of TCP is patient discomfort that is proportional to the intensity of skeletal muscle contraction and the direct electrical stimulation of cutaneous nerves (Table 8-2). The degree of discomfort varies with the device used and the stimulating current required to achieve

---

SKILL 8-1   Transcutaneous Pacing

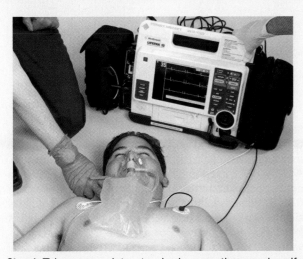

Step 1 Take appropriate standard precautions and verify that the procedure is indicated. Place the patient on oxygen, assess the patient's vital signs, establish IV access, and apply ECG electrodes. Identify the rhythm on the cardiac monitor. Record a rhythm strip and verify the presence of a paceable rhythm. Continuous monitoring of the patient's ECG is *essential* throughout the procedure.

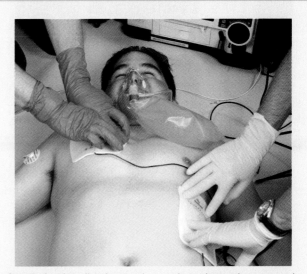

Step 2 Apply adhesive pacing pads to the patient according to the manufacturer's recommendations. Do not place the pads over open cuts, sores, or metal objects. The pacing pads should fit completely on the patient's chest; have a minimum of 1 to 2 inches of space between electrodes (pads); and not overlap bony areas of the sternum, spine, or scapula.

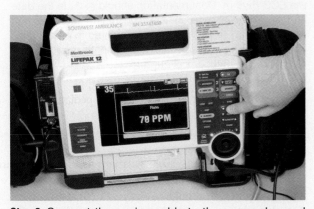

Step 3 Connect the pacing cable to the pacemaker and to the adhesive pads on the patient. Turn the power on to the pacemaker. Set the pacing rate to the desired number of paced pulses per minute (ppm). In an adult, set the initial rate at a nonbradycardic rate between 60 and 80 beats/min.

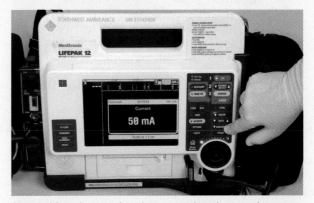

Step 4 After the rate has been regulated, start the pacemaker. Increase the stimulating current (output or milliamperes) until pacer spikes are visible before each QRS complex. Increase the current slowly but steadily until capture is achieved. Sedation or analgesia may be needed to minimize the discomfort associated with this procedure (common with currents of 50 mA or more). Give medications according to local protocol or physician instructions.

Continued

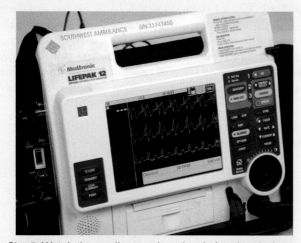

Step 5 Watch the cardiac monitor closely for *electrical* capture. This usually is seen by a wide QRS and broad T wave. In some patients electrical capture is less obvious—indicated only as a change in the shape of the QRS.

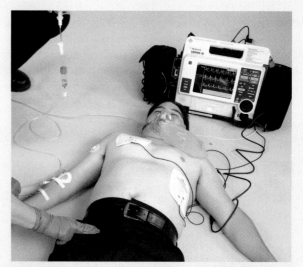

Step 6 Assess *mechanical* capture. Mechanical capture occurs when pacing produces a response that can be measured, such as a palpable pulse and blood pressure. Assess mechanical capture by assessing the patient's right upper extremity or right femoral pulses. Once capture is achieved, continue pacing at an output level slightly higher (approximately 2 mA) than the threshold of initial electrical capture. For example, if the monitor reveals 100% capture when you reached 80 mA, your final setting would be 82 mA.

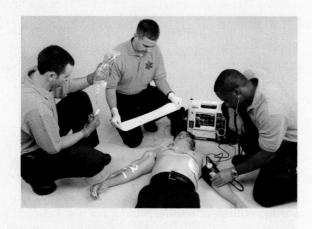

Step 7 Assess the patient's blood pressure, SpO$_2$, and level of responsiveness. Closely monitor the patient, including assessment of the skin for irritation where the pacing pads have been applied. Document and record the ECG rhythm. Documentation should include the date and time pacing was initiated (including baseline and pacing rhythm strips), the current required to obtain capture, the pacing rate selected, the patient's responses to electrical and mechanical capture, medications administered during the procedure, and the date and time pacing was terminated (if applicable).

capture. Increased chest wall muscle mass, chronic obstructive pulmonary disease (COPD), or pleural effusions may require increased stimulating current.[5]

PACEMAKER MALFUNCTION

Failure to Pace

[OBJECTIVE 12]

Failure to pace (also referred to as *failure to fire)* is a pacemaker malfunction that occurs when the pacemaker fails to deliver an electrical stimulus or when it fails to deliver the correct number of electrical stimulations per minute. Failure to pace is recognized on the ECG as an absence of pacemaker spikes (even though the patient's intrinsic rate is less than that of the pacemaker) and a return of the underlying rhythm for which the pacemaker was implanted. Patient signs and symptoms may include syncope, chest pain, bradycardia, and hypotension.

Causes of failure to pace include battery failure, fracture of the pacing lead wire, displacement of the electrode tip, pulse generator failure, a broken or loose connection between the pacing lead and the pulse generator, electromagnetic interference, and/or the sensitivity setting set too high. Treatment may include adjusting the sensitivity setting, replacing the

TABLE 8-2	Patient Responses to Current with Transcutaneous Pacing
Output (mA)*	Patient Response
20	Prickly sensation on skin
30	Slight thump on chest
40	Definite thump on chest
50	Coughing
60	Diaphragm pacing and coughing
70	Coughing and knock on chest
80	More uncomfortable than 70 mA
90	Strong, painful knock on chest
100	Leaves bed because of pain

*Responses with Zoll-NTP
From Flynn JB: *Introduction to critical care skills,* St Louis, 1993, Mosby.

pulse generator battery, replacing the pacing lead, replacing the pulse generator unit, tightening connections between the pacing lead and pulse generator, performing an electrical check, and/or removing the source of electromagnetic interference.

Failure to Capture

[OBJECTIVE 12]

Capture is successful depolarization of the atria and/or ventricles by an artificial pacemaker and is obtained after the pacemaker electrode is properly positioned in the heart. Failure to capture is the inability of the pacemaker stimulus to depolarize the myocardium and is recognized on the ECG by visible pacemaker spikes not followed by P waves (if the electrode is located in the atrium) or QRS complexes (if the electrode is located in the right ventricle) (Figure 8-7). Patient signs and symptoms may include fatigue, bradycardia, and hypotension.

Causes of failure to capture include battery failure, fracture of the pacing lead wire, displacement of pacing lead wire (common cause), perforation of the myocardium by a lead wire, edema or scar tissue formation at the electrode tip, output energy (mA) set too low (common cause), and/or increased stimulation threshold because of medications,

electrolyte imbalance, or increased fibrin formation on the catheter tip.

Treatment may include repositioning the patient, slowly increasing the output setting (mA) until capture occurs or the maximum setting is reached, replacing the pulse generator battery, replacing or repositioning of the pacing lead, or surgery.

Failure to Sense (Undersensing)

[OBJECTIVE 12]

Sensitivity is the extent to which a pacemaker recognizes intrinsic electrical activity. Failure to sense occurs when the pacemaker fails to recognize spontaneous myocardial depolarization (Figure 8-8). This pacemaker malfunction is recognized on the ECG by pacemaker spikes that follow too closely behind the patient's QRS complexes (earlier than the programmed escape interval). Because pacemaker spikes occur when they should not, this type of pacemaker malfunction may result in pacemaker spikes that fall on T waves (R-on-T phenomenon) and/or competition between the pacemaker and the patient's own cardiac rhythm. The patient may complain of palpitations or skipped beats. R-on-T phenomenon may precipitate VT or VF.

Causes of failure to sense include battery failure, fracture of pacing lead wire, displacement of the electrode tip (most common cause), decreased P wave or QRS voltage, circuitry dysfunction (generator unable to process QRS signal), increased sensing threshold from edema or fibrosis at the electrode tip, antiarrhythmic medications, severe electrolyte disturbances, and myocardial perforation. Treatment may include increasing the sensitivity setting, replacing the pulse generator battery, and/or replacing or repositioning the pacing lead.

Oversensing

[OBJECTIVE 12]

Oversensing is a pacemaker malfunction that results from inappropriate sensing of extraneous electrical signals. Atrial sensing pacemakers may inappropriately sense ventricular activity; ventricular sensing pacemakers may misidentify a tall, peaked intrinsic T wave as a QRS complex. Oversensing

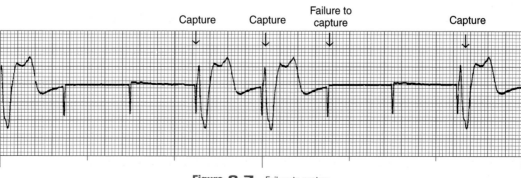

Figure 8-7 Failure to capture.

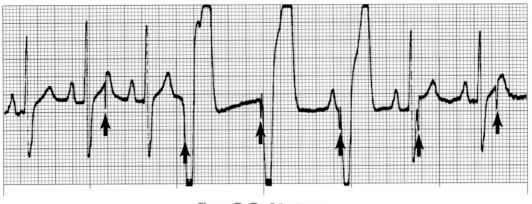

Figure 8-8   Failure to sense.

is recognized on the ECG as pacemaker spikes at a rate slower than the pacemaker's preset rate (paced QRS complexes that come later than the pacemaker's preset escape interval) or no paced beats even though the pacemaker's preset rate is greater than the patient's intrinsic rate.

The patient with a pacemaker should avoid strong electromagnetic fields such as those associated with welding equipment or a magnetic resonance imaging (MRI) machine. Treatment includes adjustment of the pacemaker's sensitivity setting or possible insertion of a bipolar lead if oversensing is caused by unipolar lead dysfunction. Some pacemakers are MRI safe. The pacemaker information contained in the patient's wallet card will indicate this.

PACEMAKER COMPLICATIONS

Complications of Transcutaneous Pacing

[OBJECTIVE 13]
Complications of TCP include the following:
- Coughing
- Skin burns
- Interference with sensing from patient agitation or muscle contractions
- Pain from electrical stimulation of the skin and muscles
- Failure to recognize that the pacemaker is not capturing
- Tissue damage, including third-degree burns (reported in pediatric patients with improper or prolonged TCP)
- When pacing is prolonged, pacing threshold changes, leading to capture failure

Complications of Temporary Transvenous Pacing

Complications of temporary transvenous pacing include bleeding, infection, pneumothorax, cardiac dysrhythmias, myocardial infarction, lead displacement, fracture of the pacing lead, hematoma at the insertion site, perforation of the right ventricle with or without pericardial tamponade,

and perforation of the inferior vena cava, pulmonary artery, or coronary arteries because of improper placement of the pacing lead.

Complications of Permanent Pacing

Complications of permanent pacing associated with the implantation procedure include bleeding, local tissue reaction, pneumothorax, cardiac dysrhythmias, air embolism, and thrombosis. Long-term complications of permanent pacing may include infection, electrode displacement, congestive heart failure, fracture of the pacing lead, pacemaker-induced dysrhythmias, externalization of the pacemaker generator, and perforation of the right ventricle with or without pericardial tamponade.

ANALYZING PACEMAKER FUNCTION ON THE ECG

[OBJECTIVE 14]
Step 1. Identify the intrinsic rate and rhythm
- Are P waves present? At what rate?
- Are QRS complexes present? At what rate?

Step 2. Is there evidence of paced activity?
- If paced atrial activity is present, evaluate the paced interval. Using calipers or paper, measure the distance between two consecutively paced atrial beats. Determine the rate and regularity of the paced interval.
- If paced ventricular activity is present, evaluate the paced interval. Using calipers or paper, measure the distance between two consecutively paced ventricular beats. Determine the rate and regularity of the paced interval.

Step 3. Evaluate the Escape Interval
- Compare the escape interval to the paced interval measured earlier. The paced interval and escape interval should measure the same.

Step 4. Analyze the Rhythm Strip
- Analyze the rhythm strip for failure to capture, failure to sense, oversensing, and failure to pace.

REFERENCES

1. Gibler WB: Emergency cardiac care, St Louis, 1994, Mosby.
2. Munter DW: Assessment of implanted pacemaker/AICD devices. In Roberts JR III, Hedges JR, eds: Clinical procedures in emergency medicine, 4th ed, 2004 Elsevier, p 257-268.
3. Vukmir RB: Emergency cardiac pacing, Am J Emerg Med 1993;11:166-176.
4. Falk RH, Ngai S: External cardiac pacing: Influence of electrode placement, Crit Care Med 1986;14:931-932.
5. Correa LF: Electrical intervention in cardiac disease. In Crawford MV, Spence MI, eds: Common sense approach to coronary care, ed 6, St Louis, 1995, Mosby, p 443-496.

STOP & REVIEW

Matching

____ **1.** Rate at which the pulse generator of a pacemaker paces when no intrinsic activity is detected; expressed in pulses per minute

____ **2.** Discharges only when the patient's heart rate drops below the pacemaker's preset rate

____ **3.** The minimum amount of voltage (mA) needed to obtain consistent capture

____ **4.** Successful depolarization of the atria and/or ventricles by an artificial pacemaker

____ **5.** Power source that houses the battery and controls for regulating a pacemaker

____ **6.** Time measured between a sensed cardiac event and the next pacemaker output

____ **7.** Pacemaker response in which the output pulse is suppressed when an intrinsic event is sensed

____ **8.** Pacemaker that stimulates the atrium and ventricle

____ **9.** Electrical stimulus delivered by a pacemaker's pulse generator

____ **10.** In dual-chamber pacing, the length of time between an atrial sensed or atrial paced event and the delivery of a ventricular pacing stimulus; analogous to the PR interval of intrinsic waveforms

____ **11.** In dual-chamber pacing, the interval between a sensed or ventricular paced event and the next atrial paced event

____ **12.** A vertical line on the ECG that indicates the pacemaker has discharged

____ **13.** ECG waveform that results when an intrinsic depolarization and a pacing stimulus occur simultaneously and both contribute to depolarization of that cardiac chamber

____ **14.** Ability of a pacemaker to increase the pacing rate in response to physical activity or metabolic demand

____ **15.** A pacing system with a lead attached to the right atrium designed to correct abnormalities in the SA node

a. Output

b. Threshold

c. Rate modulation

d. Fusion beat

e. Pulse generator

f. Demand pacemaker

g. V-A interval

h. Capture

i. Pacemaker spike

j. Base rate

k. A-V interval

l. Escape interval

m. Atrial pacemaker

n. Dual-chamber pacemaker

o. Inhibition

PACEMAKER RHYTHMS—*PRACTICE RHYTHM STRIPS*

For each of the following rhythm strips, determine the presence of atrial- and ventricular-paced activity, the paced interval rate, and then identify the rhythm. All strips lead II unless otherwise noted.

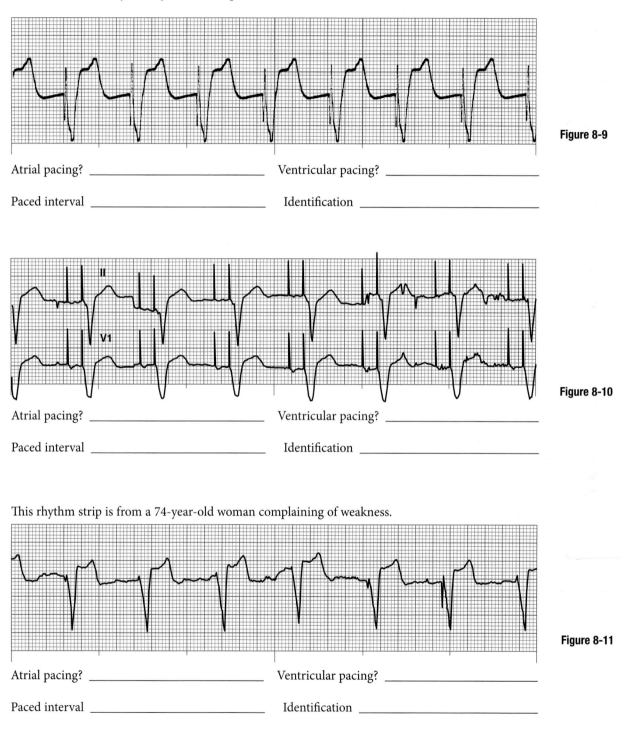

Figure 8-9

Atrial pacing? _____   Ventricular pacing? _____

Paced interval _____   Identification _____

Figure 8-10

Atrial pacing? _____   Ventricular pacing? _____

Paced interval _____   Identification _____

This rhythm strip is from a 74-year-old woman complaining of weakness.

Figure 8-11

Atrial pacing? _____   Ventricular pacing? _____

Paced interval _____   Identification _____

These rhythm strips are from a 52-year-old man with syncope.

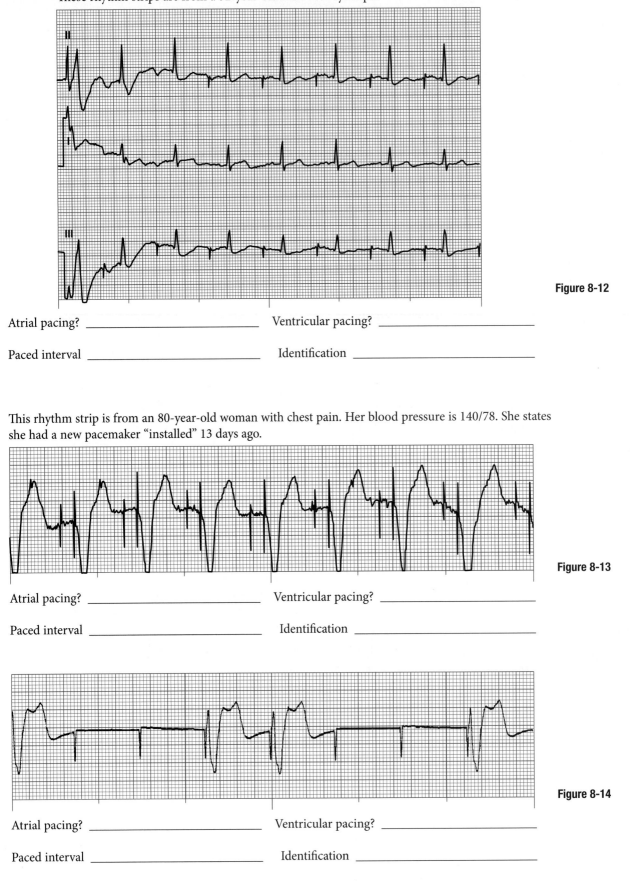

Figure 8-12

Atrial pacing? _____   Ventricular pacing? _____

Paced interval _____   Identification _____

This rhythm strip is from an 80-year-old woman with chest pain. Her blood pressure is 140/78. She states she had a new pacemaker "installed" 13 days ago.

Figure 8-13

Atrial pacing? _____   Ventricular pacing? _____

Paced interval _____   Identification _____

Figure 8-14

Atrial pacing? _____   Ventricular pacing? _____

Paced interval _____   Identification _____

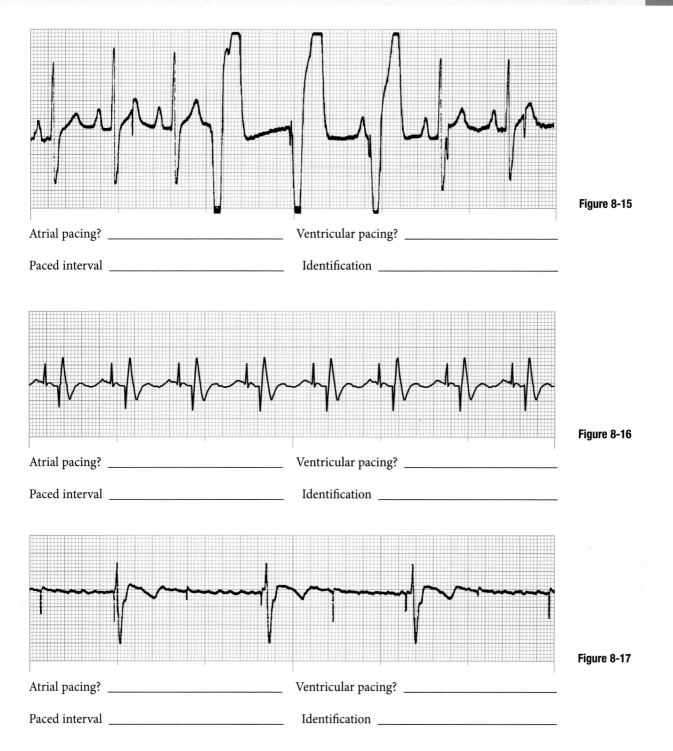

Figure 8-15

Atrial pacing? _____   Ventricular pacing? _____

Paced interval _____   Identification _____

Figure 8-16

Atrial pacing? _____   Ventricular pacing? _____

Paced interval _____   Identification _____

Figure 8-17

Atrial pacing? _____   Ventricular pacing? _____

Paced interval _____   Identification _____

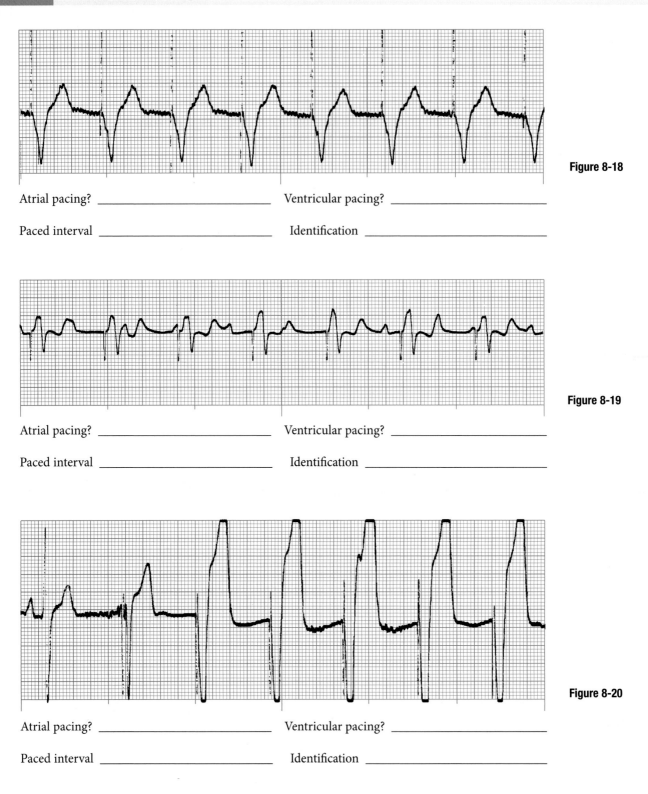

Figure 8-18

Atrial pacing? _____   Ventricular pacing? _____

Paced interval _____   Identification _____

Figure 8-19

Atrial pacing? _____   Ventricular pacing? _____

Paced interval _____   Identification _____

Figure 8-20

Atrial pacing? _____   Ventricular pacing? _____

Paced interval _____   Identification _____

STOP & REVIEW ANSWERS

Matching

1. j
2. f
3. b
4. h
5. e
6. l
7. o
8. n

9. a
10. k
11. g
12. i
13. d
14. c
15. m

Figure 8-9 answer

Atrial pacing?	No
Ventricular pacing?	Yes
Paced interval	79
Identification	100% ventricular-paced rhythm

Figure 8-10 answer

Atrial pacing?	Yes
Ventricular pacing?	Yes
Paced interval	71
Identification	100% paced rhythm – AV sequential pacemaker

Figure 8-11 answer

Atrial paced activity?	No
Ventricular paced activity?	Yes
Paced interval rate?	68
Identification	Ventricular demand pacemaker

Figure 8-12 answer

Atrial pacing?	Yes
Ventricular pacing?	No
Paced interval	79
Identification	Atrial pacemaker

Figure 8-13 answer

Atrial paced activity?	Yes
Ventricular paced activity?	Yes
Paced interval rate?	83
Identification	100% paced rhythm – AV sequential pacemaker

Figure 8-14 answer

Atrial pacing?	No
Ventricular pacing?	Yes
Paced interval	80
Identification	Ventricular paced rhythm with failure to capture

Figure 8-15 answer

Atrial pacing?	No
Ventricular pacing?	Yes
Paced interval	71
Identification	Pacemaker malfunction (failure to sense); underlying rhythm is a sinus rhythm at 88 beats/min with a PVC; note the pacer spikes in the T waves of the second and eighth beats from the left

Figure 8-16 answer

Atrial paced activity?	Yes
Ventricular paced activity?	Yes
Paced interval rate?	79
Identification	100% paced rhythm – AV sequential pacemaker

Figure 8-17 answer

Atrial pacing?	No
Ventricular pacing?	Yes
Paced interval	72
Identification	Malfunctioning ventricular demand pacemaker—failure to capture; underlying rhythm appears to be atrial flutter

Figure 8-18 answer

Atrial pacing?	No
Ventricular pacing?	Yes
Paced interval	74
Identification	100% ventricular-paced rhythm

Figure 8-19 answer

Atrial pacing?	No
Ventricular pacing?	Yes
Paced interval	71
Identification	100% ventricular-paced rhythm; underlying rhythm is a complete AV block

Figure 8-20 answer

Atrial pacing?	No
Ventricular pacing?	Yes
Paced interval	71
Identification	Normal pacemaker function-ventricular-demand pacer

Introduction to the 12-Lead ECG

OBJECTIVES

On completion of this chapter, you will be able to:

1. Discuss possible indications for use of a 12-lead ECG.
2. List the leads that make up the standard 12-lead ECG.
3. Compare bipolar, unipolar, and chest leads.
4. Describe the portion of the heart viewed by each lead of the 12-lead ECG.
5. Explain the term electrical axis and its significance.
6. Determine electrical axis using leads I and aVF.
7. Describe ECG changes that may reflect evidence of myocardial ischemia, injury, or infarction.
8. Describe a method for recognizing a posterior wall myocardial infarction.
9. Identify the ECG features of right ventricular myocardial infarction.
10. Describe the sequence of normal R wave progression.
11. Describe differentiation of right and left bundle branch block using leads V_1 and V_6.
12. Explain what is meant by the terms dilatation, hypertrophy, and enlargement.
13. Identify the ECG changes characteristically produced by electrolyte imbalances.
14. Describe a systematic method for analyzing a 12-lead ECG.

INTRODUCTION TO THE 12-LEAD ECG

[OBJECTIVE 1]

A standard 12-lead ECG provides views of the heart in both the frontal and horizontal planes and views the surfaces of the left ventricle from 12 different angles. Multiple views of the heart can provide useful information including:

- Recognition of bundle branch blocks
- Identification of ST-segment and T wave changes associated with myocardial ischemia, injury, and infarction
- Identification of ECG changes associated with certain medications and electrolyte imbalances
  Indications for using a 12-lead ECG include the following:
- Chest pain or discomfort
- Assisting in dysrhythmia interpretation
- Right and/or left ventricular failure
- Status before and after electrical therapy (defibrillation, cardioversion, pacing)
- Syncope or near syncope
- Electrical injuries
- Stroke
- Known or suspected medication overdoses
- Known or suspected electrolyte imbalances

LEADS

[OBJECTIVE 2, 3, 4]

The standard 12-lead is composed of six limb leads and six chest leads. Leads allow viewing of the heart's electrical activity in two different planes: frontal (coronal) or horizontal (transverse). Each lead records the average current flow at a specific time in a portion of the heart. Frontal plane leads view the heart from the front of the body. Directions in the frontal plane are superior, inferior, right, and left. Leads I, II, and III (bipolar leads) and leads aVR, aVL, and aVF (unipolar leads) view the heart in the frontal plane. Leads I, II, III, aVR, aVL, and aVF are obtained from electrodes placed on the patient's arms and legs.

Horizontal plane leads view the heart as if the body were sliced in half. Directions in the horizontal plane are anterior, posterior, right, and left. Six chest (precordial or V) leads view the heart in the horizontal plane, allowing a view of the front and left side of the heart. As their names suggest, the chest leads, V_1-V_6, are obtained from electrodes placed on the patient's chest.

All 12 leads are obtained from only 10 electrodes. This is possible because the four limb electrodes are used for different purposes in different leads. For example, the left arm electrode is used as a negative electrode when lead III is obtained and is used as a positive electrode when lead aVL is obtained.

Standard Limb Leads

Leads I, II, and III make up the standard limb leads. If an electrode is placed on the right arm, left arm, and left leg, three leads are formed. Remember that an imaginary line joining the positive and negative electrodes of a lead is called the axis of the lead. Since each of these three leads has a distinct negative pole and a distinct positive pole, they are considered **bipolar** leads. Lead I views the lateral surface of the left ventricle. Leads II and III view the inferior surface of the left ventricle.

Augmented Limb Leads

Leads aVR, aVL, and aVF make up the augmented limb leads. The augmented limb leads are unipolar consisting of only one electrode (a positive electrode) on the body surface (Figure 9-1). The electrical potential produced by the augmented leads is normally relatively small. The ECG machine augments (magnifies) the amplitude of the electrical potentials detected at each extremity by approximately 50% over those recorded at the bipolar leads. The "a" in aVR, aVL, and aVF refers to augmented. The "V" refers to voltage. The "R" refers to right arm, the "L" to left arm, and the "F" to left foot (leg). The position of the positive electrode corresponds to the last letter in each of these leads. The positive pole in aVR is located on the right arm, aVL has a positive pole at the left arm, and aVF has a positive electrode positioned on the left leg.

Lead aVR views the heart from the right shoulder (the positive electrode) and views the base of the heart (primarily the atria and the great vessels). This lead does not view any wall of the heart. Lead aVL views the heart from the left shoulder (the positive electrode) and is oriented to the lateral wall of the left ventricle. Lead aVF views the heart

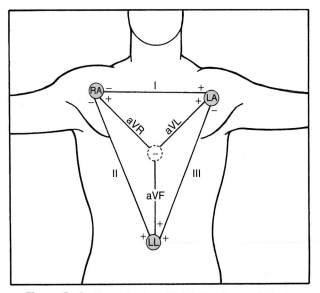

Figure 9-1   View of the standard limb leads and augmented leads.

from the left foot (leg) (positive electrode). Leads II and III, in conjunction with lead aVF, view the inferior surface of the left ventricle.

Chest Leads

The six chest leads are identified as V_1, V_2, V_3, V_4, V_5, and V_6. Each electrode placed in a "V" position is a positive electrode. Because the chest leads (also known as precordial leads) are unipolar, the positive electrode for each lead is placed at a specific location on the chest, and the heart is the theoretical negative electrode (Figure 9-2). Leads V_1 and V_2 view the interventricular septum, V_3 and V_4 view the anterior surface of the left ventricle, and V_5 and V_6 view the lateral surface of the left ventricle. The procedures for standard chest lead placement, right chest lead placement, and posterior chest lead placement are shown in Skills 2-2 to 2-4.

ECG Pearl

What Each Lead "Sees"

Leads	Heart Surface Viewed
II, III, aVF	Inferior
V_1, V_2	Septal
V_3, V_4	Anterior
I, aVL, V_5, V_6	Lateral

VECTORS

[OBJECTIVE 5]

Because the ECG does not directly measure the heart's electrical activity, it does not "see" all of the current flowing through the heart. What the ECG does see from its vantage point on the body's surface is the net result of countless individual currents competing in a tug-of-war. For example, the QRS complex is not a display of all the electrical activity occurring in the right and left ventricles. It is the net result of a tug-of-war produced by the numerous individual currents in both the right and left ventricles. Since the left ventricle is much more

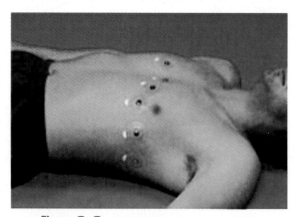

Figure 9-2 Anatomic placement of the chest leads.

massive than the right, the left overpowers the right. What is seen in the QRS complex is the remaining electrical activity of the left ventricle (i.e., the portion not used to cancel out the right ventricle). Therefore, in a normally conducted beat, the QRS complex represents the electrical activity occurring in the left ventricle. It has been estimated that 80% of the cardiac electrical activity is canceled out by the tug-of-war leaving only 20% for the ECG to sense.

Leads have a negative (−) and positive (+) electrode pole that senses the magnitude and direction of the electrical force caused by the spread of waves of depolarization and repolarization throughout the myocardium. A **vector** (arrow) is a symbol representing this force. A vector points in the direction of depolarization. Leads that face the tip or point of a vector record a positive deflection on ECG paper.

A **mean vector** identifies the average of depolarization waves in one portion of the heart. The mean P vector represents the average magnitude and direction of both right and left atrial depolarization. The mean QRS vector represents the average magnitude and direction of both right and left ventricular depolarization. The average direction of a mean vector is called the **mean axis** and is only identified in the frontal plane. An imaginary line joining the positive and negative electrodes of a lead is called the axis of the lead. **Electrical axis** refers to determining the direction (or angle in degrees) in which the main vector of depolarization is pointed. When "axis" is used by itself, it refers to the QRS axis.

Axis

[OBJECTIVE 6]

During normal ventricular depolarization, the left side of the interventricular septum is stimulated first. The electrical impulse then traverses the septum to stimulate the right side. The left and right ventricles are then depolarized simultaneously. Because the left ventricle is considerably larger than the right, right ventricular depolarization forces are overshadowed on the ECG. As a result, the mean QRS vector points down (inferior) and to the left.

The axes of leads I, II, and III form an equilateral triangle with the heart at the center (Einthoven's triangle). If the augmented limb leads are added to this configuration and the axes of the six leads moved in a way in which they bisect each other, the result is the hexaxial reference system (Figure 9-3). The hexaxial reference system represents all of the frontal plane (limb) leads with the heart in the center and is the means used to express the location of the frontal plane axis. This system forms a 360-degree circle surrounding the heart. The positive end of lead I is designated at 0 degrees. The six frontal plane leads divide the circle into segments, each representing 30 degrees. All degrees in the upper hemisphere are labeled as negative degrees, and all degrees in the lower hemisphere are labeled as positive degrees. The mean QRS vector (normal electrical axis) lies between 0 and +90 degrees.

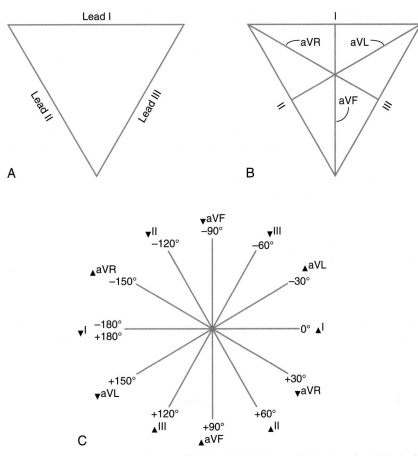

Figure 9-3 **A,** Einthoven's equilateral triangle formed by leads I, II, and III. **B,** The unipolar leads are added to the equilateral triangle. **C,** The hexaxial reference system derived from **B**.

Current flow to the right of normal is called right axis deviation (+90 to +180 degrees). Current flow in the direction opposite of normal is called indeterminate, "no man's land," northwest, or extreme right axis deviation (−91 to −179 degrees). Current flow to the left of normal is called left axis deviation (−1 to −90 degrees).

In the hexaxial reference system, the axes of some leads are perpendicular to each other. Lead I is perpendicular to lead aVF. Lead II is perpendicular to aVL, and lead III is perpendicular to lead aVR. If the electrical force moves toward a positive electrode, a positive (upright) deflection will be recorded. If the electrical force moves away from a positive electrode, a negative (downward) deflection will be recorded. If the electrical force is parallel to a given lead, the largest deflection in that lead will be recorded. If the electrical force is perpendicular to a lead axis, the resulting ECG complex will be small or biphasic in that lead. Axis determination can provide clues in the differential diagnosis of wide QRS tachycardia, hemiblocks, and localization of accessory pathways.

Leads I and aVF divide the heart into four quadrants. These two leads can be used to quickly estimate electrical axis. In leads I and aVF, the QRS complex is normally positive. If the QRS complex in either or both of these leads is negative, axis deviation is present (Table 9-1).

TABLE 9-1	Two-Lead Method of Axis Determination			
Axis	Normal	Left	Right	Indeterminate ("No Man's Land")
Lead I – QRS direction	Positive	Positive	Negative	Negative
Lead aVF – QRS direction	Positive	Negative	Positive	Negative

Right axis deviation may be a normal variant, particularly in the young and in thin individuals. Other causes of right axis deviation include mechanical shifts associated with inspiration or emphysema, right ventricular hypertrophy, chronic obstructive pulmonary disease (COPD), Wolff-Parkinson-White Syndrome (WPW), and pulmonary embolism.

Left axis deviation may be a normal variant, particularly in older individuals and obesity. Other causes of left axis deviation include mechanical shifts associated with expiration;

a high diaphragm caused by pregnancy, ascites, or abdominal tumors; hyperkalemia, inspiration or emphysema, left atrial hypertrophy, and dextrocardia.

LAYOUT OF THE 12-LEAD ECG

Most 12-lead monitors record all 12 leads simultaneously but display them in a conventional 3 row by 4-column format. The standard limb leads are recorded in the first column, the augmented limb leads in the second column, and the chest leads in the third and fourth columns (Table 9-2). All of the QRS complexes in a row are consecutive while QRS complexes that are aligned vertically represent a simultaneous recording of the same beat. Because the leads are obtained simultaneously, only 10 seconds of sampling time is required to record all 12 leads.[1]

The 12-lead ECG provides a 2.5-second view of each lead because it is assumed that 2.5 seconds is long enough

to capture at least one representative complex. However, a 2.5-second view is not long enough to properly assess rate and rhythm, so at least one continuous rhythm strip is usually included at the bottom of the tracing. A 12-lead ECG is shown in Figure 9-4. When reviewing a 12-lead ECG, intervals and duration are expressed in milliseconds (ms). Seconds can be easily converted to milliseconds by moving the decimal point three places to the right. Measurements are provided by the 12-lead computer's interpretive program, which is usually very accurate when measuring intervals and durations.

ECG Pearl

When viewing a 12-lead, keep in mind that leads that line up vertically are simultaneous recordings of the same beat. When you read the 12-lead from left to right, the ECG tracing is continuous. As you switch from one lead to the next, it is still continuous.

ACUTE CORONARY SYNDROMES

[OBJECTIVE 7]

When a temporary or permanent blockage occurs in a coronary artery, the blood supply to the heart muscle is impaired. An impaired blood supply results in a decreased supply of oxygen to the myocardium. When the heart's demand for oxygen exceeds its supply from the coronary circulation, chest discomfort or related symptoms often occur. A decreased supply of oxygenated blood to a body part or organ is called ischemia.

TABLE 9-2 Layout of the 4-Column 12-Lead ECG

LIMB LEADS		CHEST LEADS	
Standard Leads	Augmented Leads	V_1-V_3	V_4-V_6
Column I	Column II	Column III	Column IV
I: lateral	aVR: none	V_1: septum	V_4: anterior
II: inferior	aVL: lateral	V_2: septum	V_5: lateral
III: inferior	aVF: inferior	V_3: anterior	V_6: lateral

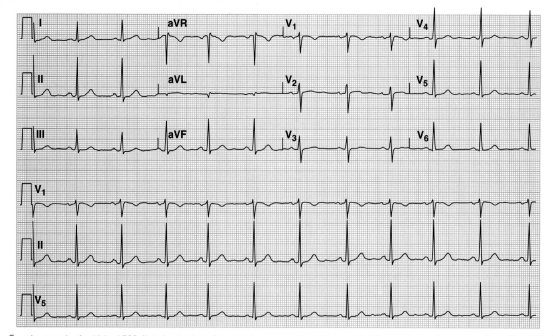

Figure 9-4 An example of a 12-lead ECG. Note the 4-column format at the upper portion of the page. In this example, continuous recordings of leads V_1, II, and V_5 are shown at the bottom of the page.

Acute coronary syndromes (ACS) are conditions caused by a similar sequence of pathologic events—a temporary or permanent blockage of a coronary artery. This sequence of events results in conditions ranging from myocardial ischemia or injury to death (necrosis) of heart muscle. ACS include unstable angina, non–ST-segment elevation MI (NSTEMI), and ST-segment elevation MI (STEMI). Sudden cardiac death can occur with any of these conditions.

The usual cause of an ACS is the rupture of an atherosclerotic plaque. To understand this process, let us quickly review relevant anatomy. Arteries consist of three layers. The outermost layer is the tunica adventitia. It consists of flexible connective tissue and helps hold the vessel open. The middle layer is the tunica media. It consists of smooth muscle tissue and elastic connective tissue. This layer is encircled by smooth muscle and innervated by fibers of the autonomic nervous system that allows constriction and dilation of the vessel. Smooth muscle cells function to maintain vascular tone and regulate local blood flow depending on the body's metabolic needs. These cells also are capable of producing collagen, elastin, and other substances important in the formation of atherosclerotic plaques. The innermost layer of an artery is the tunica intima. It is composed of endothelium that lines the vascular system. Endothelium is a single layer of cells in direct contact with the blood. The intima is at risk of damage from conditions such as hypertension, high cholesterol, smoking, and diabetes.

Arteriosclerosis is a chronic disease of the arterial system characterized by abnormal thickening and hardening of the vessel walls. Atherosclerosis (from athero, meaning gruel or paste, and sclerosis, meaning hardness) is a form of arteriosclerosis in which the thickening and hardening of the vessel walls are caused by a buildup of fatty deposits in the inner lining of large- and middle-sized muscular arteries. As the fatty deposits build up, the opening of the artery slowly narrows and blood flow to the muscle decreases (Figure 9-5).

Any artery in the body can develop atherosclerosis. If the coronary arteries are involved (coronary artery disease) and blood flow to the heart is decreased, angina or more serious signs and symptoms may result. If the arteries in the leg are involved (peripheral vascular disease), leg pain (claudication) may result. If the arteries supplying the brain are involved (carotid artery disease), a stroke or transient ischemic attack may result.

Atherosclerotic plaques differ in their makeup, vulnerability to rupture, and tendency to make blood clots. Stable plaques are unlikely to rupture. They consist mainly of collagen-rich tissue that has hardened. They have a thick, fibrous cap over the fatty center that separates it from contact with the blood, making them less likely to rupture (Figure 9-6). As these plaques increase in size, the artery can become severely narrowed. Plaques prone to rupture are called vulnerable plaques. They are soft and have a thin cap of fibrous tissue over the fatty center that separates it from the opening of the artery. If the fibrous cap tears or ruptures, the contents of the plaque are exposed to flowing blood. Platelets stick to the damaged lining of the vessel and to each other and form a plug. Sticky platelets secrete several chemicals, including thromboxane A_2. These substances stimulate vasoconstriction, reducing blood flow at the site. Aspirin blocks the production of thromboxane A_2, slowing the clumping (aggregation) of platelets.

Once platelets are activated, glycoprotein IIb/IIIa receptors needed for platelet clumping appear on the surface of the platelet. Fibrinogen molecules bind to these receptors to form bridges (cross links) between nearby platelets, allowing them to clump. Medications called glycoprotein IIb/IIIa receptor inhibitors prevent fibrinogen binding and platelet clumping. As the process continues, thrombin is made and

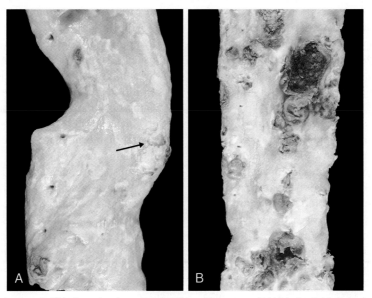

Figure 9-5   Atherosclerosis in the aorta. **A,** Mild atherosclerosis composed of fibrous plaques, one of which is denoted by the arrow. **B,** Severe disease with diffuse and complicated lesions.

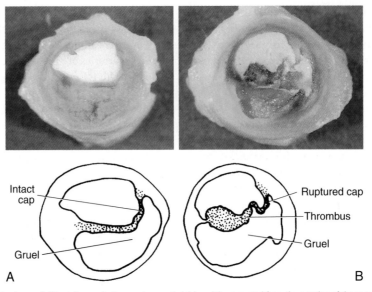

Figure 9-6   View of a vulnerable plaque. **A,** The yellow, soft atheromatous material (gruel) is separated from the opening of the vessel only by a thin, but intact, fibrous cap. The vessel opening contains white radiographic contrast medium. **B,** This specimen was just a few millimeters distal to the one shown in **A**. Here the thin fibrous cap is ruptured, a big cap fragment and some of the soft atheromatous gruel are missing (from downstream embolization), and a clot has evolved where the gruel has been exposed. White contrast medium has penetrated the soft gruel through the ruptured cap.

fibrin is formed, ultimately producing a clot. Clots can be dissolved by a process called **fibrinolysis**. Fibrinolytics (clot busters) are medications that stimulate the conversion of plasminogen to plasmin, which dissolves the clot.

Rupture of a vulnerable plaque may follow extreme physical activity (especially in someone unaccustomed to regular exercise), severe emotional trauma, sexual activity, exposure to illicit drugs (cocaine, marijuana, or amphetamines), exposure to cold, or acute infection.[2] Contributing factors to plaque rupture include the frictional force from blood flow, coronary spasm at the site of the plaque, internal plaque changes, and the effects of risk factors, such as high blood pressure and high cholesterol.

Blockage of a coronary artery by a clot may be complete or incomplete. Complete blockage of a coronary artery may result in STEMI or sudden death. Partial (incomplete) blockage of a coronary artery by a clot may result in no clinical signs and symptoms (silent MI), unstable angina, NSTEMI, or possibly sudden death.

Angina pectoris is chest discomfort that occurs when the heart muscle does not receive enough oxygen (myocardial ischemia). Ischemia can occur because of increased myocardial oxygen demand (demand ischemia), reduced myocardial oxygen supply (supply ischemia), or both. If the cause of the ischemia is not reversed and blood flow restored to the affected area of the heart muscle, ischemia may lead to cellular injury and ultimately infarction.

Angina most often occurs in patients with coronary artery disease involving at least one coronary artery. However, it can be present in patients with normal coronary arteries. Angina also occurs in persons with uncontrolled high blood pressure or valvular heart disease.

Stable (classic) angina remains relatively constant and predictable in terms of severity, signs and symptoms, precipitating events, and response to treatment. It is characterized by brief episodes of chest discomfort related to activities that increase the heart's need for oxygen, such as emotional upset, exercise or exertion, and exposure to cold weather. Related symptoms include shortness of breath, palpitations, sweating, nausea, or vomiting. Symptoms typically last 2 to 5 minutes and occasionally 5 to 15 minutes. Prolonged discomfort (more than 30 minutes) is uncommon in stable angina.

Unstable angina (also known as preinfarction angina) is a condition of intermediate severity between stable angina and acute MI. Unstable angina is characterized by one or more of the following:

- Symptoms that occur at rest (or minimal exertion) and usually last more than 20 minutes
- Symptoms that are severe and/or of new onset (i.e., within the previous 4 to 6 weeks)
- Symptoms that are more severe, prolonged, or frequent in a patient with a history of stable angina

Unlike stable angina, the discomfort associated with unstable angina may be described as painful. Patients with untreated unstable angina are at high risk of a heart attack or death. Early assessment, including a focused history, and intervention is essential to prevent worsening ischemia.

Prinzmetal's angina (also called Prinzmetal's variant angina, variant angina, or vasospastic angina) is a form of unstable angina. Patients with Prinzmetal's angina often have coronary artery plaques,[3] but some patients have normal coronary arteries. This uncommon type of angina is the result of intense spasm of a segment of a coronary artery. The spasm occurs almost exclusively at rest, often occurs at night or in the early morning hours, and may awaken the patient from sleep. It is usually not brought on by physical exertion or emotional stress. Chest discomfort may be accompanied by difficulty breathing and/or palpitations. Episodes usually last only a few minutes, but this may be long enough to produce serious dysrhythmias, including ventricular tachycardia and ventricular fibrillation as well as sudden death.

Ischemia prolonged more than just a few minutes results in myocardial injury. Injured myocardial cells are still alive but will die (infarct) if the ischemia is not quickly corrected. If blood flow is quickly restored, no tissue death occurs. Methods to restore blood flow include administration of fibrinolytic agents, coronary angioplasty, or a coronary artery bypass graft, among others.

A myocardial infarction (MI) occurs when blood flow to the heart muscle stops or is suddenly decreased long enough to cause cell death (Figure 9-7). An acute MI usually results from a thrombus. Less commonly, acute MI may occur because of coronary spasm (as in cocaine abuse) or coronary embolism (rare).

Patients with a STEMI show evidence of ST-segment elevation on their ECG. As its name implies, patients with an NSTEMI do not show signs of myocardial injury (ST-segment elevation) on their ECG. Distinguishing patients with unstable angina from those with acute MI may be impossible during initial presentation because their signs, symptoms, and ECG findings may be identical. The diagnosis of infarction is made based on the patient's signs and symptoms, ECG findings, history, and blood test results that confirm the presence of an infarction (cardiac biomarkers).

Recognition of infarction on the ECG relies on the detection of morphologic changes (i.e., changes in shape) of the QRS complex, the T wave, and the ST-segment. These changes occur in relation to certain events during the infarction. Figure 9-8 shows the ECG changes attributable to STEMI that often occur in a predictable pattern. The changes described below are not seen in every lead. They appear only in leads looking at the infarct site. The first change you might detect in the ECG is the development of a tall T wave. In addition to an increase in height, the T wave becomes more symmetric and may also become pointed (Figure 9-8, A). These T wave changes may occur within the first few minutes of infarction during what has been described as the hyperacute phase of infarction. As time progresses, signs of myocardial injury may develop. ST-segment elevation (Figure 9-8, B) provides the primary indication of myocardial injury in progress. ST-segment elevation may occur within the first hour or the first few hours of infarction and is considered to occur in the early acute phase of infarction. In the later acute phase of the infarction, one may see the presence of T wave inversion, suggesting the presence of ischemia (Figure 9-8, C). In fact, T wave inversion may precede the development of ST-segment elevation, or it may occur simultaneously. A few hours later, the ECG may give its first evidence that tissue death has occurred. That evidence comes with the development of abnormal Q waves (Figure 9-8, D). Remember that a Q wave that is 40 ms or more wide (one small box or more wide) or more than one third of the amplitude of the R wave in that lead is suggestive of infarction. An abnormal Q wave indicates the presence of dead myocardial tissue and subsequently a loss of electrical activity. Abnormal Q waves can appear within hours after occlusion of a coronary artery, but they more commonly appear several hours or days after the onset of signs and symptoms of an acute MI. When combined with ST-segment or T wave changes, the presence of abnormal Q waves suggests an acute MI. In time, the T wave regains its normal contour and the ST-segment returns to the isoelectric line. The Q wave, however, often remains as evidence that an infarct has occurred (Figure 9-8, E). When this pattern is seen, establishing the time of the infarct is impossible. It is only possible to recognize the presence of a previous MI.

Localization of Infarctions

Contiguous Leads

When ECG changes of myocardial ischemia, injury, or infarction occur, they are not found in every lead of the ECG. Findings are considered significant if viewed in two or more leads looking at the same area of the heart. If these findings

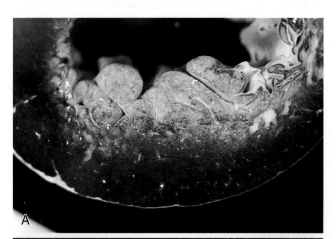
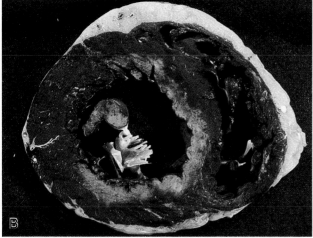

Figure 9-7 Myocardial infarction. **A,** Local infarction confined to one area of the heart. **B,** Massive infarction caused by blockage of three coronary arteries.

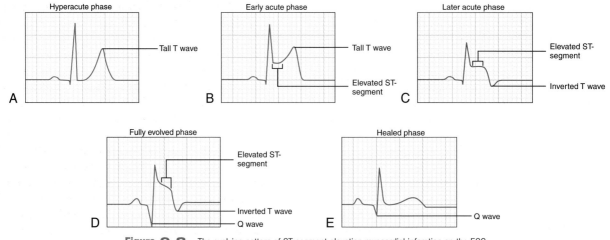

Figure 9-8   The evolving pattern of ST-segment elevation myocardial infarction on the ECG.

are seen in leads that look directly at the affected area, they are called **indicative changes**. If findings are seen in leads opposite the affected area, they are called **reciprocal changes** (also called "mirror image" changes) (Figure 9-9). Of the indicative changes, ST-segment elevation provides the strongest evidence for the early recognition of MI. ST-segment elevation is considered significant when it is elevated at least 1 mm and is viewed in two or more leads looking at the same area of the heart.

Indicative changes are significant when they are seen in two *anatomically contiguous* leads. Two leads are contiguous if they look at the same area of the heart or they are numerically consecutive chest leads. To better understand this, let us look at Figure 9-10 and Table 9-3. The colors in the table were added so that you can quickly see the areas of the heart viewed by the same leads. For example, leads II, III, and aVF appear the same color in the table because they view the inferior wall of the left ventricle. Because these leads "see" the

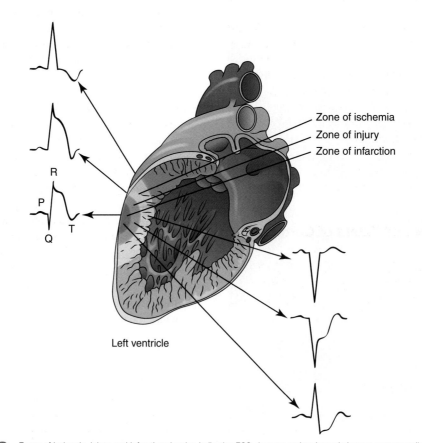

Figure 9-9   Zones of ischemia, injury, and infarction showing indicative ECG changes and reciprocal changes corresponding to each zone.

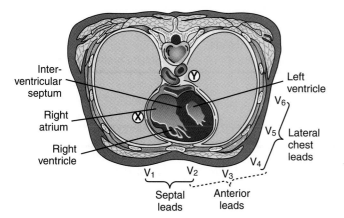

Figure 9-10 The areas of the heart as seen by the chest leads. Leads V_1, V_2, and V_3 are contiguous. Leads V_3, V_4, and V_5 are contiguous as well as V_4, V_5, and V_6. Note that neither the right ventricular wall (X) nor the posterior wall of the left ventricle (Y) is well visualized by any of the usual six chest leads.

same part of the heart, they are considered contiguous leads. Leads I, aVL, V_5, and V_6 are contiguous because they all look at adjoining tissue in the lateral wall of the left ventricle. Leads V_1 and V_2 are contiguous because both leads look at the septum. Leads V_3 and V_4 are contiguous because both leads look at the anterior wall of the left ventricle. If right chest leads such as V_4R, V_5R, and V_6R are used, they are contiguous because they view the right ventricle. Leads V_7, V_8, and V_9 are contiguous because they look at the posterior surface of the heart.

Are leads II and V_2 contiguous? No. Leads II and V_2 are not contiguous. Remember: two leads are contiguous if they look at the same area of the heart or they are numerically consecutive *chest* leads. Lead II is a *limb* lead that looks at the inferior wall. V_2 is a *chest* lead that looks at the septum.

Now look at Figure 9-10. We have already determined that V_1 and V_2 are contiguous leads. Are leads V_2 and V_3 contiguous? Yes. V_2 and V_3 are right next to each other on the patient's chest. When each of these positive electrodes "looks in" at tissue, they see adjoining tissue in the heart as well. Leads V_3, V_4, and V_5 are contiguous, as well as V_4, V_5, and V_6.

Predicting the Site and Extent of Coronary Artery Occlusion

In the standard 12-lead ECG, leads II, III, and aVF examine tissue supplied by the RCA and eight leads evaluate tissue supplied by the left coronary artery: leads I, aVL, V_1, V_2, V_3, V_4, V_5, and V_6. When evaluating the extent of infarction produced by a left coronary artery occlusion, determine how many of these leads are showing changes consistent with an acute infarction. The more of these eight leads demonstrating acute changes, the larger the infarction is presumed to be.[1]

To recognize signs of ischemia, injury, and infarction, knowing which portion of the heart each lead is viewing is necessary. To localize the site, note which leads display that evidence and consider which part of the heart that those leads "see." If an ECG shows changes in leads II, III, and aVF, the inferior wall is affected. Because the inferior wall of the left ventricle is supplied by the RCA in most people, assuming that these ECG changes are from partial or complete blockage of the RCA is reasonable. When indicative changes are seen in the leads viewing the septal, anterior, and/or lateral walls of the left ventricle (V_1 to V_6, I, and aVL), suspecting that these ECG changes are from partial or complete blockage of the left coronary artery is reasonable.

Although ECG localization of the infarct site is possible, it is not perfect. For example, what appears to be a lateral wall infarction on the ECG may actually be an anterior wall infarction. This can occur with any location of infarction and is because the ECG is simply a measurement of current flow on the patient's skin. Factors including anatomic variations, patient position, and other underlying conditions may affect the perceived locations versus the actual location. The patient's unique pattern of coronary artery distribution also can affect the location of infarct, as can the presence of collateral circulation. For these reasons, you may occasionally encounter infarctions that are difficult to localize into the previously mentioned regions. Table 9-4 summarizes the pattern in which coronary arteries most commonly supply the myocardium.

Anterior Wall Infarctions

Leads V_3 and V_4 face the anterior wall of the left ventricle. The left main coronary artery supplies the LAD artery and the circumflex artery. Blockage of the left main coronary artery (the "widow maker") often leads to cardiogenic shock and death without prompt reperfusion (Figures 9-11 and 9-12). Because the LAD artery supplies approximately 40% of the heart's blood and a critical section of the left ventricle, a blockage in this area can lead to complications such as left ventricular dysfunction, including heart failure and cardiogenic shock. Increased sympathetic nervous system activity is common with anterior MIs with resulting sinus tachycardia and/or high blood pressure.

TABLE 9-3	Localizing ECG Changes			
I Lateral	aVR —	V1 septum	V4 anterior	V4R right ventricle
II Inferior	aVL lateral	V2 septum	V5 lateral	V5R right ventricle
III Inferior	aVF inferior	V3 anterior	V6 lateral	V6R right ventricle

TABLE **9-4**	Localization of a MI			
Location of MI	**Indicative Changes (Leads Facing Affected Area)**	**Reciprocal Changes (Leads Opposite Affected Area)**	**Affected Coronary Artery**
Anterior	V_3, V_4	V_7, V_8, V_9	Left coronary artery LAD, diagonal branch
Anteroseptal	V_1, V_2, V_3, V_4	V_7, V_8, V_9	Left coronary artery LAD, diagonal branch LAD, septal branch
Anterolateral	I, aVL, V_3, V_4, V_5, V_6	II, III, aVF, V_7, V_8, V_9	Left coronary artery LAD, diagonal branch and/or circumflex branch
Inferior	II, III, aVF	I, aVL	RCA (most common), posterior descending branch or left coronary artery, circumflex branch
Lateral	I, aVL, V_5, V_6	II, III, aVF	Left coronary artery LAD, diagonal branch and/or circumflex branch RCA
Septum	V_1, V_2	V_7, V_8, V_9	Left coronary artery LAD, septal branch
Posterior	V_7, V_8, V_9	V_1, V_2, V_3	RCA or circumflex artery
Right ventricle	V_1R-V_6R	I, aVL	RCA, proximal branches

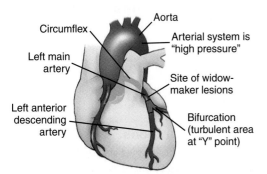

Figure 9-11 The left main coronary artery supplies the left anterior descending artery and the circumflex artery. Blockage of the left main coronary artery (the "widow maker") often leads to cardiogenic shock and death without prompt reperfusion.

An anterior wall MI may cause dysrhythmias including PVCs, atrial flutter, or AFib. Although some portions of the bundle branches are supplied by the RCA, the left coronary artery supplies most of the bundle branch tissue. Thus bundle branch blocks may occur if the left coronary artery is blocked. An example of an anterior wall infarction is shown in Figure 9-13.

Inferior Wall Infarctions

Leads II, III, and aVF view the inferior surface of the left ventricle. In most individuals the inferior wall of the left ventricle is supplied by the posterior descending branch of the RCA (Figure 9-14). Increased parasympathetic

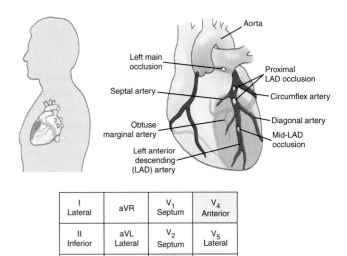

I Lateral	aVR	V_1 Septum	V_4 Anterior
II Inferior	aVL Lateral	V_2 Septum	V_5 Lateral
III Inferior	aVF Inferior	V_3 Anterior	V_6 Lateral

Figure 9-12 Anterior wall infarction. Occlusion of the midportion of the left anterior descending (LAD) artery results in an anterior infarction. Proximal occlusion of the LAD may become an anteroseptal infarction if the septal branch is involved or an anterolateral infarction if the marginal branch is involved. If the occlusion occurs proximal to both the septal and diagonal branches, an extensive anterior infarction (anteroseptal-lateral myocardial infarction) will result.

nervous system activity is common with inferior wall MIs, resulting in bradydysrhythmias. Conduction delays such as first-degree AV block and second-degree AV block type I are common and usually transient. An example of an infarction involving the inferior wall is shown in Figure 9-15.

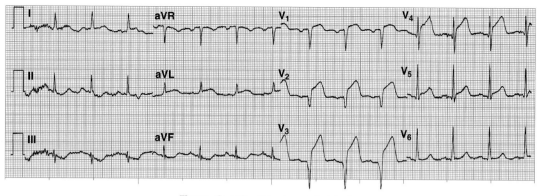

Figure 9-13   Extensive anterior infarction.

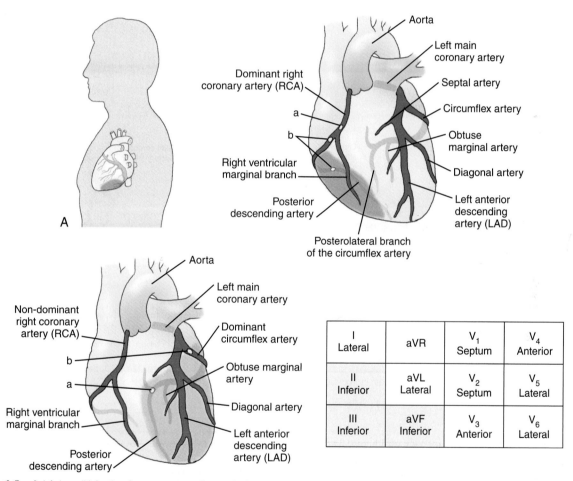

I Lateral	aVR	V_1 Septum	V_4 Anterior
II Inferior	aVL Lateral	V_2 Septum	V_5 Lateral
III Inferior	aVF Inferior	V_3 Anterior	V_6 Lateral

Figure 9-14   **A,** Inferior wall infarction. Coronary anatomy shows a dominant right coronary artery (RCA). Occlusion at point *a* results in an inferior and right ventricular infarction. Occlusion at point *b* is limited to the inferior wall, sparing the right ventricle. **B,** Inferior wall infarction. Coronary anatomy shows a dominant circumflex artery. Occlusion at point *a* results in an inferior infarction. An occlusion at *b* may result in infarction in the lateral and posterior walls.

Lateral Wall Infarctions

Leads I, aVL, V_5, and V_6 view the lateral wall of the left ventricle. The lateral wall of the left ventricle may be supplied by the circumflex artery, the LAD artery, or a branch of the RCA (Figure 9-16).

Septal Infarctions

Leads V_1 and V_2 face the septal area of the left ventricle. The septum, which contains the bundle of His and bundle branches, is normally supplied by the LAD artery (Figure 9-17). If the site of infarction is limited to the septum, ECG changes are

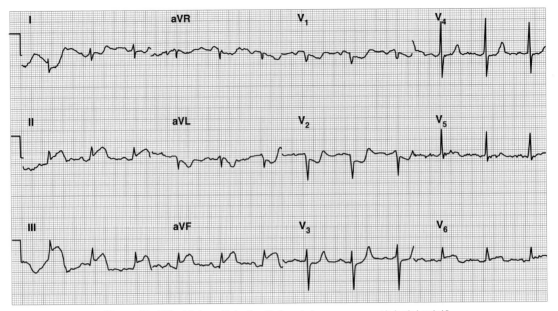

Figure 9-15   Inferior wall infarction. Reciprocal changes are present in leads I and aVL.

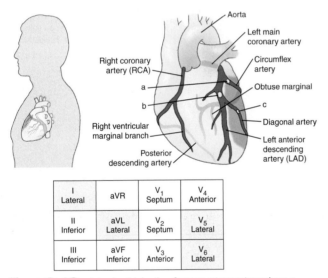

I Lateral	aVR	V₁ Septum	V₄ Anterior
II Inferior	aVL Lateral	V₂ Septum	V₅ Lateral
III Inferior	aVF Inferior	V₃ Anterior	V₆ Lateral

Figure 9-16   Lateral wall infarction. Coronary artery anatomy shows *a* occlusion of the circumflex, *b* occlusion of the proximal LAD artery, and *c* occlusion of the diagonal artery.

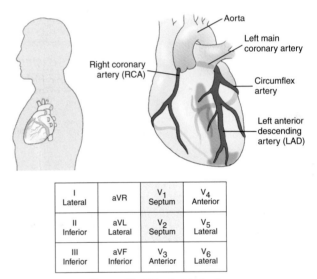

I Lateral	aVR	V₁ Septum	V₄ Anterior
II Inferior	aVL Lateral	V₂ Septum	V₅ Lateral
III Inferior	aVF Inferior	V₃ Anterior	V₆ Lateral

Figure 9-17   Septal infarction.

seen in V_1 and V_2. If the entire anterior wall is involved, ECG changes will be visible in V_1, V_2, V_3, and V_4. A blockage in this area may result in both right and left (more common) bundle branch blocks, second-degree AV block type II, and complete AV block.

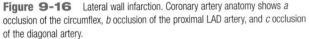

ECG Pearl

Lead aVR is useful in determining if the limb lead electrodes have been correctly positioned. Current normally moves away from aVR. So, under normal conditions you would expect the QRS complex in lead aVR to be predominantly negative (upside down). If the QRS complex is predominantly

negative, continue with your interpretation of the 12-lead. If the QRS complex is predominantly positive (upright), there are two possible causes—there has been a change in current flow and the current is now moving toward the patient's right arm (significant axis deviation) or a cable has been incorrectly placed on the wrong limb. If the cables are incorrectly positioned, reposition the cables and run another 12-lead.[1]

Posterior Wall Infarctions

[OBJECTIVE 8]

The posterior wall of the left ventricle is supplied by the circumflex artery in most patients; however, in some patients it is supplied by the RCA (Figure 9-18). Because no leads of a

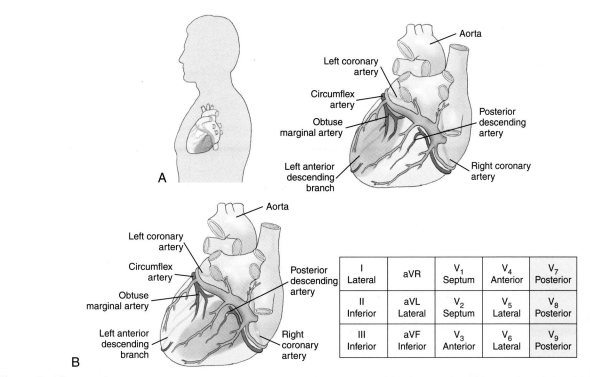

I Lateral	aVR	V₁ Septum	V₄ Anterior	V₇ Posterior
II Inferior	aVL Lateral	V₂ Septum	V₅ Lateral	V₈ Posterior
III Inferior	aVF Inferior	V₃ Anterior	V₆ Lateral	V₉ Posterior

Figure 9-18   **A,** Posterior infarction. Coronary anatomy shows a dominant right coronary artery (RCA). Occlusion of the RCA commonly results in an inferior and posterior infarction. **B,** Coronary anatomy shows a dominant circumflex artery. Occlusion of a marginal branch is the cause of most isolated posterior infarctions.

standard 12-lead ECG directly view the posterior wall of the left ventricle, additional chest leads (V₇ to V₉) may be used to view the heart's posterior surface. Indicative changes of a posterior wall infarction include ST-segment elevation in these leads.

If placement of posterior chest leads is not feasible, changes in the opposite (anterior) wall of the heart can be viewed as reciprocal changes. A posterior wall MI usually produces tall R waves and ST-segment depression in leads V₁, V₂, and to a lesser extent in lead V₃. To assist in the recognition of ECG changes suggesting a posterior wall MI, the "mirror test" is helpful. Flip over the ECG to the blank side and turn it upside down. When held up to the light, the tall R waves become deep Q waves and ST-segment depression becomes ST-segment elevation—the "classic" indicative changes associated with MI.

Complications of a posterior wall MI may include left ventricular dysfunction. If the posterior wall is supplied by the RCA, complications may include dysrhythmias involving the SA node, AV node, and bundle of His.

Right Ventricular Infarctions

[OBJECTIVE 9]

About 50% of patients with inferior infarction have some involvement of the right ventricle.[1] The right ventricle is supplied by the right ventricular marginal branch of the RCA (Figure 9-19). An occlusion of the right ventricular marginal branch results in an isolated right ventricular infarction (RVI). Occlusion of the RCA proximal to the

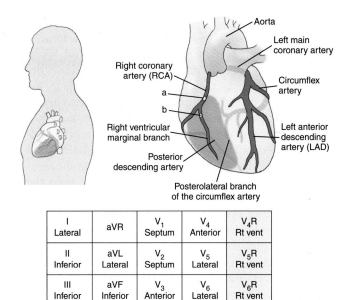

I Lateral	aVR	V₁ Septum	V₄ Anterior	V₄R Rt vent
II Inferior	aVL Lateral	V₂ Septum	V₅ Lateral	V₅R Rt vent
III Inferior	aVF Inferior	V₃ Anterior	V₆ Lateral	V₆R Rt vent

Figure 9-19   Right ventricular infarction (RVI). Occlusion of the right coronary artery (RCA) proximal to the right ventricular marginal branch results in an inferior and RVI. An occlusion of the right ventricular marginal branch results in an isolated RVI.

right ventricular marginal branch results in an inferior and right ventricular infarction. RVI should be suspected when ECG changes suggesting an inferior infarction (ST-segment elevation in leads II, III, and/or aVF) are seen. An example of an infarction involving the right ventricle is shown in Figure 9-20.

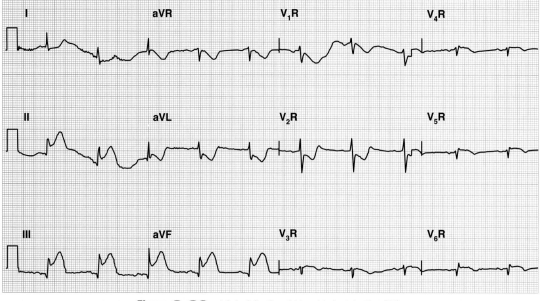

Figure 9-20 Inferior infarction, right ventricular infarction (RVI).

In addition to ECG evidence, certain clinical signs also support the suspicion of RVI. The clinical evidence of RVI involves three main areas: hypotension, jugular venous distention, and clear breath sounds. This triad of signs is estimated to be present in only 10% to 15% of patients with RVI.

In the setting of RVI, the right ventricle may lose some of its ability to pump blood into the pulmonary circuit. When this happens, blood stalls in the right ventricle and may begin to back up. (Technically, the blood does not back up; the venous return exceeds ventricular output and blood begins to build up). This stalling and backing up produce the hypotension, jugular venous distention, and absence of pulmonary edema (clear lung sounds) considered the clinical triad of RVI. As blood backs up from the right ventricle, the jugular veins become enlarged. Hypotension results from the decrease in blood volume moving into the lungs and left ventricle. The left ventricle can only pump as much blood as it receives, and if less blood reaches the left ventricle, less blood is pumped into the systemic circulation. The net effect of this reduction in left ventricular output is a decrease in blood pressure. Complications associated with RVI include hypotension, cardiogenic shock, AV blocks, atrial flutter or fibrillation, and PACs.

R Wave Progression

[OBJECTIVE 10]
Depolarization of the interventricular septum normally occurs from left to right and posteriorly to anteriorly. The wave of ventricular depolarization in the major portions of the ventricles is normally from right to left and in an anterior to posterior direction. When viewing the chest leads in a normal heart, the R wave becomes taller and the S wave

becomes smaller as the electrode is moved from right to left. This pattern is called *R wave progression* (Figure 9-21).

In V_1 and V_2, the QRS deflection is predominantly negative (moving away from the positive chest electrode), reflecting depolarization of the septum and right ventricle (small R wave) and the left ventricle (large S wave). As the chest electrode is placed further left, the wave of depolarization is moving toward the positive electrode. V_3 and V_4 normally record an equiphasic (equally positive and negative) RS complex. The area in which this equiphasic complex occurs is called the transitional zone. V_5 and V_6

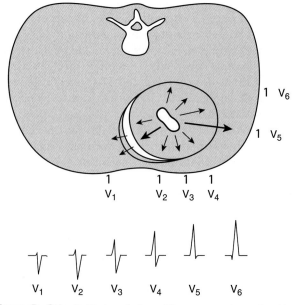

Figure 9-21 Ventricular activation and R wave progression as viewed in the chest leads.

normally record a QR complex in which the Q wave is small, reflecting depolarization of the septum, and the R wave is tall, reflecting ventricular depolarization.

Poor R wave progression (Figure 9-22) is a phrase used to describe R waves that decrease in size from V_1 to V_4. This is often seen in an anteroseptal infarction but may be a normal variant in young persons, particularly in young women. Other causes of poor R wave progression include left bundle branch block, left ventricular hypertrophy, severe chronic obstructive pulmonary disease (particularly emphysema), and old anteroseptal and anterior infarction.

INTRAVENTRICULAR CONDUCTION DELAYS

[OBJECTIVE 11]

During normal ventricular depolarization, the left side of the interventricular septum (stimulated by the left posterior fascicle) is stimulated first. The electrical impulse (wave of depolarization) then traverses the septum to stimulate the right side. The left and right ventricles are then depolarized at the same time. If a delay or block occurs in one of the bundle branches, the ventricles will not be depolarized at the same time. The impulse first travels down the unblocked branch and stimulates that ventricle. Because of the block, the impulse must then travel from cell to cell through the myocardium (rather than through the normal conduction pathway) to stimulate the other ventricle. This means of conduction is slower than normal, and the QRS complex appears widened on the ECG. The ventricle with the blocked bundle branch is the last to be depolarized.

A delay or block can occur in any part of the intraventricular conduction system. A block in only one of the fascicles of the bundle branches is called a **monofascicular block**. A block in any two divisions of the bundle branches is a **bifascicular block**. Although this term may be used to describe a block in both the anterior and posterior branches of the left bundle branch, it is more commonly used to describe a combination of a right bundle branch block and either a left anterior fascicular block (LAFB) or a left posterior fascicular block (LPFB). A **trifascicular block** is a block in the three primary divisions of the bundle branches (i.e., right bundle branch, left anterior fascicle, and left posterior fascicle). A hemiblock is a block in either of the fascicles of the left bundle branch (e.g., left anterior hemiblock, left posterior hemiblock). A hemiblock can be complete or intermittent. Because

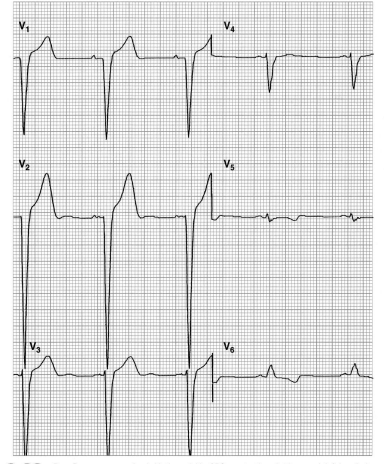

Figure 9-22   Poor R wave progression in V_1 through V_4; QRS greater than 0.12 second: left bundle branch block.

the right bundle branch has only one fascicle, there is no right hemiblock.

The following are ECG criteria for identification of a right or left bundle branch block (BBB):

- QRS duration of more than 0.12 second (if a complete BBB)
- QRS complexes produced by supraventricular activity (i.e., the QRS complex is not a paced beat, and it did not originate in the ventricles)

When measuring for BBB, select the widest QRS complex with a discernible beginning and end. Lead V_1 is probably the single best lead to use when differentiating between right and left BBB.

A QRS measuring 0.10 to 0.12 second is called an incomplete right or left BBB. A QRS measuring more than 0.12 seconds is called a complete right or left BBB. If the QRS is wide but no BBB pattern is discernable, the term wide QRS or intraventricular conduction delay is used to describe the QRS.

In right BBB, the electrical impulse travels through the AV node and down the left bundle branch into the interventricular septum. The septum is activated by the left posterior fascicle and is depolarized in a left-to-right direction. Thus septal depolarization moves in a left-to-right direction, which is toward V_1, and produces an initial small R wave (Figure 9-23). As the left bundle continues to conduct impulses, the entire left ventricle is depolarized from right to left. This produces movement away from V_1 and results in a negative deflection (S wave). The impulses that depolarized the left ventricle conduct through the myocardial cells and depolarize the right ventricle. This depolarization creates a movement of electrical activity in the direction of V_1, and so a second positive deflection is recorded (R'). The rSR' pattern is characteristic of right BBB. Whenever the two criteria for BBB have been met, and V_1 displays an rSR' pattern, right BBB is suspected. The rSR' pattern is sometimes referred to as an M or "rabbit ear" pattern.

In left BBB, the septum is depolarized by the right bundle branch, as is the right ventricle. The septum is part of the left ventricle, and thus the wave of depolarization has begun with the net movement of current going away from V_1. This movement of current continues to move away from V_1 as the rest of the left ventricle is depolarized, and the QRS complex continues in its negative direction. Thus left BBB produces a QS pattern in V_1 (Figure 9-24). When BBB is known to exist and a QS pattern is seen in V_1, left BBB is suspected.

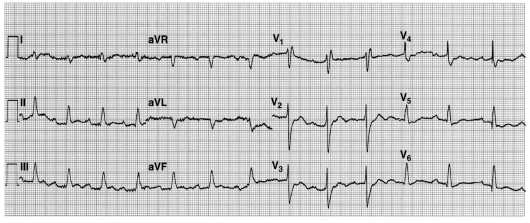

Figure 9-23   The rSR' pattern, characteristic of right bundle branch block.

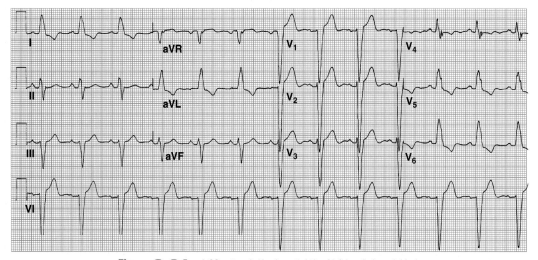

Figure 9-24   A QS pattern in V_1, characteristic of left bundle branch block.

Unfortunately, not every BBB presents with a clear rSR' or QS pattern in V_1. Often the pattern more closely resembles a qR pattern or an rS pattern, making the differentiation less clear. When this occurs, focus should be on the terminal force of the QRS complex. Examination of the terminal force (final portion) of the QRS complex reveals the ventricle that was depolarized last, and therefore the bundle that was blocked. To identify the terminal force, first look at lead V_1 and locate the J-point. Move from the J-point backward into the QRS complex and determine if the terminal portion (last 0.04 sec) of the QRS complex is a positive (upright) or negative (downward) deflection (Figure 9-25). If it is directed upward, a right BBB is present (the current is moving toward the right ventricle and toward V_1). A left BBB is present when the terminal force of the QRS complex is directed downward (the current is moving away from V_1 and toward the left ventricle). A simple way to remember this rule is demonstrated in Figure 9-26. As shown in the figure, this rule is similar to the turn indicator on a vehicle. When a right turn is made, the turn indicator is lifted up. Likewise, when a right BBB is present, the terminal force of the QRS complex points up. Conversely, left turns and left BBB are directed downward.

Two notable exceptions must be mentioned to complete the discussion of BBB. The first involves the criteria used to recognized BBB, while the second relates to differentiating LBBB from RBBB. The criteria used to recognize BBB are valid, but lack some sensitivity and specificity. The sensitivity can be limited by junctional rhythms because there may be no discernible P waves when the AV junction is the pacemaker site. While the AV junction is a supraventricular pacemaker, this presents as an exception to the two-part rule of BBB recognition. Specificity is limited by Wolff-Parkinson-White syndrome (WPW) and other conditions that produce wide QRS complexes resulting from atrial activity. If the

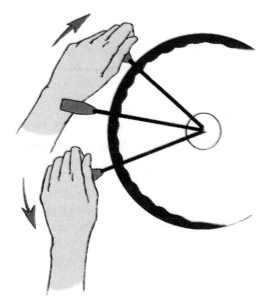

Figure 9-26   Differentiating right versus left BBB. The "turn signal theory:" right is up, left is down.

characteristic delta wave and shortened PR interval are recognized, then WPW can be suspected. Similarly, hyperkalemia and other conditions that can widen the QRS are relatively infrequent.[1]

As for differentiating LBBB from RBBB, a third category exists—Nonspecific Intraventricular Conduction Delay (NSIVCD). These blocks do not display the typical V_1 morphologies generally produced by BBB. Their origin may not be due to a complete BBB, but are often the result of several factors, of which incomplete BBB may be one. Atypical patterns of BBB can be attributed to NSIVCD.[1]

CHAMBER ENLARGEMENT

[OBJECTIVE 12]

Enlargement of the atrial and/or ventricular chambers of the heart may occur if there is a volume or pressure overload in the heart. **Dilatation** is an increase in the diameter of a chamber of the heart caused by volume overload. Dilatation may be acute or chronic. **Hypertrophy** is an increase in the thickness of a heart chamber because of chronic pressure overload. Hypertrophy is commonly accompanied by dilatation. **Enlargement** is a term that implies the presence of dilatation or hypertrophy or both.

The vertical axis of ECG graph paper represents voltage or amplitude of the ECG waveforms or deflections. The size or amplitude of a waveform is measured in millivolts (mV) or millimeters (mm). The ECG machine's sensitivity must be calibrated so that a 1-mV electrical signal will produce a deflection measuring exactly 10 mm tall. Clinically, the height of a waveform is usually stated in millimeters not millivolts.

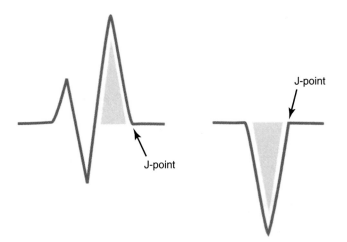

Figure 9-25   Move from the J-point back into the QRS complex and determine if the terminal portion (last 0.04 sec) of the QRS complex is a positive (upright) or negative (downward) deflection. If the criteria for bundle branch block are met and the terminal portion of the QRS is positive, a RBBB is most likely present. If the terminal portion of the QRS is negative, a LBBB is most likely present.

Atrial Enlargement

The first half of the P wave is recorded when the electrical impulse that originated in the SA node stimulates the right atrium and reaches the AV node. The downslope of the P wave reflects stimulation of the left atrium. A normal P wave is smooth and rounded, no more than 2.5 mm in height, and no more than 0.11 sec in duration (width). Normal P waves are positive (upright) in leads I, II, aVF, and V_4 through V_6.

Enlargement of the right atrium produces an abnormally tall initial part of the P wave. The P wave is tall (2.5 mm or more in height in leads II, III, and aVF), peaked, and of normal duration. This type of P wave is called P pulmonale because right atrial enlargement (RAE) is usually caused by conditions that increase the work of the right atrium, such as chronic obstructive pulmonary disease with or without

pulmonary hypertension, congenital heart disease, or right ventricular failure of any cause (Figure 9-27). The P wave may be biphasic in lead V_1 with a more prominent positive portion.

The latter part of the P wave is prominent in left atrial enlargement (LAE). This is because the impulse starts in the right atrium where the SA node is located and chamber size is normal. The electrical impulse then travels to the left to depolarize the left atrium. The waveform inscribed on the ECG is widened (latter part of the P wave) because it takes longer to depolarize an enlarged muscle. The P wave is more than 0.11 second in duration and often notched in leads I, II, aVL, and V_4, V_5, and V_6 (Figure 9-28). The P wave may be biphasic in lead V_1 with a more prominent negative portion. LAE occurs because of conditions that increase left atrial pressure or volume overload or both. These conditions

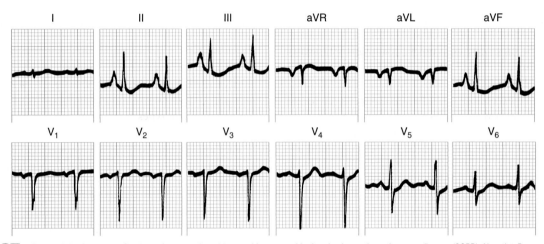

Figure 9-27   Right atrial enlargement. P pulmonale pattern in a 44-year-old woman with chronic obstructive pulmonary disease (COPD). Negative P waves are visible in leads V_1 and V_2.

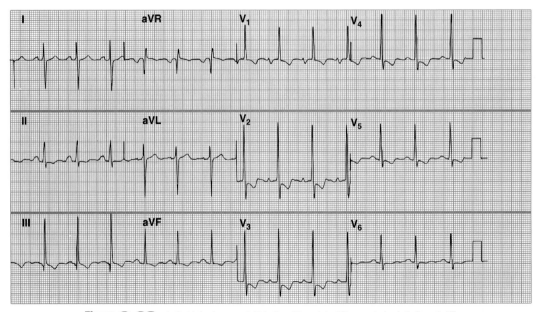

Figure 9-28   Left atrial enlargement. Note the wide, notched P waves in leads II, III, and aVF.

include mitral regurgitation, mitral stenosis, left ventricular failure, and systemic hypertension. Because of the frequent association of LAE with mitral valve disease, the wide, notched P wave that is usually seen is called P mitrale.

Ventricular Enlargement

Ventricular muscle thickens (hypertrophies) when it sustains a persistent pressure overload. Dilatation occurs because of persistent volume overload. The two often go hand in hand. Hypertrophy increases the QRS amplitude and is often associated with ST-segment depression and asymmetric T wave inversion. The ST-segment depression and T wave inversion pattern is called *ventricular strain* or *secondary repolarization changes.*

The amplitude (voltage) of the QRS complex can be affected by various factors, including age, body weight, and lung disease. Increased QRS amplitude may occur normally in thin-chested individuals or young adults because the chest electrodes are closer to the heart in these patients.

Because the right ventricle is normally considerably smaller than the left, it must become extremely enlarged before changes are visible on the ECG. Right axis deviation is one of the earliest and most reliable findings of right ventricular hypertrophy (RVH). Further, normal R wave progression is reversed in the chest leads, revealing taller than normal R waves and small S waves in V_1 and V_2 and deeper than normal S waves and small R waves in V_5 and V_6. Ventricular activation time (VAT) is delayed in V_1. Causes of RVH include pulmonary hypertension and chronic lung diseases, valvular heart disease, and congenital heart disease (Figure 9-29).

Recognition of left ventricular hypertrophy (LVH) on the ECG is not always obvious, and many methods to assist in its recognition have been suggested. ECG signs of LVH include deeper than normal S waves and small R waves in V_1 and V_2 and taller than normal R waves and small S waves in V_5 and V_6. If S wave amplitude in lead V_1 added to the R wave amplitude in V_5 is greater than or equal to 35 mV, LVH should be suspected (Figure 9-30). Causes of LVH include systemic hypertension, hypertrophic cardiomyopathy, aortic stenosis, and aortic insufficiency. LVH may be accompanied by left axis deviation.

ECG Pearl

While bundle branch block increases the *width* of the QRS complex, LVH increases the *amplitude* because of the increase in electrical activity.

ECG CHANGES ASSOCIATED WITH ELECTROLYTE DISTURBANCES

[OBJECTIVE 13]

The primary ions involved in propagation of impulses from cell to cell in the myocardium are sodium, calcium, magnesium, and potassium.

There are two types of action potentials in the heart: fast and slow. This classification is based on the rate of voltage change during depolarization of cardiac cells. Fast-response action potentials occur in the cells of the atria, ventricles, and Purkinje fibers. The fast-response action potential occurs because of the presence of many voltage-sensitive sodium channels that allow a rapid influx of sodium when these channels are open and prevent influx when they are closed. Myocardial fibers with a fast-response action potential can conduct impulses at relatively rapid rates.

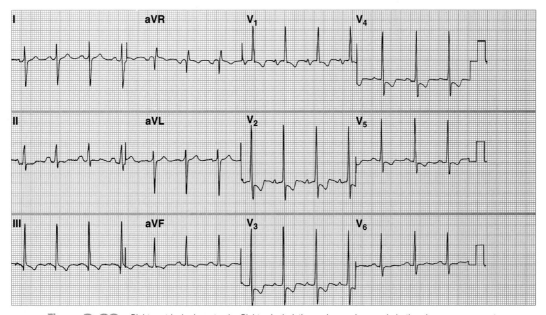

Figure 9-29 Right ventricular hypertrophy. Right axis deviation and secondary repolarization changes are present.

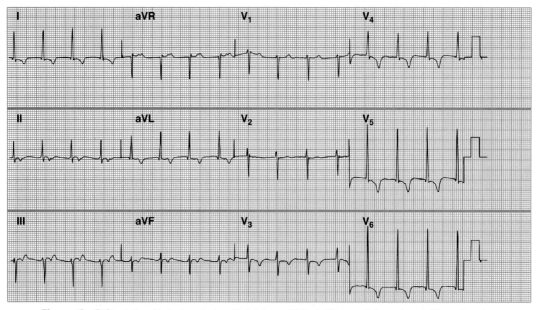

Figure 9-30 Left ventricular hypertrophy with first-degree AV block, ST-segment depression, and T wave inversion.

Slow-response action potentials normally occur in cells such as the SA and AV nodes. These cells do not have fast sodium channels but have slow calcium and slow sodium channels that result in a slower rate of depolarization compared to the depolarization of cardiac cells with fast sodium channels. Slow-response action potentials can occur abnormally anywhere in the heart, usually secondary to ischemia, injury, or an electrolyte imbalance.

Sodium

Normal values: 135 to 145 mEq/L. Causes of hypernatremia (sodium excess) include hypertonic parenteral fluid administration, significantly deficient water intake, excessive salt ingestion, high-protein liquid diets without adequate fluid intake, severe watery diarrhea, or severe insensible water losses (e.g., heat stroke, prolonged high fever). Hypernatremia does not cause any significant changes on the ECG.

Hyponatremia (sodium deficit) may occur because of prolonged diuretic therapy, excessive diaphoresis, and excessive loss of sodium from trauma (e.g., burns); adrenal insufficiency; severe gastrointestinal fluid losses from gastric suctioning or lavage; prolonged vomiting or diarrhea or laxative use; and an insufficient intake of sodium. Hyponatremia does not cause any significant changes on the ECG.

Calcium

Normal values: 4.5 to 5.5 mEq/L or 9 to 11 mg/dL. Causes of hypercalcemia (calcium excess) include prolonged immobility, excessive vitamin D intake, thyrotoxicosis, metastatic carcinoma, excessive use of calcium-containing antacids, and an excessive intake of calcium supplements. ECG changes include a prolonged PR interval, prolonged QRS

complex, and shortened QT interval (because of shortening of the ST-segment).

Hypocalcemia (calcium deficit) may occur because of acute or chronic renal failure, vitamin D deficiency, hyperphosphatemia, hypomagnesemia, and inadequate exposure to ultraviolet light. ECG changes include a long, flattened ST-segment and prolonged QT interval.

Magnesium

Normal values: 1.2 to 2.6 mEq/L. Causes of hypermagnesemia (magnesium excess) include renal failure, excessive use of parenteral magnesium, and excessive use of magnesium-containing antacids or laxatives. ECG changes include a prolonged PR interval, prolonged QRS complex, and elevated T wave.

Hypomagnesemia (magnesium deficit) may occur because of prolonged or excessive diuretic therapy, excessive calcium or vitamin D intake, administration of intravenous fluids or total parenteral nutrition without magnesium replacement, hypercalcemia, high-dose steroid use, cancer chemotherapy, and sepsis. ECG changes include diminished voltage of P waves and QRS complexes, flattened T waves, slightly widened QRS complexes, and prominent U waves.

Potassium

Normal values: 3.5 to 5.0 mEq/L. Hyperkalemia (potassium excess) may occur because of an excessive administration of potassium supplements, excessive use of salt substitutes, potassium-sparing diuretics (e.g., spironolactone), widespread cell damage (e.g., crush injuries, burns), metabolic or respiratory acidosis, and acute or chronic renal failure. ECG changes include tall, peaked (tented) T waves; widened QRS complexes, prolonged PR intervals, flattened ST-segments, and flattened or absent P waves. Hyperkalemia may lead to ventricular dysrhythmias and asystole if not reversed.

Hypokalemia (potassium deficit) may be the result of prolonged diuretic therapy with thiazide diuretics or furosemide, an inadequate dietary intake of potassium, administration of potassium-deficient parenteral fluids, severe gastrointestinal fluid losses from gastric suctioning or lavage, prolonged vomiting or diarrhea, or laxative use without replacement of potassium. ECG changes include a depressed ST-segment, flattened T wave, and prominent U wave (Figure 9-31). Hypokalemia may increase the patient's sensitivity to digitalis toxicity.

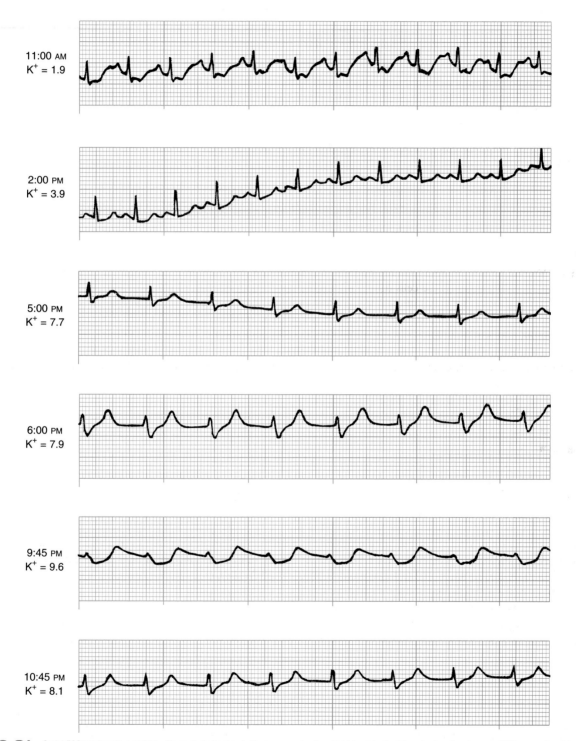

Figure 9-31 Serial ECG tracings in a patient with marked changes in the serum potassium (K+) level. In the 11 AM tracing, the depressed ST-segment and low amplitude T wave blending into a probable U wave (this cannot be seen with clarity because of the superimposed P waves) indicate the presence of hypokalemia. After administration of K+, the 2 PM tracing becomes relatively normal. Continued K+ administration results in hyperkalemia with the disappearance of atrial activity on the ECG and some prolongation of the QRS complex. By 6 PM, the QRS complex is more prolonged, and by 9:45 PM, the QRS complex is greatly prolonged. Secondary ST T wave changes are present. Improvement follows the administration of bicarbonate, glucose, and insulin at 10:45 PM with reduction in the serum K+ level; improvement in the ECG results.

A summary of the ECG changes associated with electrolyte disturbances can be found in Table 9-5.

ANALYZING THE 12-LEAD ECG

[OBJECTIVE 14]

When analyzing a 12-lead ECG, it is important to use a systematic method. Begin by assessing the quality of the tracing. If baseline wander or artifact is present to any significant degree, note it. If the presence of either of these conditions interferes with the assessment of any lead, use a modifier such as "possible" or "apparent" in your interpretation. Next, identify the rate and underlying rhythm. Evaluate intervals—PR interval, QRS duration, and the QT interval and then evaluate waveforms— P waves, Q waves, R waves (R wave progression), T waves, and U waves. If a Q wave is present, express the duration in milliseconds. Examine each lead for the presence of ST-segment displacement (elevation or depression). If ST-segment elevation is present, express it in millimeters. Assess the areas of ischemia or injury by assessing lead groupings. Examine the T waves for any changes in orientation, shape, and size.

Determine axis, look for evidence of hypertrophy/chamber enlargement, and look for effects of medications and electrolyte imbalances. Interpret your findings.

TABLE 9-5   ECG Changes Associated With Electrolyte Disturbances

Electrolyte Disturbance	P Wave	PR Interval	QRS Complex	ST-Segment	T Wave	QT Interval	Heart Rate
Hypocalcemia				Long, flattened		Prolonged	
Hypercalcemia		Prolonged		Shortened		Shortened	
Hypokalemia			Widens as level decreases	Depressed	Flattened; U wave present	Prolonged	
Hyperkalemia	Disappear as level increases	Normal or prolonged	Widens as level increases	Disappear as level increases	Tall, peaked, or tented		Slows
Hypomagnesemia	Diminished voltage (amplitude)		Widens as level decreases; diminished voltage	Depressed	Flattened; U wave present	Prolonged	
Hypermagnesemia		Prolonged	Widened		Tall or elevated		

REFERENCES

1. Phalen T, Aehlert B: The 12-lead ECG in acute coronary syndromes, St Louis, 2006, Elsevier.
2. Shah PK: Mechanisms of plaque vulnerability and rupture, J Am Coll Cardiol 2003;41(4 Suppl S), 15S-22S.
3. Braunwald E, Antman EM, Beasley JW et al: (2002). ACC/ AHA 2002 guideline update for the management of patients with unstable angina and non-ST segment elevation myocardial infarction: A report of the American College of Cardiology/ American Heart Association Task Force on Practice Guidelines (Committee on the Management of Patients With Unstable Angina). Retrieved on June 9, 2006 from http://www.acc.org/ qualityandscience/clinical/guidelines/unstable/incorporated/ US_incorporated.pdf

STOP & REVIEW

True/False

Decide whether each statement is true or false. In the space provided, write T for true or F for false.

_____ 1. Placement of right precordial leads is identical to the standard precordial leads except on the right side of the chest.

_____ 2. In a patient experiencing an acute coronary syndrome, ST-segment elevation in the shape of a "smiley" face (upward concavity) is usually associated with an acute injury pattern.

_____ 3. Consider the presence of right ventricular infarction if a patient with an inferior wall infarction becomes hypotensive after administration of nitrates.

_____ 4. In most patients, the posterior wall of the left ventricle is supplied by the right coronary artery.

_____ 5. An abnormal (pathologic) Q wave indicates the presence of dead myocardial tissue.

_____ 6. Leads V_4R, V_5R, and V_6R are used to view the posterior wall of the left ventricle.

_____ 7. When you read a 12-lead ECG from left to right, the ECG tracing is continuous.

_____ 8. "Poor R wave progression" is a phrase used to describe R waves that decrease in size from V_1 to V_4.

_____ 9. The six limb leads view the heart in the frontal plane as if the body were flat.

Completion

Complete each statement.

10. Each electrode placed on the chest in a "V" position is a _____ (positive/negative) electrode.

11. 0.12 second = _____ milliseconds

12. The axes of leads I, II, and III form an equilateral triangle with the heart at the center (Einthoven's triangle). If the augmented limb leads are added to this configuration and the axes of the six leads moved in a way in which they bisect each other, the result is the _____ _____ _____.

13. Complete the following.

Lead	Heart surface viewed
V_1	_____
V_2	_____
V_3	_____
V_4	_____
V_5	_____
V_6	_____

Matching

Match each item with the correct statement below.

____ 14. Lead located at the fourth intercostal space, left sternal border

____ 15. Common ECG finding in hyperkalemia

____ 16. The zone of _____ is typically characterized by ST-segment elevation.

____ 17. Lead I + Lead III = _____

____ 18. Occlusion of the left anterior descending coronary artery may result in a(n) _____ myocardial infarction.

____ 19. Leads that view the heart in the horizontal plane

____ 20. Leads that view the inferior wall of the heart

____ 21. Lead I is perpendicular to lead _____.

____ 22. Occlusion of the right coronary artery may result in a(n) _____ myocardial infarction.

____ 23. Leads used to view the right ventricle

____ 24. Lead located at the fourth intercostal space, right sternal border

____ 25. Lead II is perpendicular to lead _____.

____ 26. Leads that view the heart in the frontal plane

____ 27. Lead located at the fifth intercostal space, left midclavicular line

____ 28. Direction of the mean QRS vector

____ 29. Lead III is perpendicular to lead _____.

____ 30. Leads that view the lateral wall of the heart

____ 31. The zone of _____ is typically characterized by Q waves.

____ 32. Indicator of the magnitude and direction of current flow

____ 33. Leads that view the septum

a. Lead II

b. aVR

c. Vector

d. Chest

e. V_1-V_2

f. Inferior

g. Electrical axis

h. Injury

i. V_1

j. I, aVL, V_5, V_6

k. Anterior

l. Infarction

m. aVF

n. Tall, tented T waves

o. II, III, aVF

p. V_2

q. Limb

r. aVL

s. V_1R-V_6R

t. V_4

Short Answer

34. List two (2) other names for the "chest" leads.

1.

2.

35. Complete the following table.

Axis	Normal	Left	Right	Indeterminate
Lead I – QRS direction				
Lead aVF – QRS direction				

36. List three (3) acute coronary syndromes.
   1.

   2.

   3.

37. List "the three 'I's" of an acute coronary event.
   1.

   2.

   3.

38. List four (4) causes of ST-segment elevation other than myocardial infarction.
   1.

   2.

   3.

   4.

39. Explain what is meant by the phrase, "Poor R wave progression."

40. In a 12-lead ECG, how long (in seconds) is the view of each lead?

41. Differentiate a physiologic Q wave from a pathologic Q wave.

42. When is the term "intraventricular conduction delay" used?

43. What causes the ST-segment elevation seen in acute myocardial infarction?

44. Explain what is meant by the phrase "anatomically contiguous leads."

12-lead ECGs—*PRACTICE RHYTHM STRIPS*

This 12-lead ECG is from a 42-year-old Caucasian woman.

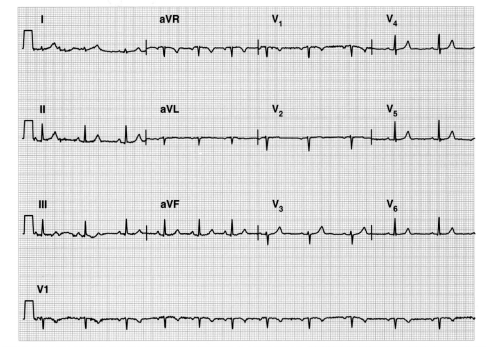

I Lateral	aVR —	V1 septum	V4 anterior	V4R right ventricle
II Inferior	aVL lateral	V2 septum	V5 lateral	V5R right ventricle
III Inferior	aVF inferior	V3 anterior	V6 lateral	V6R right ventricle
Baseline wander or artifact? Yes ☐ No ☐		ST-segment elevation?	Leads: _____	
Underlying rhythm? _____		ST-segment depression?	Leads: _____	
Pathologic Q waves Leads: _____		T wave changes?	Leads: _____	
Poor R-wave progression? Leads: _____		Interpretation: _____		

Figure 9-32

This 12-lead ECG is from a 58-year-old Caucasian man.

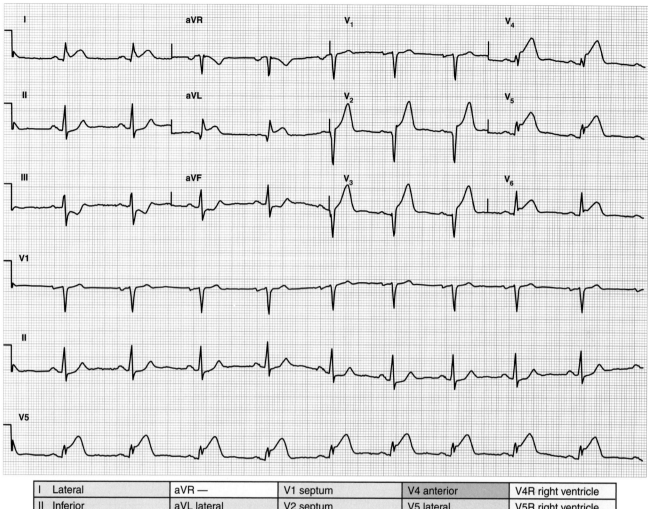

I Lateral	aVR —	V1 septum	V4 anterior	V4R right ventricle
II Inferior	aVL lateral	V2 septum	V5 lateral	V5R right ventricle
III Inferior	aVF inferior	V3 anterior	V6 lateral	V6R right ventricle
Baseline wander or artifact? Yes ☐ No ☐		ST-segment elevation?	Leads: _____	
Underlying rhythm? _____		ST-segment depression?	Leads: _____	
Pathologic Q waves Leads: _____		T wave changes?	Leads: _____	
Poor R-wave progression? Leads: _____		Interpretation: _____		

Figure 9-33

This 12-lead ECG is from a 71-year-old Caucasian woman.

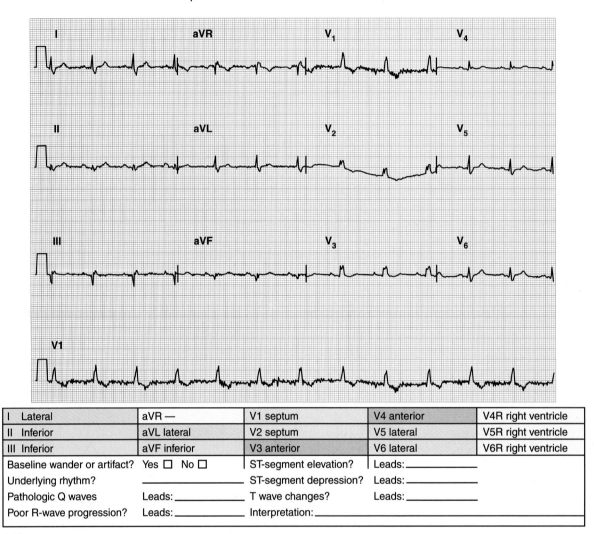

I Lateral	aVR —	V1 septum	V4 anterior	V4R right ventricle
II Inferior	aVL lateral	V2 septum	V5 lateral	V5R right ventricle
III Inferior	aVF inferior	V3 anterior	V6 lateral	V6R right ventricle
Baseline wander or artifact? Yes ☐ No ☐		ST-segment elevation?	Leads: _____	
Underlying rhythm? _____		ST-segment depression?	Leads: _____	
Pathologic Q waves Leads: _____		T wave changes?	Leads: _____	
Poor R-wave progression? Leads: _____		Interpretation: _____		

Figure 9-34

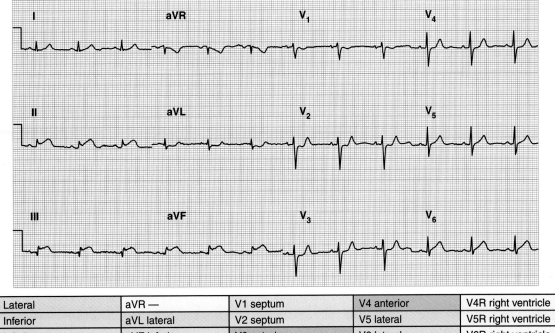

I Lateral	aVR —	V1 septum	V4 anterior	V4R right ventricle
II Inferior	aVL lateral	V2 septum	V5 lateral	V5R right ventricle
III Inferior	aVF inferior	V3 anterior	V6 lateral	V6R right ventricle
Baseline wander or artifact? Yes ☐ No ☐		ST-segment elevation?	Leads: _____	
Underlying rhythm? _____		ST-segment depression?	Leads: _____	
Pathologic Q waves Leads: _____		T wave changes?	Leads: _____	
Poor R-wave progression? Leads: _____		Interpretation: _____		

Figure 9-35

This 12-lead ECG is from an 88-year-old Caucasian man.

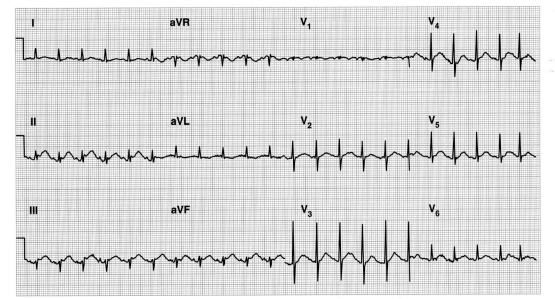

I Lateral	aVR —	V1 septum	V4 anterior	V4R right ventricle
II Inferior	aVL lateral	V2 septum	V5 lateral	V5R right ventricle
III Inferior	aVF inferior	V3 anterior	V6 lateral	V6R right ventricle
Baseline wander or artifact? Yes ☐ No ☐		ST-segment elevation?	Leads: _____	
Underlying rhythm? _____		ST-segment depression?	Leads: _____	
Pathologic Q waves Leads: _____		T wave changes?	Leads: _____	
Poor R-wave progression? Leads: _____		Interpretation: _____		

Figure 9-36

This 12-lead ECG is from a 59-year-old Caucasian woman.

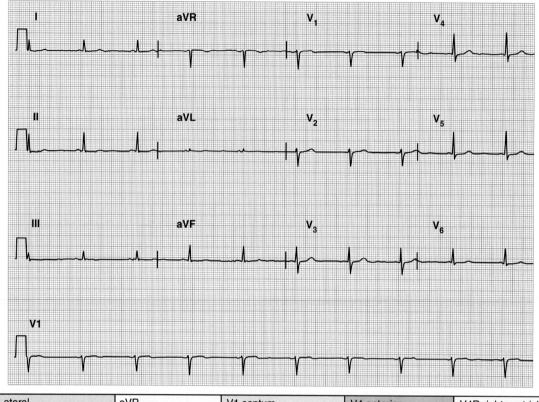

I Lateral	aVR —	V1 septum	V4 anterior	V4R right ventricle
II Inferior	aVL lateral	V2 septum	V5 lateral	V5R right ventricle
III Inferior	aVF inferior	V3 anterior	V6 lateral	V6R right ventricle

Baseline wander or artifact?	Yes ☐ No ☐	ST-segment elevation?	Leads:_____	
Underlying rhythm?	_____	ST-segment depression?	Leads:_____	
Pathologic Q waves	Leads:_____	T wave changes?	Leads:_____	
Poor R-wave progression?	Leads:_____	Interpretation:_____		

Figure 9-37

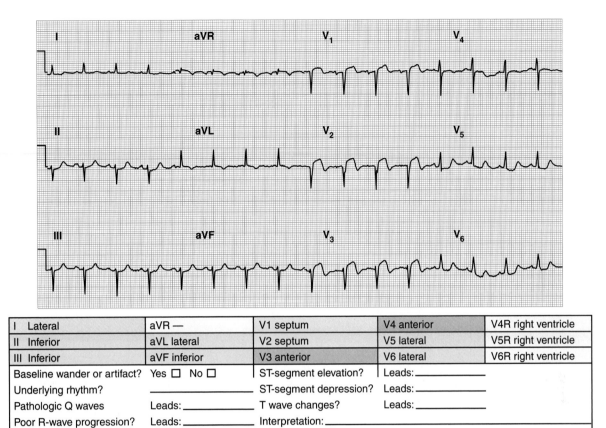

I Lateral	aVR —	V1 septum	V4 anterior	V4R right ventricle
II Inferior	aVL lateral	V2 septum	V5 lateral	V5R right ventricle
III Inferior	aVF inferior	V3 anterior	V6 lateral	V6R right ventricle

Baseline wander or artifact?	Yes ☐ No ☐	ST-segment elevation?	Leads: _____
Underlying rhythm?	_____	ST-segment depression?	Leads: _____
Pathologic Q waves	Leads: _____	T wave changes?	Leads: _____
Poor R-wave progression?	Leads: _____	Interpretation:	_____

Figure 9-38

This 12-lead ECG is from an 86-year-old Caucasian woman.

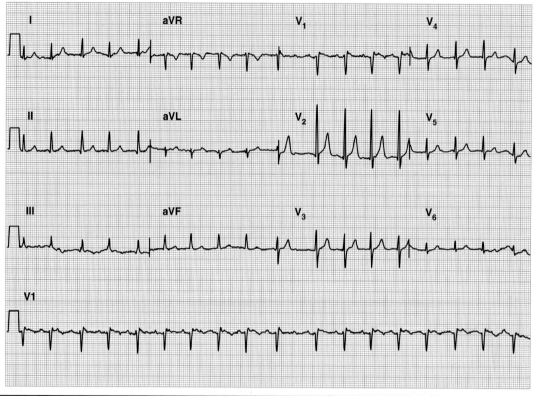

I	Lateral	aVR —	V1 septum	V4 anterior	V4R right ventricle
II	Inferior	aVL lateral	V2 septum	V5 lateral	V5R right ventricle
III	Inferior	aVF inferior	V3 anterior	V6 lateral	V6R right ventricle

Baseline wander or artifact?	Yes ☐ No ☐	ST-segment elevation?	Leads: _____	
Underlying rhythm?	_____	ST-segment depression?	Leads: _____	
Pathologic Q waves	Leads: _____	T wave changes?	Leads: _____	
Poor R-wave progression?	Leads: _____	Interpretation: _____		

Figure 9-39

This 12-lead ECG is from a 69-year-old Caucasian woman.

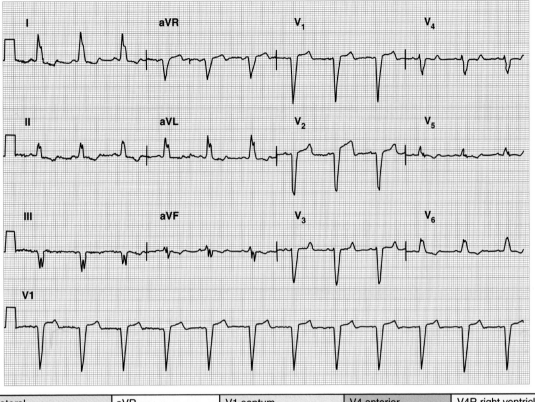

I Lateral	aVR —	V1 septum	V4 anterior	V4R right ventricle
II Inferior	aVL lateral	V2 septum	V5 lateral	V5R right ventricle
III Inferior	aVF inferior	V3 anterior	V6 lateral	V6R right ventricle
Baseline wander or artifact? Yes ☐ No ☐		ST-segment elevation?	Leads: _____	
Underlying rhythm? _____		ST-segment depression?	Leads: _____	
Pathologic Q waves Leads: _____		T wave changes?	Leads: _____	
Poor R-wave progression? Leads: _____		Interpretation: _____		

Figure 9-40

STOP & REVIEW ANSWERS

True/False

1. T
2. F
3. T
4. F

   The posterior wall of the left ventricle is supplied by the circumflex coronary artery in most patients; however, in some patients it is supplied by the right coronary artery.

5. T
6. F

   The leads corresponding to the posterior wall of the left ventricle are V_7, V_8, and V_9.

7. T
8. T
9. T

Completion

10. Each electrode placed on the chest in a "V" position is a *positive* electrode.
11. 0.12 second = *120* milliseconds
12. The axes of leads I, II, and III form an equilateral triangle with the heart at the center (Einthoven's triangle). If the augmented limb leads are added to this configuration and the axes of the six leads moved in a way in which they bisect each other, the result is the *hexaxial reference system.*

13.

Lead	Heart surface viewed
V_1	Septum
V_2	Septum
V_3	Anterior
V_4	Anterior
V_5	Lateral
V_6	Lateral

Matching

14. p
15. n
16. h
17. a
18. k
19. d
20. o
21. m
22. f
23. s

24. i
25. r
26. q
27. t
28. g
29. b
30. j
31. l
32. c
33. e

Short Answer

34. The chest leads are also known as precordial or V leads.
35.

Axis	Normal	Left	Right	Indeterminate ("No Man's Land")
Lead I - QRS Direction	Positive	Positive	Negative	Negative
Lead aVF - QRS Direction	Positive	Negative	Positive	Negative

36. ACS include unstable angina, non–ST-segment elevation myocardial infarction (MI), and ST-segment elevation MI.

37. The processes of ischemia, injury, and infarction are called "the three 'I's" of an acute coronary event.
38. ST-segment elevation may be present in ventricular hypertrophy, conduction abnormalities, pulmonary embolism, spontaneous pneumothorax, intracranial hemorrhage, hyperkalemia, and pericarditis.
39. *Poor R wave progression* is a phrase used to describe R waves that decrease in size from V_1 to V_4.
40. The 12-lead ECG provides a 2.5-second view of each lead because it is assumed that 2.5 seconds is long enough to capture at least one representative complex. However, a 2.5-second view is not long enough to properly assess rate and rhythm, so at least one continuous rhythm strip is usually included at the bottom of the tracing.

41. A physiologic Q wave (present as a normal part of the QRS) in the limb leads is less than 40 ms (less than 0.04 second, or one small box) in duration and less than one third of the amplitude of the R wave in that lead. An abnormal (pathologic) Q wave is more than 40 ms (0.04 sec) in duration and equal to or more than one third of the amplitude of the following R wave in that lead.

42. A QRS measuring 100 to 120 ms is called an incomplete right or left bundle branch block. A QRS measuring more than 120 ms is called a complete right or left bundle branch block. If the QRS is wide but there is no BBB pattern, the term "wide QRS" or "intraventricular conduction delay" is used to describe the QRS.

43. ST-segment elevation is not caused by myocardial infarction per se. While the theories are complex, suffice it to say that ST-segment elevation is caused by changes that affect ventricular repolarization and/or ventricular depolarization. Myocardial infarction produces ST-segment elevation because the infarction affects ventricular repolarization and/or depolarization.

44. *Anatomically contiguous leads* refers to those leads that "see" the same area of the heart. Two leads are contiguous if they look at the same area of the heart or they are numerically consecutive *chest* leads.

Figure 9-32 answer

Underlying rhythm?	Sinus arrhythmia at 67 beats/min
ST-segment depression?	Leads: III
T wave changes?	Leads: Inversion in V_1
Interpretation	Normal ECG
PR interval	164 ms, QRS 66 ms
QT/Q-Tc	392/414 ms
P-R-T axes	81 84 61

Figure 9-33 answer

Underlying rhythm?	Sinus bradycardia at 58 beats/min
ST-segment elevation?	Leads: I, aVL, V_2-V_6
ST-segment depression?	Leads: II, III, aVF
Interpretation	Extensive anterior infarction
PR interval	184 ms, QRS 92 ms
QT/Q-Tc	416/409 ms
P-R-T axes	39 16 16

Figure 9-34 answer

Baseline wander or artifact?	Artifact V_1, baseline wander V_2
Underlying rhythm?	Sinus rhythm at 74 beats/min
Pathologic Q waves?	Leads: III, aVF
T wave changes?	Leads: Inverted V_1, V_2
Interpretation	Right bundle branch block, inferior infarction-age undetermined
PR interval	168 ms, QRS 130 ms
Q-T/Q-Tc	388/430 ms
P-R-T axes	60 −21 46

Figure 9-35 answer

Underlying rhythm?	Sinus rhythm at 71 beats/min
ST-segment elevation?	Leads: II, III, aVF
ST-segment depression?	Leads: V1-V4
Interpretation	Inferior infarction; low QRS voltage (less than 0.5 mV) in limb leads
PR interval	144 ms, QRS 108 ms
QT/Q-Tc	376/398 ms
P-R-T axes	43 44 38

Figure 9-36 answer

Underlying rhythm?	Sinus tachycardia at 136 beats/min with short PR interval, short QT interval
ST-segment elevation?	Leads: II, III, aVF
ST-segment depression?	Leads: I, aVL
T wave changes?	Leads: Inverted in aVL, V_1
Interpretation	Inferior infarction
PR interval	116 ms, QRS 76 ms
Q-T/Q-Tc	228/306 ms
P-R-T axes	59 2 77

Figure 9-37 answer

Underlying rhythm?	Sinus bradycardia at 58 beats/min
ST-segment elevation?	Leads:
ST-segment depression?	Leads:
T wave changes?	Leads:
Interpretation	Sinus bradycardia, otherwise normal ECG
PR interval	122 ms, QRS 86 ms
QT/Q-Tc	416/408 ms
P-R-T axes	41 54 22

Figure 9-38 answer

Baseline wander or artifact?	Baseline wander V_5, V_6
Underlying rhythm?	Sinus rhythm at 95 beats/min
ST-segment elevation?	Leads: V_1-V_3
ST-segment depression?	Leads: II, III, V_5, V_6
T wave changes?	Leads: Inverted in aVL
Interpretation	Septal infarction, possible anterior epicardial injury
PR interval	164 ms, QRS 96 ms
QT/Q-Tc	380/433 ms
P-R-T axes	62 −62 83

Figure 9-39 answer

Baseline wander or artifact?	Baseline wander V_4-V_6
Underlying rhythm?	Atrial fibrillation at 107 beats/min
ST-segment depression?	Leads: V_6
T wave changes?	Leads: Tall in V_2
Interpretation	Atrial fibrillation with rapid ventricular response
PR interval	None, QRS 90 ms
QT/Q-Tc	304/405 ms
P-R-T axes	None 69 17

Figure 9-40 answer

Underlying rhythm?	Sinus rhythm at 73 beats/min
ST-segment elevation?	Leads: V_1-V_2
ST-segment depression?	Leads: I, II, aVL, aVF, V_5-V_6
Interpretation	Left bundle branch block
PR interval	136 ms, QRS 144 ms
QT/Q-Tc	438/482 ms
P-R-T axes	28 −5 238

Post-Test

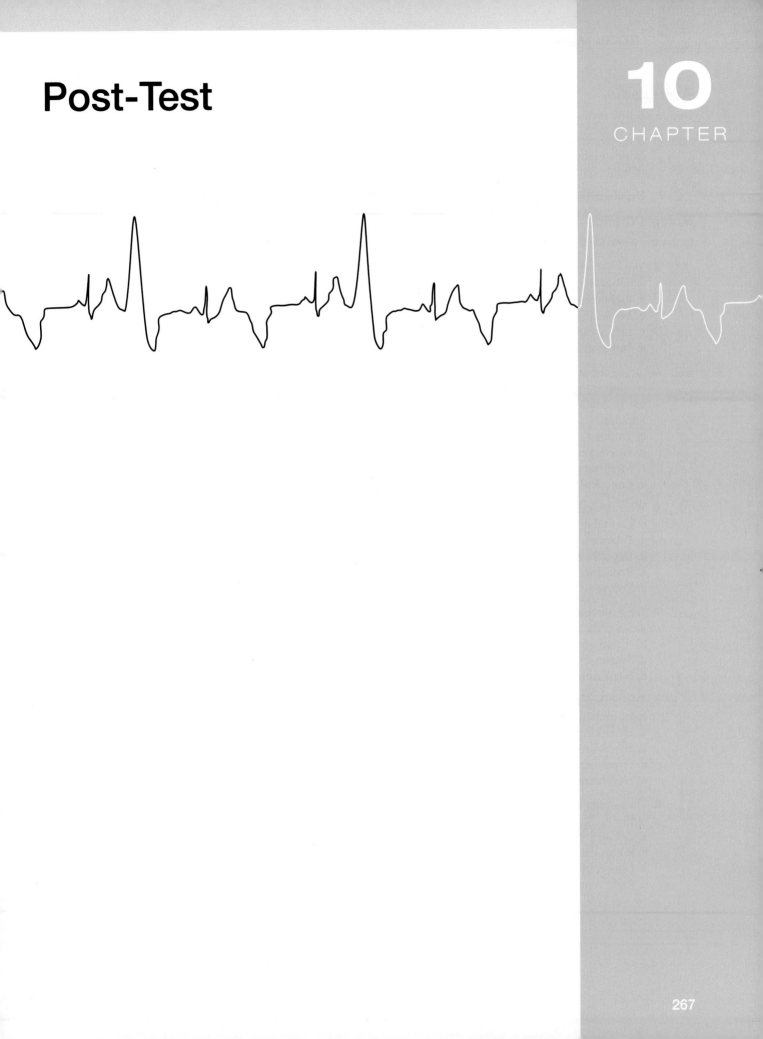

True/False

Decide whether each statement is true or false. In the space provided, write T for true or F for false.

____ **1.** A macroreentrant circuit is one that involves a small area of heart tissue, usually a few centimeters or less.

____ **2.** Depolarization is the same as contraction.

____ **3.** Proper positioning of the electrodes for leads I, II, and III requires placement on the patient's torso.

Multiple Choice

In the space provided, identify the letter of the choice that best completes each statement or answers each question.

____ **4.** The _____ supplies the right atrium and ventricle with blood.
   a. Right coronary artery
   b. Left main coronary artery
   c. Left circumflex artery
   d. Left anterior descending artery

____ **5.** _____ cells are specialized cells of the electrical conduction system responsible for the spontaneous generation and conduction of electrical impulses.
   a. Working
   b. Pacemaker
   c. Mechanical
   d. Contractile

____ **6.** When the cardiac muscle cell is stimulated, the cell is said to:
   a. Polarize
   b. Depolarize
   c. Repolarize
   d. Recover

____ **7.** The basic contractile unit of a myofibril is the:
   a. Sinoatrial (SA) node
   b. Action potential
   c. Sarcomere
   d. Intercalated disk

____ **8.** Tall, peaked T waves observed on the ECG are most commonly seen in patients with:
   a. Hyperkalemia
   b. Hypokalemia
   c. Hypernatremia
   d. Hyponatremia

____ **9.** The anterior surface of the heart consists primarily of the:
   a. Left atrium
   b. Right atrium
   c. Left ventricle
   d. Right ventricle

____ **10.** The absolute refractory period:
   a. Begins with the onset of the P wave and terminates with the end of the QRS complex
   b. Begins with the onset of the QRS complex and terminates at approximately the apex of the T wave
   c. Begins with the onset of the QRS complex and terminates with the end of the T wave
   d. Begins with the onset of the P wave and terminates with the beginning of the QRS complex

____ **11.** How do you determine whether the atrial rhythm on an ECG tracing is regular or irregular?
   a. Compare QT intervals
   b. Compare PR intervals
   c. Compare R to R intervals
   d. Compare P to P intervals

____ **12.** Which of the following ECG leads are bipolar leads?
   a. Leads aVR, aVL, and aVF
   b. Leads V_4, V_5, and V_6
   c. Leads V_1, V_2, and V_3
   d. Leads I, II, and III

____ **13.** Which of the following are chest leads?
   a. Leads I, II, and III
   b. Leads I and aVL
   c. Leads V_1, V_2, V_3, V_4, V_5, V_6
   d. Leads I, II, III, aVR, aVL, and aVF

____ **14.** U waves are thought to represent:
   a. Repolarization of the Purkinje fibers
   b. Ventricular depolarization
   c. Repolarization of the bundle of His
   d. Atrial depolarization

____ **15.** In sinus arrhythmia, a gradual decreasing of the heart rate is usually associated with:
   a. Expiration
   b. Inspiration
   c. Excessive caffeine intake
   d. Early signs of congestive heart failure

____ **16.** An ECG rhythm strip shows a ventricular rate of 46, a regular rhythm, a PR interval of 0.14 second, a QRS duration of 0.06, and one upright P wave before each QRS. This rhythm is:
  a. Sinus rhythm
  b. Sinus bradycardia
  c. Sinus arrest
  d. Sinoatrial block

____ **17.** What is meant by the term "uncontrolled" atrial fibrillation?
  a. The overall ventricular rate is less than 100 beats/min.
  b. The atrial rate is less than 100 beats/min.
  c. The overall ventricular rate is greater than 100 beats/min.
  d. The atrial rate is greater than 100 beats/min.

____ **18.** Which of the following correctly describes multifocal atrial tachycardia?
  a. Atrial rhythm is regular.
  b. Ventricular rhythm is irregular.
  c. Atrial and ventricular rhythms are regular.
  d. Atrial and ventricular rhythms are irregular.

____ **19.** The most common type of supraventricular tachycardia (SVT) is:
  a. Atrial tachycardia
  b. Atrial flutter
  c. AV reentrant tachycardia (AVRT)
  d. AV nodal reentrant tachycardia (AVNRT)

____ **20.** Wolff-Parkinson-White syndrome is associated with a:
  a. Long PR interval, delta wave, and wide QRS complex
  b. Short PR interval, flutter waves, and narrow QRS complex
  c. Long PR interval, flutter waves, and narrow QRS complex
  d. Short PR interval, delta wave, and wide QRS complex

____ **21.** Signs and symptoms experienced during a tachydysrhythmia are usually primarily related to:
  a. Slowed conduction through the AV node
  b. Vasoconstriction
  c. Atrial irritability
  d. Decreased ventricular filling time and stroke volume

____ **22.** How are frequent PACs usually managed?
  a. Synchronized cardioversion
  b. Defibrillation
  c. Administration of medications such as atropine or epinephrine
  d. Correcting the underlying cause

____ **23.** Which of the following ECG characteristics distinguishes atrial flutter from other atrial dysrhythmias?
  a. The presence of fibrillatory waves
  b. The presence of delta waves before the QRS
  c. The sawtooth or "picket-fence" appearance of waveforms before the QRS
  d. P waves of varying size and amplitude

____ **24.** In a junctional rhythm viewed in lead II, where is the location of the P wave on the ECG if atrial and ventricular depolarization occur simultaneously?
  a. Before the QRS complex
  b. During the QRS complex
  c. After the QRS complex

____ **25.** The usual rate of nonparoxysmal junctional tachycardia is:
  a. 50 to 80 beats/min
  b. 80 to 120 beats/min
  c. 101 to 140 beats/min
  d. 150 to 300 beats/min

____ **26.** Depending on the severity of the patient's signs and symptoms, management of slow rhythms originating from the AV junction may require intervention including:
  a. Defibrillation
  b. Vagal maneuvers and/or adenosine
  c. Atropine and/or transcutaneous pacing
  d. Synchronized cardioversion

____ **27.** The term for three or more premature ventricular complexes (PVCs) occurring in a row at a rate of more than 100/min is:
  a. Ventricular trigeminy
  b. A run of ventricular tachycardia
  c. A run of ventricular escape beats
  d. Ventricular fibrillation

____ **28.** The PR interval of a first-degree AV block:
  a. Is constant and greater than 0.20 second in duration
  b. Is completely variable in duration
  c. Gradually decreases in duration until a P wave appears without a QRS complex
  d. Gradually lengthens until a P wave appears without a QRS complex

____ **29.** In 2:1 AV block, the PR interval:
  a. Is completely variable
  b. Shortens
  c. Remains the same
  d. Lengthens

____ **30.** Capture is:
   a. The time measured between a sensed cardiac event and the next pacemaker output
   b. A vertical line on the ECG that indicates the pacemaker has discharged
   c. The ability of a pacing stimulus to successfully depolarize the cardiac chamber that is being paced
   d. The electrical stimulus delivered by a pacemaker's pulse generator

____ **31.** Myocardial ischemia delays the process of repolarization; thus, the ECG changes characteristic of ischemia include:
   a. Changes in the ST-segment and T wave
   b. Widening of the QRS complex
   c. Changes in the QRS complex and ST-segment
   d. Prolongation of the PR interval

____ **32.** Poor R wave progression is a phrase used to describe R waves that decrease in size from V_1 to V_4. This is often seen in a(n) _____ infarction.
   a. Anteroseptal
   b. Anterolateral
   c. Inferolateral
   d. Inferoposterior

____ **33.** The QT interval is measured from the:
   a. Beginning of the QRS complex to the beginning of the T wave
   b. End of the Q wave to the beginning of the P wave
   c. Beginning of the QRS complex to the end of the T wave
   d. End of the T wave to the beginning of the P wave

Completion

Complete each statement.

34. A beat originating from the AV junction that appears later than the next expected sinus beat is called a _____ _____ _____.

35. A rapid, wide-QRS rhythm associated with pulselessness, shock, or congestive heart failure should be presumed to be _____ _____.

36. PACs associated with a wide QRS complex are called _____ _____ PACs, indicating that conduction through the ventricles is abnormal.

37. The right atrium receives deoxygenated blood from the _____ _____ _____ (which carries blood from the head and upper extremities), the _____ _____ _____ (which carries blood from the lower body), and the _____ _____ (which receives blood from the intracardiac circulation).

38. _____ is the period of relaxation during which a heart chamber is filling.

39. The thick, muscular middle layer of the heart wall that contains the atrial and ventricular muscle fibers necessary for contraction is the _____.

40. An ECG lead that has a positive and negative electrode is called a(n) _____ lead.

41. The appearance of coved ("frowny face") ST segment elevation is called a(n) _____ _____ _____.

42. Delivery of an electrical current timed for delivery during the QRS complex is called _____ _____.

43. Sometimes, when a premature atrial complex (PAC) occurs very prematurely and close to the T wave of the preceding beat, only a P wave may be seen with no QRS after it (appearing as a pause). This type of PAC is termed a(n) _____ _____ PAC.

44. If the AV junction paces the heart, the electrical impulse must travel in a(n) _____ direction to activate the atria.

45. A _____ _____ occurs as a result of an electrical impulse from a supraventricular site (such as the SA node) discharging at the same time as an ectopic site in the ventricles.

46. A _____ _____ is a vertical line on the ECG that indicates the pacemaker has discharged.

47. A demand pacemaker is also known as a _____ pacemaker.

48. A _____ bundle branch block produces an rSR' pattern in lead V_1.

49. Indicate the heart surface viewed by each of the following.

Leads II, III, aVF: _____

Leads V_1, V_2:   _____

Leads V_3, V_4:   _____

Leads I, aVL, V_5, V_6:   _____

50. The axes of leads I, II, and III form an equilateral triangle with the heart at the center (Einthoven's triangle). If the augmented limb leads are added to this configuration and the axes of the six leads moved in a way in which they bisect each other, the result is the _____ _____ _____.

51. The area supplied by an obstructed coronary artery goes through a characteristic sequence of events that have been identified as zones of _____, _____, and _____.

52. Indicate the inherent rates for each of the following pacemaker sites:

Sinoatrial (SA) node: _____

Atrioventricular (AV) junction: _____

Ventricles: _____

Short Answer

53. List four (4) properties of cardiac cells.
  1.

  2.

  3.

  4.

54. List five (5) signs or symptoms of hemodynamic compromise.

  1.

  2.

  3.

  4.

  5.

55. Explain what is meant by the phrase "anatomically contiguous leads."

56. Indicate the ECG criteria for the following dysrhythmias:

	Second-degree AV block type I	*Third-degree AV block*	*Ventricular*
Rhythm		_____	_____
PR interval		_____	_____
QRS width		_____	_____

57. List four (4) reasons why the AV junction may assume responsibility for pacing the heart.
   1.

   2.

   3.

   4.

58. List four (4) common causes of premature ventricular complexes.

   1.

   2.

   3.

   4.

59. What is the name given to polymorphic VT that occurs in the presence of a long QT interval?

60. Complete the following ECG criteria for second-degree AV block type II.

Rate: _____

Rhythm: _____

P waves: _____

PR interval: _____

QRS duration: _____

61. What is the most important difference between sinus rhythm and sinus tachycardia?

62. On the ECG, what do the ST-segment and T wave represent?

63. What is a biphasic waveform?

64. List three (3) causes of artifact on an ECG tracing.
   1.

   2.

   3.

65. Describe the appearance of a pathologic Q wave.

66. List three (3) uses for ECG monitoring.

67. Your patient has a VVI pacemaker. Briefly explain the meaning of each of these letters.

68. Explain the Frank-Starling law of the heart.

TEST RHYTHM STRIPS

For each of the following rhythm strips, determine the atrial and ventricular rates, measure the PR interval and QRS duration, and then identify the rhythm. All strips are lead II unless otherwise noted.

This rhythm strip is from an 85-year-old woman complaining of dizziness and feeling faint. BP 132/80, R 12, O_2 sat 96% on room air. Blood sugar is 118. She has a history of hypertension and Parkinson's disease. Medications include aspirin, Plavix, Depakote, Lexapro, Zocor, diltiazem, and amiodarone.

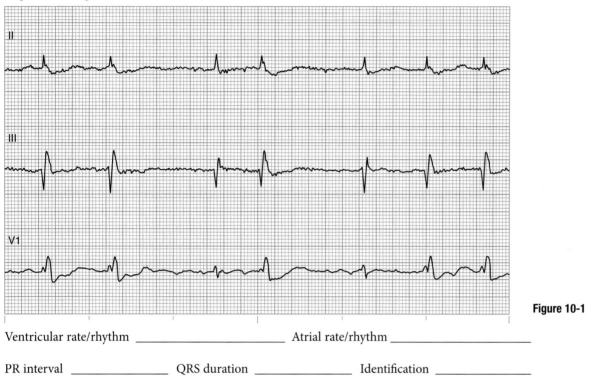

Figure 10-1

Ventricular rate/rhythm _____   Atrial rate/rhythm _____

PR interval _____   QRS duration _____   Identification _____

This rhythm strip is from a 68-year-old woman complaining of dizziness. BP 142/81, R 32. She has a history of diabetes and diverticulitis. Blood sugar is 176.

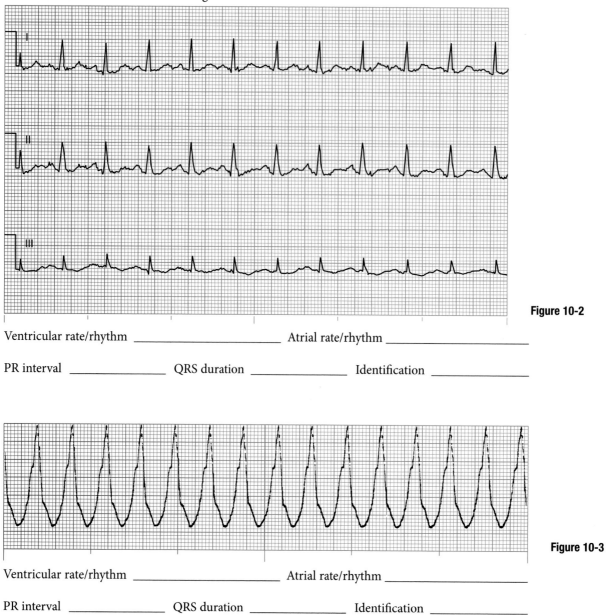

Figure 10-2

Ventricular rate/rhythm _____ Atrial rate/rhythm _____

PR interval _____ QRS duration _____ Identification _____

Figure 10-3

Ventricular rate/rhythm _____ Atrial rate/rhythm _____

PR interval _____ QRS duration _____ Identification _____

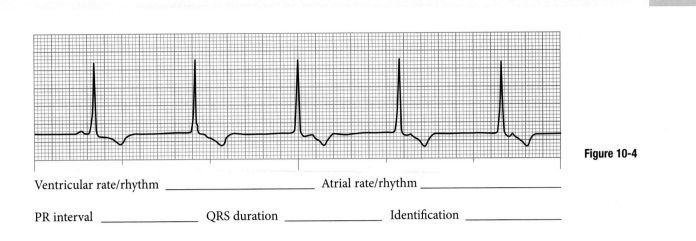

Figure 10-4

Ventricular rate/rhythm _____ Atrial rate/rhythm _____

PR interval _____ QRS duration _____ Identification _____

This rhythm strip is from a 33-year-old man who is seeking medical attention because he wants "the voices in my head to stop." Blood pressure 144/72, blood glucose 99 mg/dL.

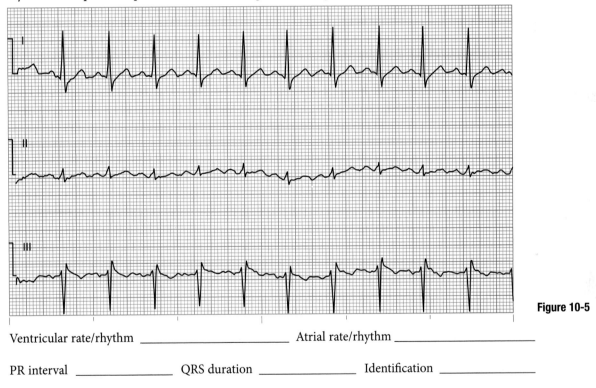

Figure 10-5

Ventricular rate/rhythm _____ Atrial rate/rhythm _____

PR interval _____ QRS duration _____ Identification _____

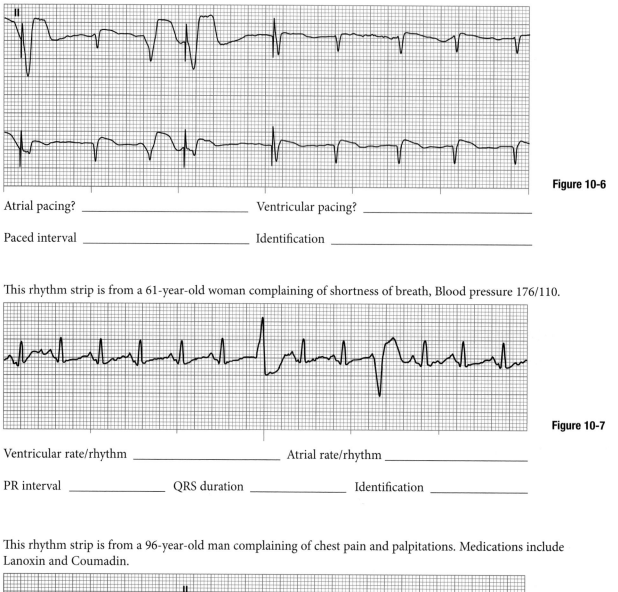

Figure 10-6

Atrial pacing? _____   Ventricular pacing? _____

Paced interval _____   Identification _____

This rhythm strip is from a 61-year-old woman complaining of shortness of breath, Blood pressure 176/110.

Figure 10-7

Ventricular rate/rhythm _____   Atrial rate/rhythm _____

PR interval _____   QRS duration _____   Identification _____

This rhythm strip is from a 96-year-old man complaining of chest pain and palpitations. Medications include Lanoxin and Coumadin.

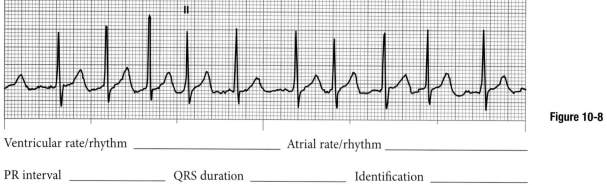

Figure 10-8

Ventricular rate/rhythm _____   Atrial rate/rhythm _____

PR interval _____   QRS duration _____   Identification _____

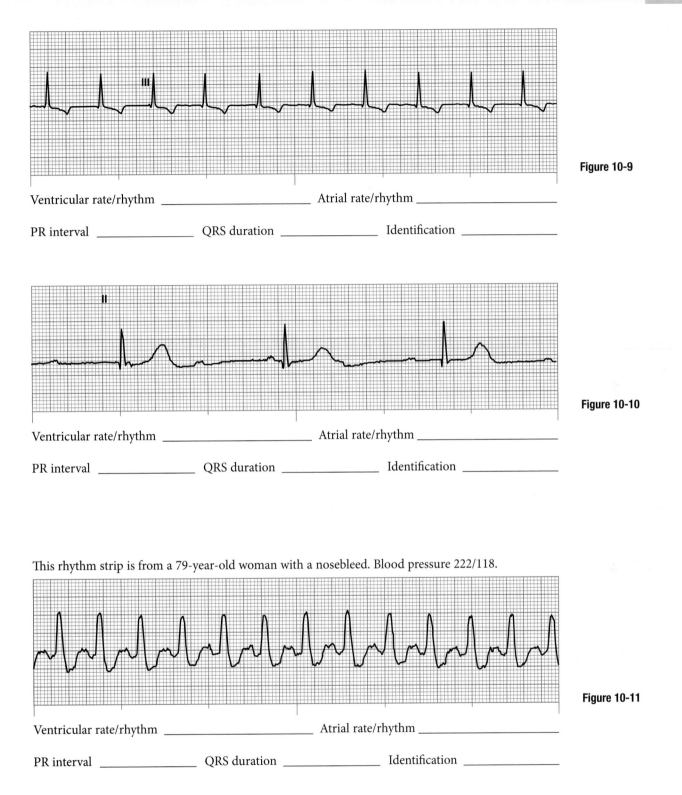

Figure 10-9

Ventricular rate/rhythm _____   Atrial rate/rhythm _____

PR interval _____   QRS duration _____   Identification _____

Figure 10-10

Ventricular rate/rhythm _____   Atrial rate/rhythm _____

PR interval _____   QRS duration _____   Identification _____

This rhythm strip is from a 79-year-old woman with a nosebleed. Blood pressure 222/118.

Figure 10-11

Ventricular rate/rhythm _____   Atrial rate/rhythm _____

PR interval _____   QRS duration _____   Identification _____

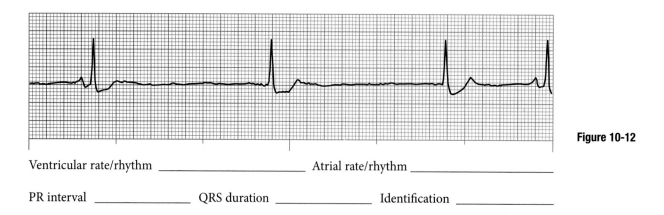

Figure 10-12

Ventricular rate/rhythm _____ Atrial rate/rhythm _____

PR interval _____ QRS duration _____ Identification _____

This rhythm strip is from a 79-year-old man after choking on a piece of meat. The foreign body was removed. BP 119/83, R 20.

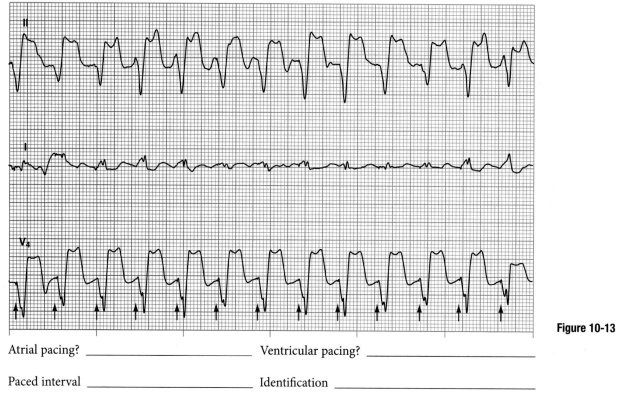

Figure 10-13

Atrial pacing? _____ Ventricular pacing? _____

Paced interval _____ Identification _____

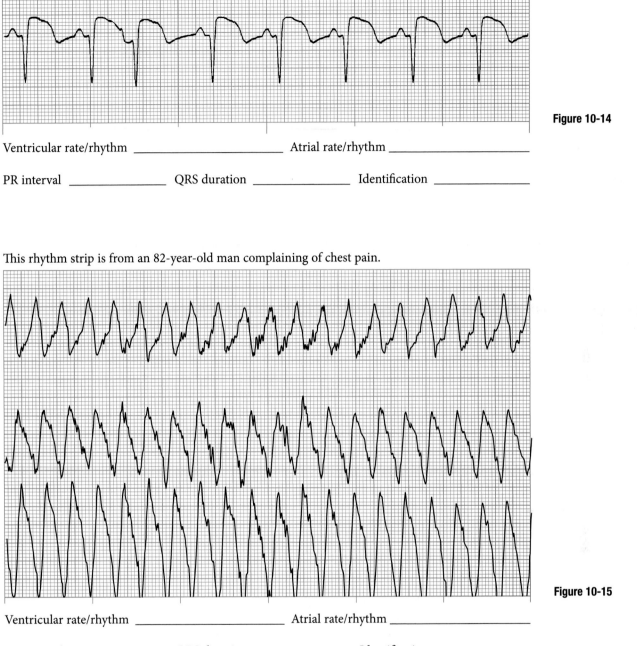

Figure 10-14

Ventricular rate/rhythm _____ Atrial rate/rhythm _____

PR interval _____ QRS duration _____ Identification _____

This rhythm strip is from an 82-year-old man complaining of chest pain.

Figure 10-15

Ventricular rate/rhythm _____ Atrial rate/rhythm _____

PR interval _____ QRS duration _____ Identification _____

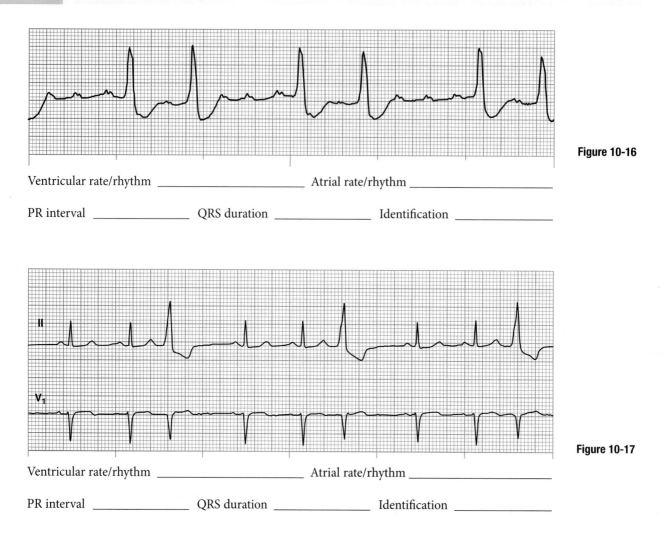

Figure 10-16

Ventricular rate/rhythm _____ Atrial rate/rhythm _____

PR interval _____ QRS duration _____ Identification _____

Ventricular rate/rhythm _____ Atrial rate/rhythm _____

PR interval _____ QRS duration _____ Identification _____

Figure 10-17

These rhythm strips are from a 52-year-old man with syncope.

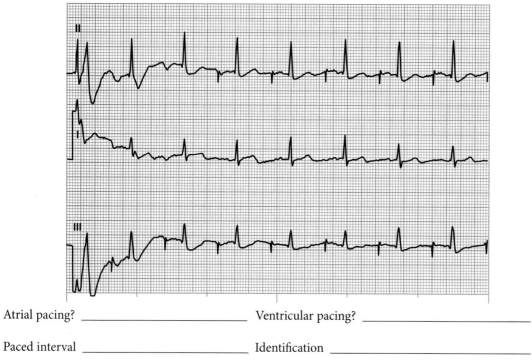

Figure 10-18

Atrial pacing? _____ Ventricular pacing? _____

Paced interval _____ Identification _____

These rhythm strips are from a 68-year-old man who has an altered level of consciousness following a dialysis treatment 7 hours ago. Blood pressure 134/69, blood glucose level 62 mg/dL.

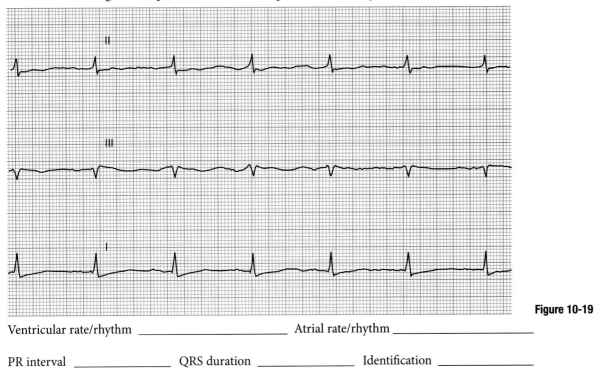

Figure 10-19

Ventricular rate/rhythm _____ Atrial rate/rhythm _____

PR interval _____ QRS duration _____ Identification _____

These rhythm strips are from a 49-year-old woman complaining of nausea and vomiting × 24 hours and chest pain. BP 179/109. Oxygen saturation 93% on room air. She has a history of hypertension, stroke, and asthma. She takes Lopressor daily.

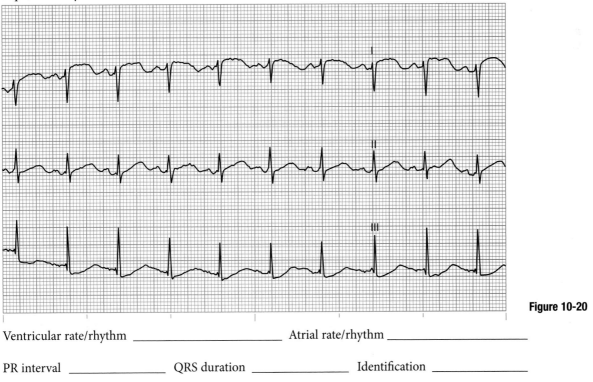

Figure 10-20

Ventricular rate/rhythm _____ Atrial rate/rhythm _____

PR interval _____ QRS duration _____ Identification _____

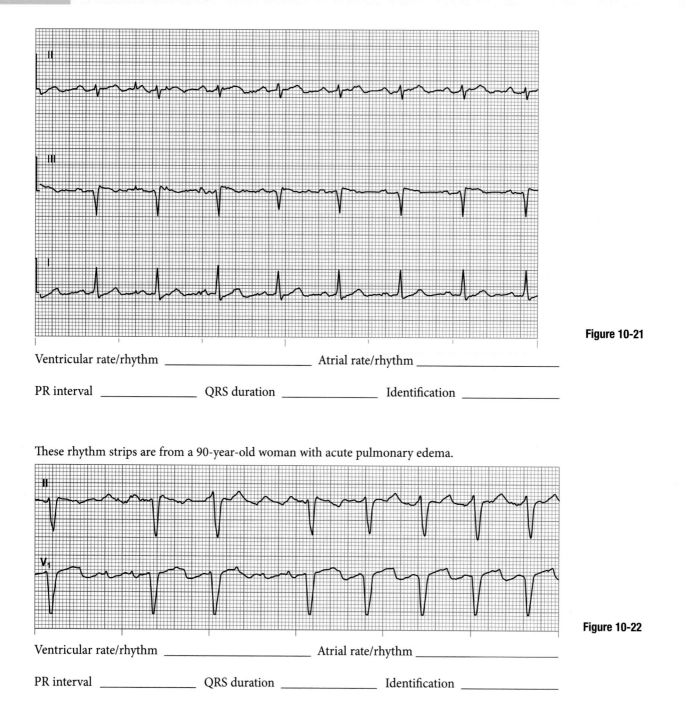

Figure 10-21

Ventricular rate/rhythm _____ Atrial rate/rhythm _____

PR interval _____ QRS duration _____ Identification _____

These rhythm strips are from a 90-year-old woman with acute pulmonary edema.

Figure 10-22

Ventricular rate/rhythm _____ Atrial rate/rhythm _____

PR interval _____ QRS duration _____ Identification _____

This rhythm strip is from a 76-year-old woman complaining of back pain. Her medical history includes a myocardial infarction 2 years ago.

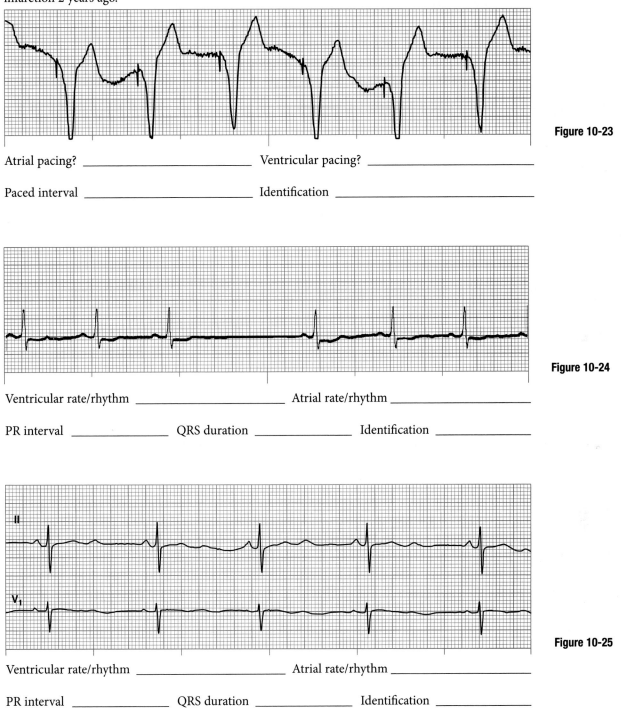

Figure 10-23

Atrial pacing? _____   Ventricular pacing? _____

Paced interval _____   Identification _____

Figure 10-24

Ventricular rate/rhythm _____   Atrial rate/rhythm _____

PR interval _____   QRS duration _____   Identification _____

Figure 10-25

Ventricular rate/rhythm _____   Atrial rate/rhythm _____

PR interval _____   QRS duration _____   Identification _____

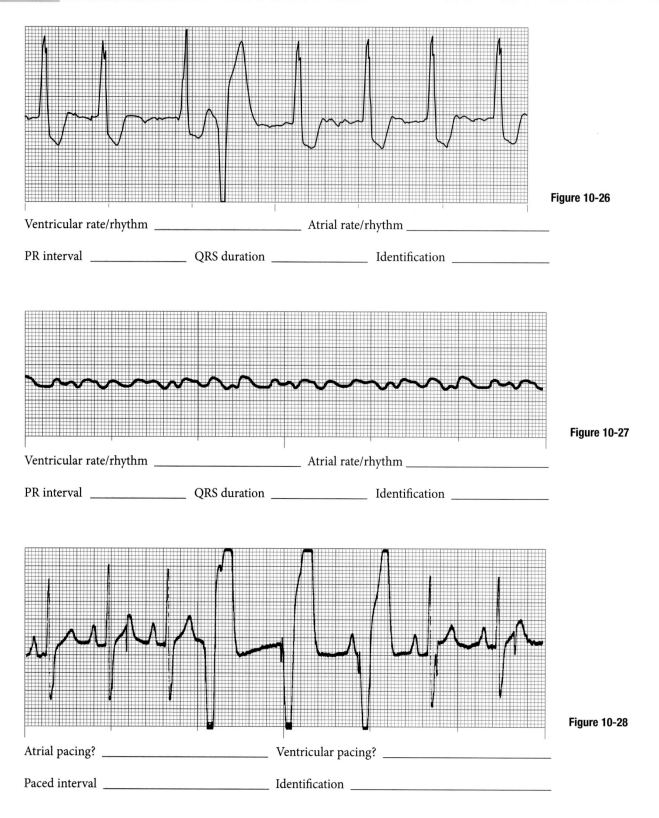

Figure 10-26

Ventricular rate/rhythm _____ Atrial rate/rhythm _____

PR interval _____ QRS duration _____ Identification _____

Figure 10-27

Ventricular rate/rhythm _____ Atrial rate/rhythm _____

PR interval _____ QRS duration _____ Identification _____

Figure 10-28

Atrial pacing? _____ Ventricular pacing? _____

Paced interval _____ Identification _____

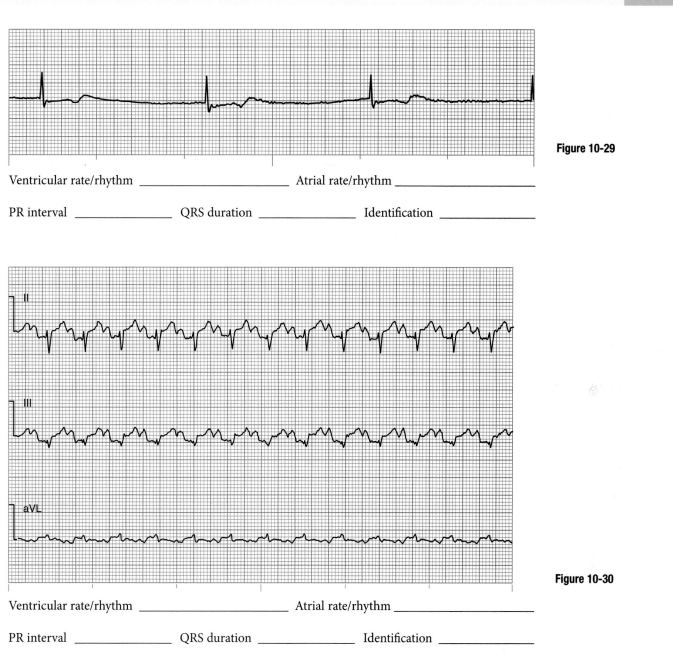

Figure 10-29

Ventricular rate/rhythm _____ Atrial rate/rhythm _____

PR interval _____ QRS duration _____ Identification _____

Figure 10-30

Ventricular rate/rhythm _____ Atrial rate/rhythm _____

PR interval _____ QRS duration _____ Identification _____

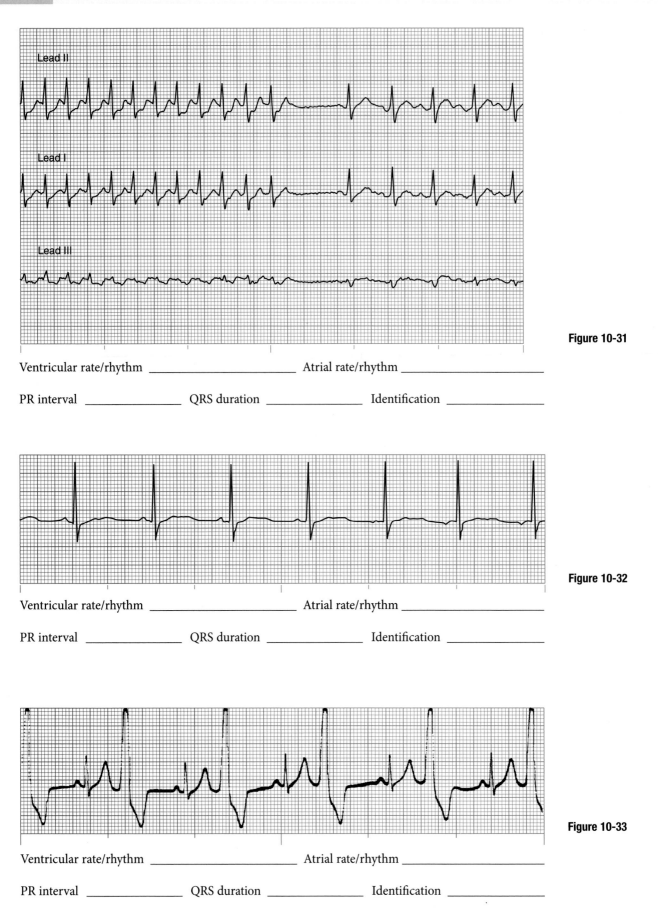

Figure 10-31

Ventricular rate/rhythm _____ Atrial rate/rhythm _____

PR interval _____ QRS duration _____ Identification _____

Figure 10-32

Ventricular rate/rhythm _____ Atrial rate/rhythm _____

PR interval _____ QRS duration _____ Identification _____

Figure 10-33

Ventricular rate/rhythm _____ Atrial rate/rhythm _____

PR interval _____ QRS duration _____ Identification _____

This rhythm strip is from a 51-year-old man complaining of "dull chest pain" that began about 2 hours ago. He rates his discomfort 6/10. BP 70/48, R 24. His skin is cool, pale, and diaphoretic.

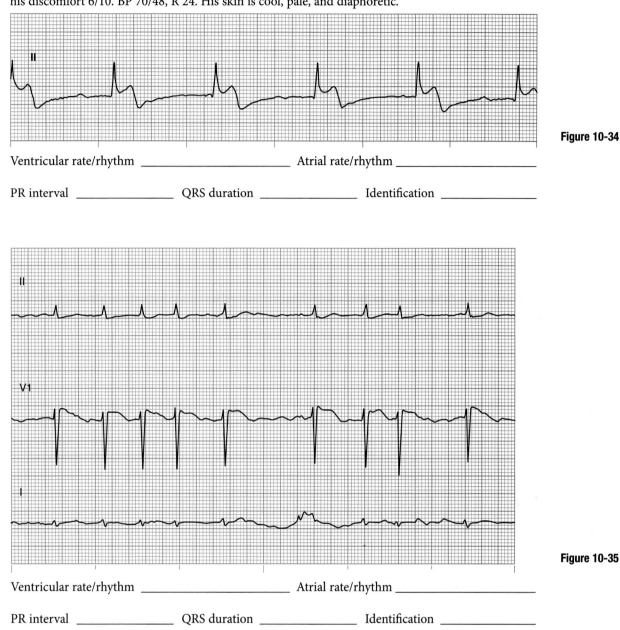

Figure 10-34

Ventricular rate/rhythm _____ Atrial rate/rhythm _____

PR interval _____ QRS duration _____ Identification _____

Figure 10-35

Ventricular rate/rhythm _____ Atrial rate/rhythm _____

PR interval _____ QRS duration _____ Identification _____

This rhythm strip is from a patient who was found apneic and pulseless. No history is available.

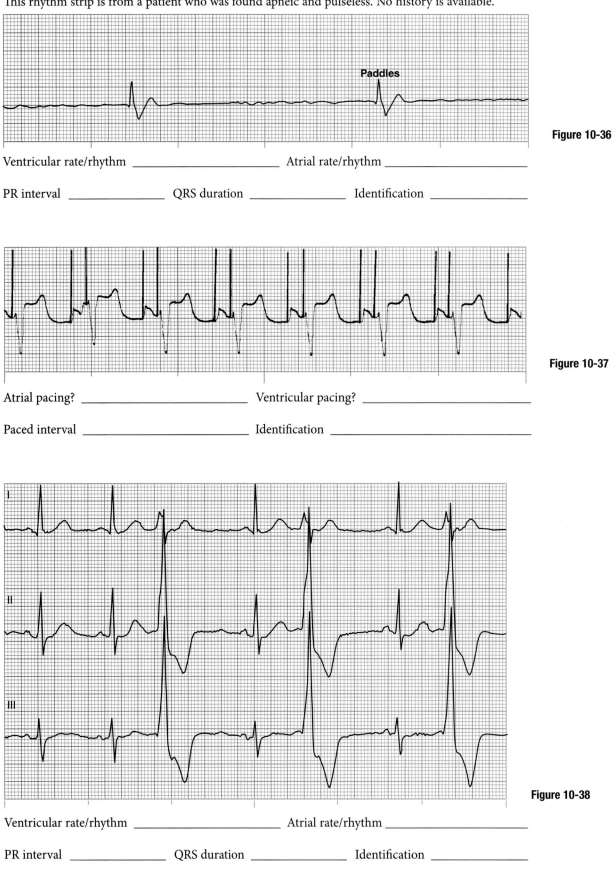

Figure 10-36

Ventricular rate/rhythm _____ Atrial rate/rhythm _____

PR interval _____ QRS duration _____ Identification _____

Figure 10-37

Atrial pacing? _____ Ventricular pacing? _____

Paced interval _____ Identification _____

Figure 10-38

Ventricular rate/rhythm _____ Atrial rate/rhythm _____

PR interval _____ QRS duration _____ Identification _____

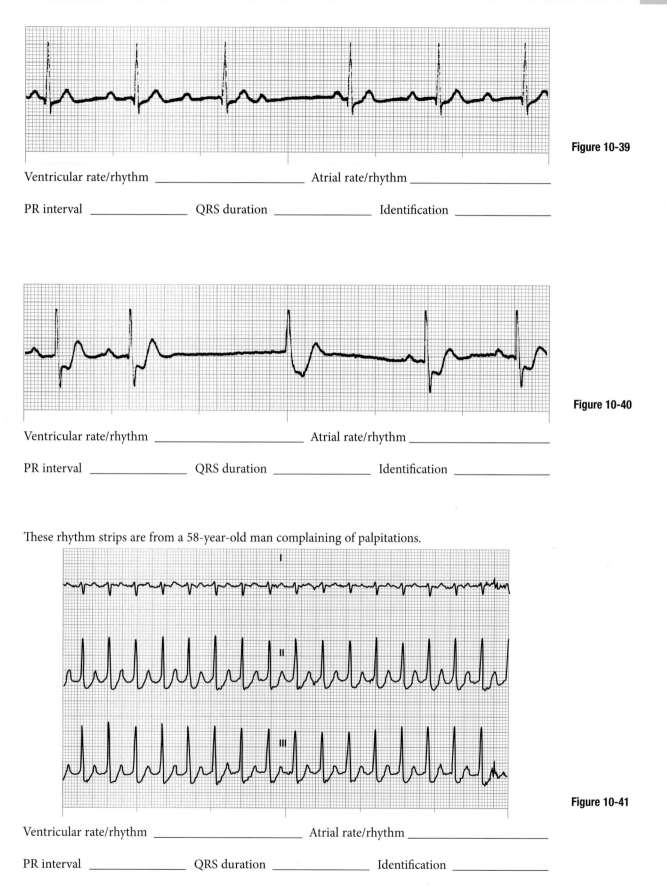

Figure 10-39

Ventricular rate/rhythm _____ Atrial rate/rhythm _____

PR interval _____ QRS duration _____ Identification _____

Figure 10-40

Ventricular rate/rhythm _____ Atrial rate/rhythm _____

PR interval _____ QRS duration _____ Identification _____

These rhythm strips are from a 58-year-old man complaining of palpitations.

Figure 10-41

Ventricular rate/rhythm _____ Atrial rate/rhythm _____

PR interval _____ QRS duration _____ Identification _____

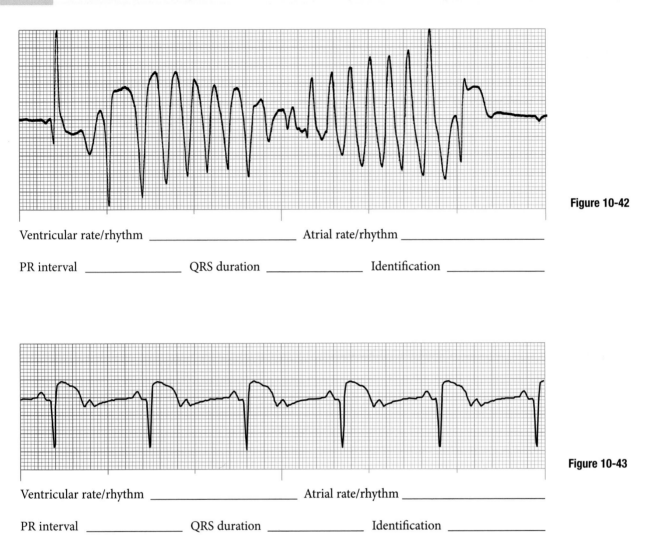

Figure 10-42

Ventricular rate/rhythm _____ Atrial rate/rhythm _____

PR interval _____ QRS duration _____ Identification _____

Figure 10-43

Ventricular rate/rhythm _____ Atrial rate/rhythm _____

PR interval _____ QRS duration _____ Identification _____

These rhythm strips are from a 57-year-old man who experienced an altered level of consciousness while being moved from a chair to his bed. Blood pressure 112/76, blood glucose level 123 mg/dL. Oxygen saturation on room air was 93%.

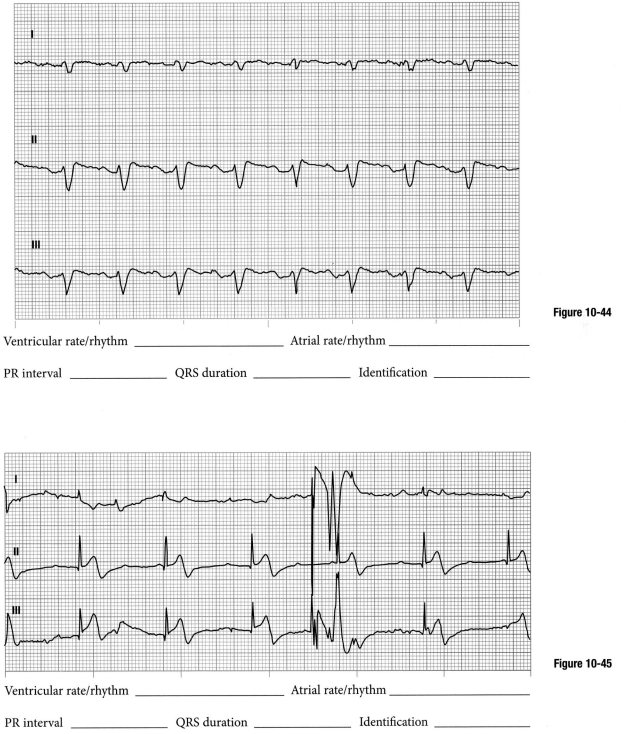

Figure 10-44

Ventricular rate/rhythm _____ Atrial rate/rhythm _____

PR interval _____ QRS duration _____ Identification _____

Figure 10-45

Ventricular rate/rhythm _____ Atrial rate/rhythm _____

PR interval _____ QRS duration _____ Identification _____

This rhythm strip is from an 82-year-old man complaining of back pain.

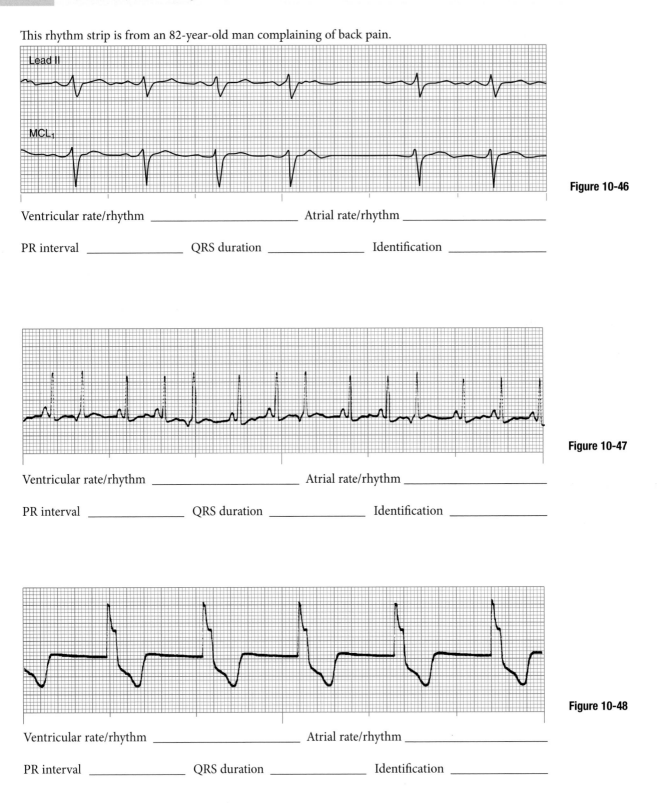

Figure 10-46

Ventricular rate/rhythm _____ Atrial rate/rhythm _____

PR interval _____ QRS duration _____ Identification _____

Figure 10-47

Ventricular rate/rhythm _____ Atrial rate/rhythm _____

PR interval _____ QRS duration _____ Identification _____

Figure 10-48

Ventricular rate/rhythm _____ Atrial rate/rhythm _____

PR interval _____ QRS duration _____ Identification _____

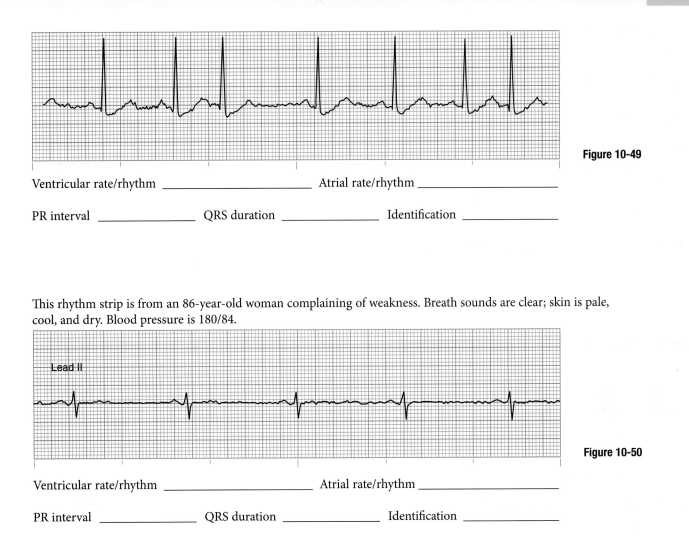

Figure 10-49

Ventricular rate/rhythm _____ Atrial rate/rhythm _____

PR interval _____ QRS duration _____ Identification _____

This rhythm strip is from an 86-year-old woman complaining of weakness. Breath sounds are clear; skin is pale, cool, and dry. Blood pressure is 180/84.

Lead II

Figure 10-50

Ventricular rate/rhythm _____ Atrial rate/rhythm _____

PR interval _____ QRS duration _____ Identification _____

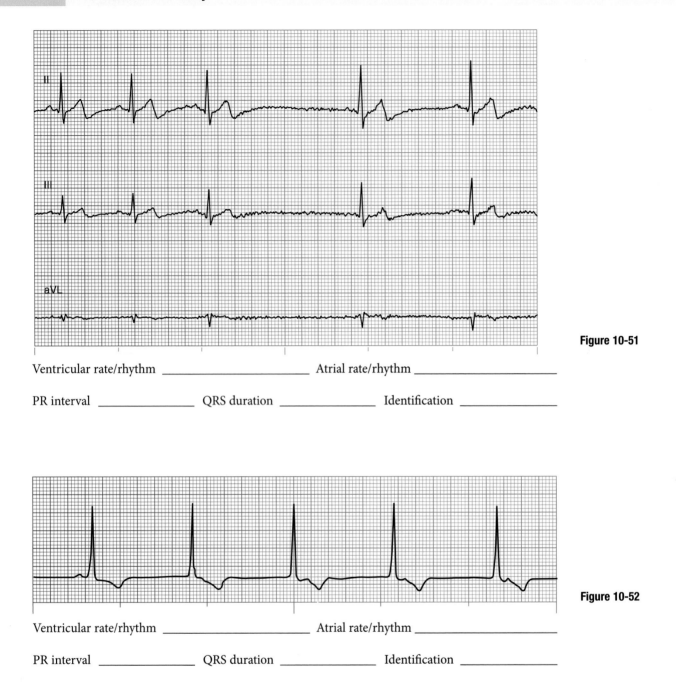

Figure 10-51

Ventricular rate/rhythm _____ Atrial rate/rhythm _____

PR interval _____ QRS duration _____ Identification _____

Figure 10-52

Ventricular rate/rhythm _____ Atrial rate/rhythm _____

PR interval _____ QRS duration _____ Identification _____

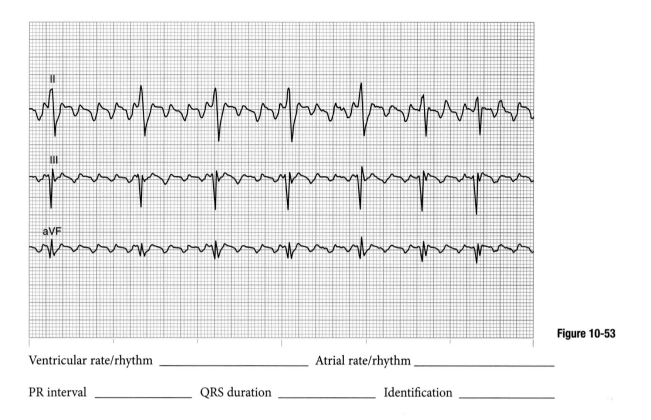

Figure 10-53

Ventricular rate/rhythm _____ Atrial rate/rhythm _____

PR interval _____ QRS duration _____ Identification _____

These rhythm strips are from a 67-year-old woman complaining of dizziness and chest pain. Blood pressure is 90/60, breath sounds are clear. She has a history of a three-vessel coronary artery bypass graft and hypertension.

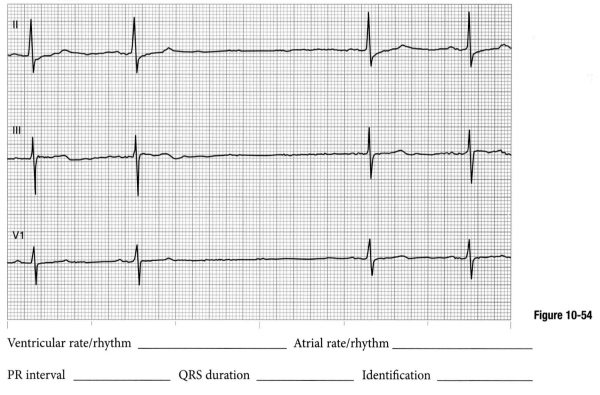

Figure 10-54

Ventricular rate/rhythm _____ Atrial rate/rhythm _____

PR interval _____ QRS duration _____ Identification _____

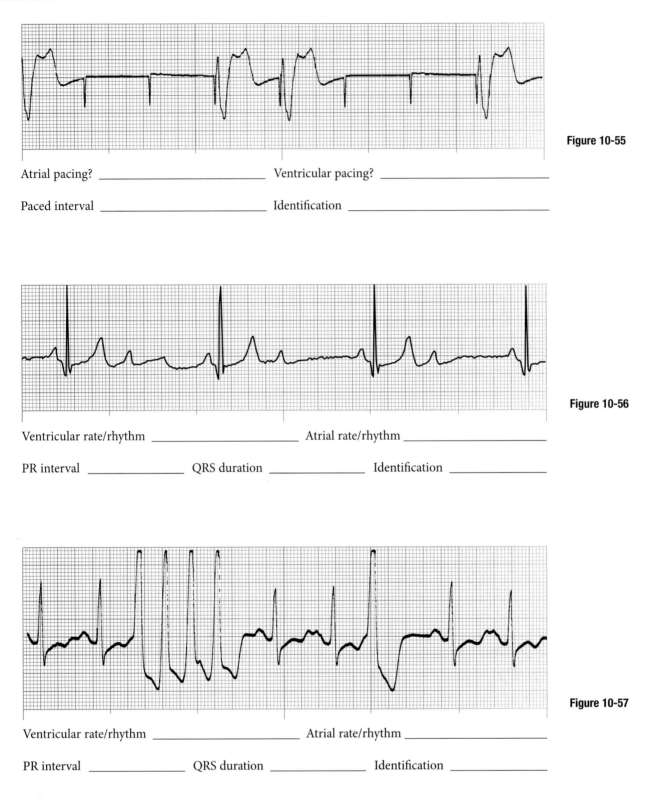

Figure 10-55

Atrial pacing? _____   Ventricular pacing? _____

Paced interval _____   Identification _____

Figure 10-56

Ventricular rate/rhythm _____   Atrial rate/rhythm _____

PR interval _____   QRS duration _____   Identification _____

Figure 10-57

Ventricular rate/rhythm _____   Atrial rate/rhythm _____

PR interval _____   QRS duration _____   Identification _____

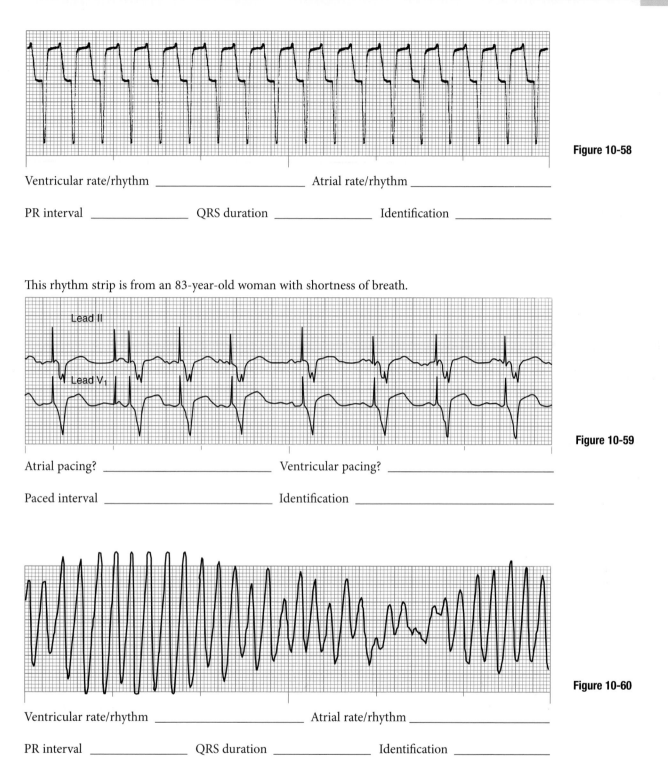

Figure 10-58

Ventricular rate/rhythm _____ Atrial rate/rhythm _____

PR interval _____ QRS duration _____ Identification _____

This rhythm strip is from an 83-year-old woman with shortness of breath.

Lead II

Lead V₁

Figure 10-59

Atrial pacing? _____ Ventricular pacing? _____

Paced interval _____ Identification _____

Figure 10-60

Ventricular rate/rhythm _____ Atrial rate/rhythm _____

PR interval _____ QRS duration _____ Identification _____

This rhythm strip is from a 69-year-old man who is disoriented. He knows his name but has no idea where he is or how he got there. BP 172/98, R 20. Blood sugar 127 mg/dL.

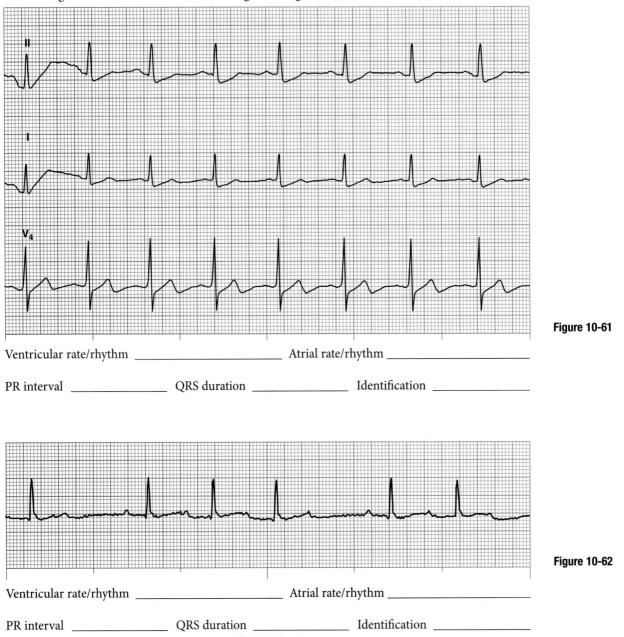

Figure 10-61

Ventricular rate/rhythm _____ Atrial rate/rhythm _____

PR interval _____ QRS duration _____ Identification _____

Figure 10-62

Ventricular rate/rhythm _____ Atrial rate/rhythm _____

PR interval _____ QRS duration _____ Identification _____

This rhythm strip is from an 18-year-old man with a gunshot wound to his chest.

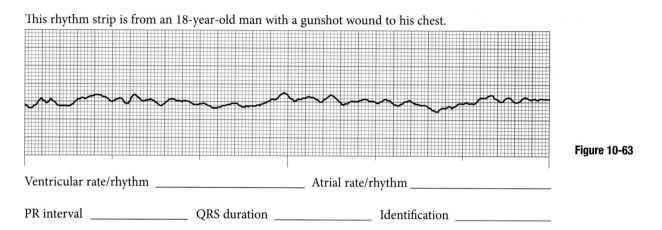

Figure 10-63

Ventricular rate/rhythm _____ Atrial rate/rhythm _____

PR interval _____ QRS duration _____ Identification _____

This rhythm strip is from an 89-year-old man complaining of weakness and nausea for 3 to 4 days. BP is 122/82. He has a history of diabetes.

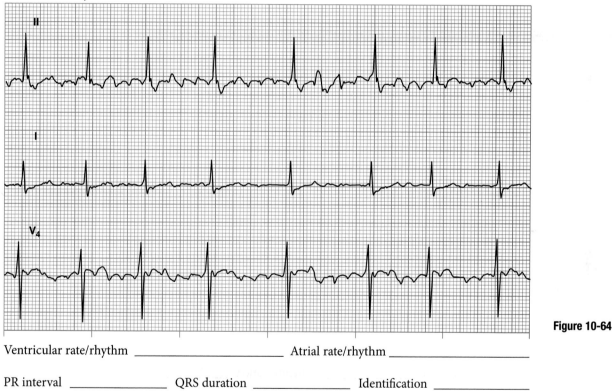

Figure 10-64

Ventricular rate/rhythm _____ Atrial rate/rhythm _____

PR interval _____ QRS duration _____ Identification _____

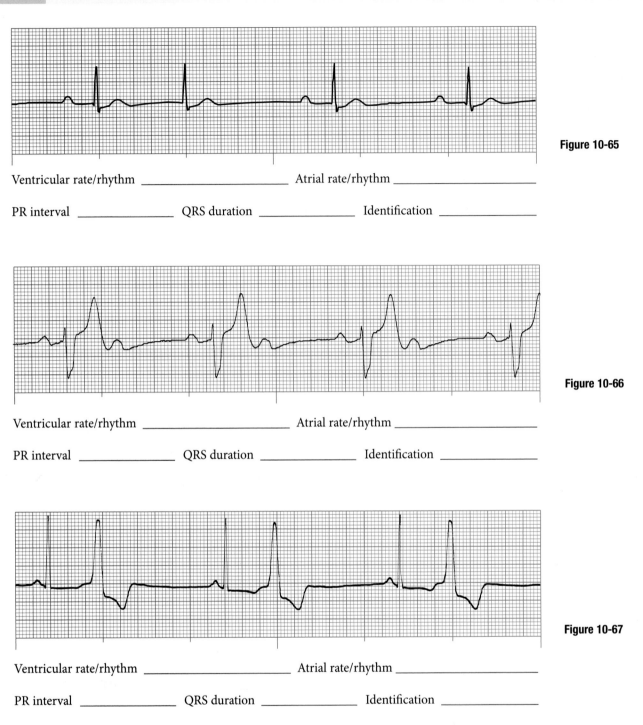

Figure 10-65

Ventricular rate/rhythm _____ Atrial rate/rhythm _____

PR interval _____ QRS duration _____ Identification _____

Figure 10-66

Ventricular rate/rhythm _____ Atrial rate/rhythm _____

PR interval _____ QRS duration _____ Identification _____

Figure 10-67

Ventricular rate/rhythm _____ Atrial rate/rhythm _____

PR interval _____ QRS duration _____ Identification _____

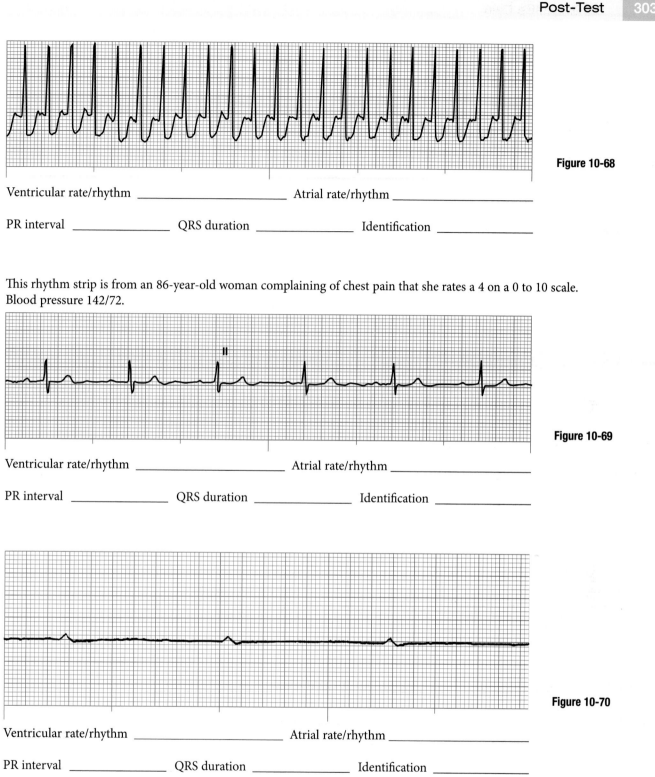

Figure 10-68

Ventricular rate/rhythm _____ Atrial rate/rhythm _____

PR interval _____ QRS duration _____ Identification _____

This rhythm strip is from an 86-year-old woman complaining of chest pain that she rates a 4 on a 0 to 10 scale. Blood pressure 142/72.

Figure 10-69

Ventricular rate/rhythm _____ Atrial rate/rhythm _____

PR interval _____ QRS duration _____ Identification _____

Figure 10-70

Ventricular rate/rhythm _____ Atrial rate/rhythm _____

PR interval _____ QRS duration _____ Identification _____

This rhythm strip is from a 44-year-old construction worker with a sudden onset of chest pressure.

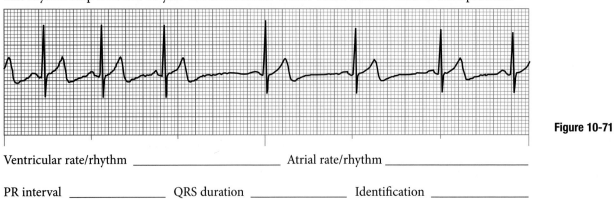

Figure 10-71

Ventricular rate/rhythm _____ Atrial rate/rhythm _____

PR interval _____ QRS duration _____ Identification _____

This rhythm strip is from a 1-year-old girl. Mom says the infant suddenly went limp and her limbs began shaking. The episode lasted about 45 seconds. Temperature normal.

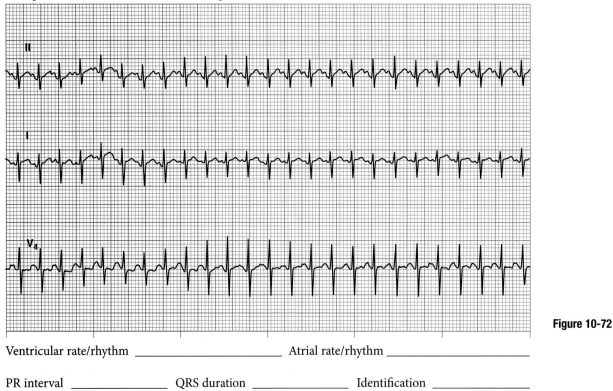

Figure 10-72

Ventricular rate/rhythm _____ Atrial rate/rhythm _____

PR interval _____ QRS duration _____ Identification _____

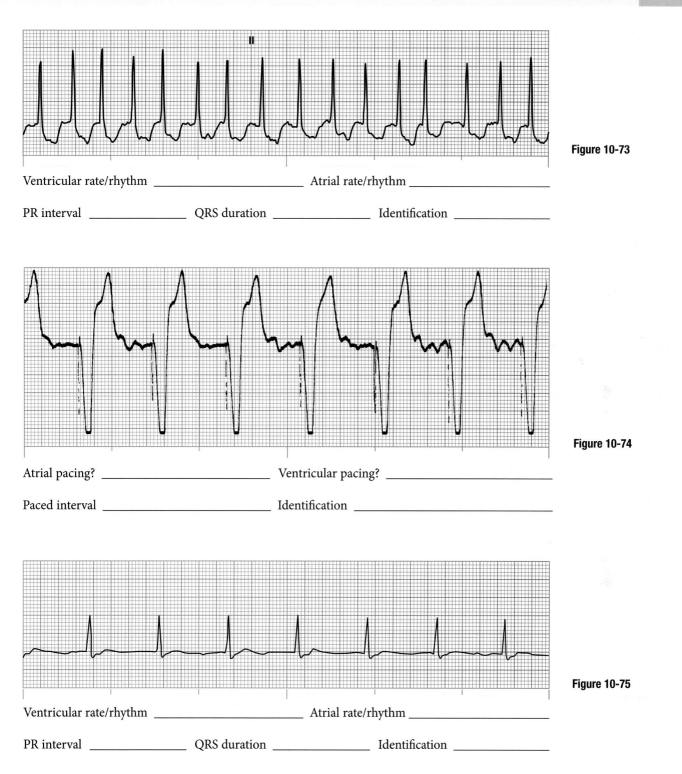

Figure 10-73

Ventricular rate/rhythm _____ Atrial rate/rhythm _____

PR interval _____ QRS duration _____ Identification _____

Figure 10-74

Atrial pacing? _____ Ventricular pacing? _____

Paced interval _____ Identification _____

Figure 10-75

Ventricular rate/rhythm _____ Atrial rate/rhythm _____

PR interval _____ QRS duration _____ Identification _____

POST-TEST ANSWERS

True/False

1. F
2. F

3. F
Always place limb leads on the limbs and palpate the inter-costal spaces to position the chest leads.

Multiple Choice

4. a
5. b
6. b
7. c
8. a
9. d
10. b
11. d
12. d
13. c
14. a
15. a
16. b
17. c
18. d

19. d
20. d
21. d
22. d
23. c
24. b
25. c
26. c
27. b
28. a
29. c
30. c
31. a
32. a
33. c

Completion

34. A beat originating from the AV junction that appears later than the next expected sinus beat is called a *junctional escape beat*.

35. A rapid, wide-QRS rhythm associated with pulselessness, shock, or congestive heart failure should be presumed to be *ventricular tachycardia*.

36. PACs associated with a wide QRS complex are called *aberrantly conducted* PACs, indicating conduction through the ventricles is abnormal.

37. The right atrium receives deoxygenated blood from the *superior vena cava* (which carries blood from the head and upper extremities), the *inferior vena cava* (which carries blood from the lower body), and the *coronary sinus* (which receives blood from the intracardiac circulation).

38. *Diastole* is the period of relaxation during which a heart chamber is filling.

39. The thick, muscular middle layer of the heart wall that contains the atrial and ventricular muscle fibers necessary for contraction is the *myocardium*.

40. An ECG lead that has a positive and negative electrode is called a *bipolar* lead.

41. The appearance of coved ("frowny face") ST segment elevation is called an *acute injury pattern*.

42. Delivery of an electrical current timed for delivery during the QRS complex is called *synchronized cardioversion*.

43. Sometimes, when a PAC occurs very prematurely and close to the T wave of the preceding beat, only a P wave may be seen with no QRS after it (appearing as a pause). This type of PAC is termed a "*nonconducted*" (or "blocked") PAC.

44. If the AV junction paces the heart, the electrical impulse must travel in a *backward* (retrograde) direction to activate the atria.

45. A *fusion beat* occurs as a result of an electrical impulse from a supraventricular site (such as the SA node), discharging at the same time as an ectopic site in the ventricles.

46. A *pacemaker spike* is a vertical line on the ECG that indicates the pacemaker has discharged.

47. A demand pacemaker is also known as a *synchronous* or *noncompetitive* pacemaker.

48. A *right* bundle branch block produces an rSR' pattern in lead V_1.

49.

Leads	Heart surface viewed
II, III, aVF	Inferior
V_1, V_2	Septal
V_3, V_4	Anterior
I, aVL, V_5, V_6	Lateral

50. The axes of leads I, II, and III form an equilateral triangle with the heart at the center (Einthoven's triangle). If the augmented limb leads are added to this configuration and the axes of the six leads moved in a way in which they bisect each other, the result is the *hexaxial reference system*.

51. The area supplied by an obstructed coronary artery goes through a characteristic sequence of events that have been identified as zones of *ischemia*, *injury*, and *infarction*.

52.

SA node:	60 to 100 beats/min
AV junction:	40 to 60 beats/min
Ventricles:	20 to 40 beats/min

Short Answer

53. The four properties of cardiac cells are: (1) automaticity, (2) excitability (or irritability), (3) conductivity, and (4) contractility.

54. Signs and symptoms of hemodynamic compromise
- Changes in mental status (restlessness, confusion, possible loss of consciousness)
- Low blood pressure
- Chest pain
- Shortness of breath
- Signs of shock
- Congestive heart failure
- Pulmonary congestion
- Fall in urine output
- Cold, clammy skin

55. The term *anatomically contiguous leads* refers to those leads that "see" the same area of the heart. Two leads are contiguous if they look at the same area of the heart or if they are numerically consecutive *chest* leads.

56.

	Second-degree AV block type I	Third-degree AV block	Ventricular
Rhythm	Irregular	Regular	
PR interval	Progressively lengthening	None	
QRS width	Usually narrow	Narrow or wide	

57. The AV junction may assume responsibility for pacing the heart if:
- The SA node fails to discharge (such as sinus arrest)
- An impulse from the SA node is generated but blocked as it exits the SA node (such as SA block)
- The rate of discharge of the SA node is slower than that of the AV junction (such as a sinus bradycardia or the slower phase of a sinus arrhythmia)
- An impulse from the SA node is generated and is conducted through the atria but is not conducted to the ventricles (such as an AV block)

58. Common causes of PVCs include normal variant, hypoxia, stress/anxiety, exercise, digitalis toxicity, acid-base imbalance, myocardial ischemia, electrolyte imbalance (hypokalemia, hypocalcemia, hypercalcemia, hypomagnesemia), congestive heart failure, increased sympathetic tone, acute myocardial infarction, stimulants (alcohol, caffeine, tobacco), and medications (sympathomimetics, cyclic antidepressants, phenothiazines).

59. Polymorphic VT that occurs in the presence of a long QT interval is called "torsades de pointes."

60.

Rate:	Atrial rate is greater than the ventricular rate; ventricular rate is often slow
Rhythm:	Atrial regular (Ps plot through); ventricular irregular
P waves:	Normal in size and shape; some P waves are not followed by a QRS complex (more Ps than QRSs)
PR interval:	Within normal limits or slightly prolonged but constant for the conducted beats; there may be some shortening of the PR interval that follows a non-conducted P wave
QRS duration:	Usually 0.10 second or greater, periodically absent after P waves

61. A sinus rhythm has a rate of 60 to 100 beats/min. A sinus tachycardia has a rate of 101 to 180 beats/min.

62. On the ECG, the ST-segment represents early ventricular repolarization and the T wave represents ventricular repolarization.

63. A biphasic waveform is partly positive and partly negative and is recorded when the wave of depolarization moves perpendicularly to the positive electrode.

64. Artifact may be due to loose electrodes, broken wires or ECG cables, muscle tremor, patient movement, external chest compressions, or 60-cycle interference.

65. A Q wave that is 40 ms or more wide (one small box or more wide) or more than one third of the amplitude of the R wave in that lead is suggestive of infarction.

66. ECG monitoring may be used to (1) monitor a patient's heart rate, (2) evaluate the effects of disease or injury on heart function, (3) evaluate pacemaker function, (4) evaluate the response to medications (e.g., antiarrhythmics), and/or (5) obtain a baseline recording before, during, and after a medical procedure.

67. A ventricular demand (VVI) pacemaker is a common type of pacemaker. With this device, the pacemaker electrode is placed in the right ventricle (V); the ventricle is sensed (V) and the pacemaker is inhibited (I) when spontaneous ventricular depolarization occurs within a preset interval. When spontaneous ventricular depolarization does not occur within this preset interval, the pacemaker fires and stimulates ventricular depolarization at a preset rate.

68. According to the Frank-Starling law of the heart, to a point, the greater the volume of blood in the heart during diastole, the more forceful the cardiac contraction, and the more blood the ventricle will pump (stroke volume). This is important so that the heart can adjust its pumping capacity in response to changes in venous return, such as during exercise. If, however, the ventricle is stretched beyond its physiological limit, cardiac output may fall due to volume overload and overstretching of the muscle fibers.

Figure answer 10-1

Ventricular rate/rhythm	48 to 115 beats/min, irregular
Atrial rate/rhythm	Unable to determine
PR interval	Unable to determine
QRS duration	0.06 to 0.08 sec
Identification	Atrial fibrillation at 48 to 115 beats/min

Figure answer 10-2

Ventricular rate/rhythm	115 beats/min, regular
Atrial rate/rhythm	115 beats/min, regular
PR interval	0.16 sec
QRS duration	0.08 sec
Identification	Sinus tachycardia at 115 beats/min

Figure answer 10-3

Ventricular rate/rhythm	150 beats/min, regular
Atrial rate/rhythm	Unable to determine
PR interval	Unable to determine
QRS duration	0.16 sec
Identification	Monomorphic ventricular tachycardia at 150 beats/min

Figure answer 10-4

Ventricular rate/rhythm	52 beats/min, regular
Atrial rate/rhythm	None
PR interval	None
QRS duration	0.06 sec
Identification	Sinus beat to junctional rhythm at 52 beats/min; inverted T waves

Figure answer 10-5

Ventricular rate/rhythm	115 beats/min, regular
Atrial rate/rhythm	115 beats/min, regular
PR interval	0.16 to 0.20 sec
QRS duration	0.08 sec
Identification	Sinus tachycardia at 115 beats/min

Figure answer 10-6

Atrial pacing?	No
Ventricular pacing?	Yes
Paced interval	60
Identification	Atrial fibrillation with a ventricular demand pacemaker

Figure answer 10-7

Ventricular rate/rhythm	125 beats/min, essentially regular except for events
Atrial rate/rhythm	125 beats/min, essentially regular except for events
PR interval	0.12 sec (sinus beats)
QRS duration	0.06 sec (sinus beats)
Identification	Sinus tachycardia at 125 beats/min with multiform PVCs

Figure answer 10-8

Ventricular rate/rhythm	8 to 130 beats/min, irregular
Atrial rate/rhythm	Unable to determine
PR interval	Unable to determine
QRS duration	0.08 sec
Identification	Atrial fibrillation at 88 to 130 beats/min

Figure answer 10-9

Ventricular rate/rhythm	100 beats/min, regular
Atrial rate/rhythm	None
PR interval	None
QRS duration	0.08 sec
Identification	Accelerated junctional rhythm at 100 beats/min; inverted T waves

Figure answer 10-10

Ventricular rate/rhythm	32 beats/min, regular
Atrial rate/rhythm	79 beats/min, regular
PR interval	Varies
QRS duration	0.10 to 12 sec
Identification	Third-degree AV block at 32 beats/min

Figure answer 10-11

Ventricular rate/rhythm	130 beats/min, regular
Atrial rate/rhythm	130 beats/min, regular
PR interval	0.16 sec
QRS duration	0.12 sec
Identification	Sinus tachycardia at 130 beats/min with a wide-QRS and ST-segment depression

Figure answer 10-12

Ventricular rate/rhythm	30 beats/min (junctional beats), irregular
Atrial rate/rhythm	None (junctional beats), irregular
PR interval	0.16 sec (sinus beats); none (junctional beats)
QRS duration	0.06 to 0.08 sec
Identification	Sinus beat, two junctional beats, sinus beat; ST-segment depression

Figure answer 10-13

Atrial pacing?	No
Ventricular pacing?	Yes
Paced interval	115
Identification	Normal functioning ventricular pacemaker

Figure answer 10-14

Ventricular rate/rhythm	78 beats/min, regular except for the event
Atrial rate/rhythm	78 beats/min, regular except for the event
PR interval	0.16 sec
QRS duration	0.06 sec
Identification	Sinus rhythm at 78 beats/min with a PAC, ST-segment elevation (PAC is the third complex from left)

Figure answer 10-15

Ventricular rate/rhythm	245 beats/min, regular
Atrial rate/rhythm	245 beats/min, regular
PR interval	None
QRS duration	0.28 sec
Identification	Monomorphic ventricular tachycardia at 245 beats/min

Figure answer 10-16

Ventricular rate/rhythm	48 to 83 beats/min, irregular
Atrial rate/rhythm	167 beats/min, regular
PR interval	0.24 sec
QRS duration	0.12 sec
Identification	Second-degree AV block type II at 48 to 83 beats/min with ST-segment depression

Figure answer 10-17

Ventricular rate/rhythm	91 beats/min (sinus beats), regular except for the event(s)
Atrial rate/rhythm	91 beats/min (sinus beats), regular except for the event(s)
PR interval	0.16 sec
QRS duration	0.06 sec
Identification	Sinus rhythm at 91 beats/min with ventricular trigeminy

Figure answer 10-18

Atrial pacing?	Yes
Ventricular pacing?	No
Paced interval	79
Identification	Atrial pacemaker

Figure answer 10-19

Ventricular rate/rhythm	65 beats/min, regular
Atrial rate/rhythm	None
PR interval	None
QRS duration	0.06 sec
Identification	Accelerated junctional rhythm at 65 beats/min

Figure answer 10-20

Ventricular rate/rhythm	96 beats/min, regular
Atrial rate/rhythm	96 beats/min, regular
PR interval	0.16 sec
QRS duration	0.08 to 0.10 sec
Identification	Sinus rhythm at 96 beats/min, ST-segment elevation in leads I and II

Figure answer 10-21

Ventricular rate/rhythm	81 beats/min, regular
Atrial rate/rhythm	81 beats/min, regular
PR interval	0.20 to 0.22 sec
QRS duration	0.06 to 0.08 sec
Identification	Sinus rhythm at 81 beats/min, borderline first-degree AV block

Figure answer 10-22

Ventricular rate/rhythm	54 to 94 beats/min, irregular
Atrial rate/rhythm	Unable to determine
PR interval	Unable to determine
QRS duration	0.10 to 0.12 sec
Identification	Atrial flutter at 54 to 94 beats/min

Figure answer 10-23

Atrial pacing?	No
Ventricular pacing?	Yes
Paced interval	65
Identification	100% ventricular paced rhythm

Figure answer 10-24

Ventricular rate/rhythm	36 to 71 beats/min, regular except for the event
Atrial rate/rhythm	36 to 71 beats/min, regular except for the event
PR interval	0.16 sec
QRS duration	0.06 sec
Identification	Sinus rhythm at a rate of 36 to 71 beats/min with an episode of sinoatrial (SA) block

Figure answer 10-25

Ventricular rate/rhythm	44 beats/min, regular
Atrial rate/rhythm	83 beats/min, regular
PR interval	0.16 sec
QRS duration	0.08 sec
Identification	2:1 AV block, probably type 1 at 44 beats/min

Figure answer 10-26

Identification	2:1 AV block, probably type 1 at 44 beats/min
Ventricular rate/rhythm	75 to 88 beats/min, irregular
Atrial rate/rhythm	Unable to determine
PR interval	None
QRS duration	0.10 to 0.12 sec
Identification	Atrial fibrillation at 75 to 88 beats/min with a ventricular complex and wide, notched QRS

Figure answer 10-27

Ventricular rate/rhythm	Unable to determine
Atrial rate/rhythm	None
PR interval	None
QRS duration	Unable to determine
Identification	Ventricular fibrillation

Figure answer 10-28

Atrial pacing?	No
Ventricular pacing?	Yes
Paced interval	71
Identification	Pacemaker malfunction (failure to sense); underlying rhythm is a sinus rhythm at 88 beats/min; note the pacer spikes in the T waves of the second and eighth beats from the left

Figure answer 10-29

Ventricular rate/rhythm	32 beats/min, regular
Atrial rate/rhythm	None
PR interval	None
QRS	0.06 to 0.08 sec
Identification	Junctional bradycardia at 32 beats/min; ST-segment depression, inverted T waves

Figure answer 10-30

Ventricular rate/rhythm	136 beats/min, regular
Atrial rate/rhythm	136 beats/min, regular
PR interval	0.16 sec
QRS duration	0.08 sec
Identification	Sinus tachycardia at 136 beats/min; ST-segment elevation

Figure answer 10-31

Ventricular rate/rhythm	214 beats/min (atrial beats), 125 beats/min (sinus beats)
Atrial rate/rhythm	Unable to determine (atrial beats), 125 beats/min (sinus beats)
PR interval	0.16 sec (sinus beats)
QRS duration	0.08 sec
Identification	Supraventricular tachycardia at 214 beats/min to a sinus tachycardia at 125 beats/min

Figure answer 10-32

Ventricular rate/rhythm	68 beats/min (sinus beats), 57 beats/min (junctional beats)
Atrial rate/rhythm	68 beats/min (sinus beats), 57 beats/min (junctional beats)
PR interval	0.16 sec
QRS duration	0.08 sec
Identification	Sinus rhythm at 68 beats/min to junctional rhythm at 57 beats/min

Figure answer 10-33

Ventricular rate/rhythm	54 beats/min, regular (sinus beats)
Atrial rate/rhythm	54 beats/min, regular (sinus beats)
PR interval	0.12 sec (sinus beats)
QRS duration	0.06 to 0.08 sec (sinus beats)
Identification	Sinus bradycardia at 54 beats/min with ventricular bigeminy; ventricular rate approximately 100 beats/min if PVCs counted in the rate

Figure answer 10-34

Ventricular rate/rhythm	48 beats/min, regular
Atrial rate/rhythm	71 beats/min, slightly irregular
PR interval	Varies
QRS duration	0.08 to 0.10 sec
Identification	Third-degree AV block at 48 beats/min with ST-segment elevation

Figure answer 10-35

Ventricular rate/rhythm	56 to 150 beats/min, irregular
Atrial rate/rhythm	Unable to determine
PR interval	None
QRS duration	0.08 sec
Identification	Atrial fibrillation at 56 to 150 beats/min

Figure answer 10-36

Ventricular rate/rhythm	20 beats/min, regular
Atrial rate/rhythm	None
PR interval	None
QRS duration	0.14 sec
Identification	Idioventricular/agonal rhythm at 20 beats/min

Figure answer 10-37

Atrial pacing?	Yes
Ventricular pacing?	Yes
Paced interval	71
Identification	Normal functioning AV sequential pacemaker

Figure answer 10-38

Ventricular rate/rhythm	70 beats/min (sinus beats), irregular
Atrial rate/rhythm	70 beats/min (sinus beats), irregular
PR interval	0.16 sec
QRS duration	0.08 sec
Identification	Sinus rhythm at 70 beats/min with frequent uniform PVCs

Figure answer 10-39

Ventricular rate/rhythm	43 to 60 beats/min, irregular
Atrial rate/rhythm	68 beats/min, regular
PR interval	Lengthens
QRS duration	0.06 sec
Identification	Second-degree AV block type I at 43 to 60 beats/min

Figure answer 10-40

Ventricular rate/rhythm	71 beats/min (sinus beats), regular except for the event
Atrial rate/rhythm	71 beats/min (sinus beats), regular except for the event
PR interval	0.24 sec
QRS duration	0.08 sec
Identification	Sinus rhythm at 71 beats/min with a first-degree AV block, an episode of sinus arrest and a junctional escape beat; ST-segment depression

Figure answer 10-41

Ventricular rate/rhythm	167 beats/min, regular
Atrial rate/rhythm	Unable to determine
PR interval	Unable to determine
QRS duration	0.06 sec
Identification	AV nodal reentrant tachycardia (AVNRT) at 167 beats/min with ST-segment depression

Figure answer 10-42

Ventricular rate/rhythm	230 to 300, irregular
Atrial rate/rhythm	Unable to determine
PR interval	Unable to determine
QRS duration	Varies
Identification	Supraventricular beat followed by polymorphic ventricular tachycardia at 230 to 300 beats/min

Figure answer 10-43

Ventricular rate/rhythm	55 beats/min, regular
Atrial rate/rhythm	107 beats/min, regular
PR interval	0.16 sec
QRS duration	0.06 sec
Identification	2:1 AV block, probably type I at 55 beats/min, with ST-segment elevation

Figure answer 10-44

Ventricular rate/rhythm	85 beats/min, regular
Atrial rate/rhythm	85 beats/min, regular
PR interval	0.24 to 0.28 sec
QRS duration	0.12 to 0.14 sec
Identification	Sinus rhythm at 85 beats/min with first-degree AV block, wide QRS

Figure answer 10-45

Ventricular rate/rhythm	36 beats/min, regular
Atrial rate/rhythm	94 beats/min, regular
PR interval	Varies
QRS duration	0.14 sec
Identification	Third-degree AV block at 36 beats/min with artifact

Figure answer 10-46

Ventricular rate/rhythm	41 to 73 beats/min, irregular
Atrial rate/rhythm	56 to 125 beats/min, irregular
PR interval	0.20 sec
QRS duration	0.12 sec
Identification	Sinus rhythm at 41 to 73 beats/min with a nonconducted PAC

Figure answer 10-47

Ventricular rate/rhythm	136 beats/min (sinus beats), regular except for the event(s)
Atrial rate/rhythm	136 beats/min (sinus beats), regular except for the event(s)
PR interval	0.10 sec
QRS duration	0.06 sec
Identification	Sinus tachycardia at 136 beats/min with frequent PJCs (the PJCs are beats 2, 5, 8, and 11 from the left)

Figure answer 10-48

Ventricular rate/rhythm	56 beats/min, regular
Atrial rate/rhythm	None
PR interval	None
QRS duration	0.12 sec
Identification	Accelerated idioventricular rhythm (AIVR) at 56 beats/min; ST-segment depression

Figure answer 10-49

Ventricular rate/rhythm	71 beats/min (sinus beats), regular except for the event(s)
Atrial rate/rhythm	71 beats/min (sinus beats), regular except for the event(s)
PR interval	0.16 sec
QRS duration	0.08 sec
Identification	Sinus rhythm at 71 beats/min with two PACs; ST-segment depression

Figure answer 10-50

Ventricular rate/rhythm	51 beats/min, essentially regular
Atrial rate/rhythm	51 beats/min, essentially regular
PR interval	0.16 sec
QRS duration	0.08 sec
Identification	Sinus bradycardia at 51 beats/min

Figure answer 10-51

Ventricular rate/rhythm	65 beats/min, regular except for the event
Atrial rate/rhythm	65 beats/min, regular except for the event
PR interval	0.16 sec
QRS duration	0.08 sec
Identification	Sinus rhythm at 65 beats/min with an episode of sinoatrial block

Figure answer 10-52

Ventricular rate/rhythm	52 beats/min, regular
Atrial rate/rhythm	None
PR interval	None
QRS duration	0.06 sec
Identification	Sinus beat to a junction escape rhythm at 52 beats/min; inverted T waves

Figure answer 10-53

Ventricular rate/rhythm	58 to 68 beats/min, irregular
Atrial rate/rhythm	About 300 beats/min, regular
PR interval	None
QRS duration	0.12 sec
Identification	Atrial flutter at 58 to 68 beats/min

Figure answer 10-54

Ventricular rate/rhythm	49 beats/min, regular except for the event
Atrial rate/rhythm	49 beats/min, regular except for the event
PR interval	0.20 sec
QRS	0.08 sec
Identification	Sinus bradycardia at 49 beats/min with an episode of sinus arrest

Figure answer 10-55

Atrial pacing?	No
Ventricular pacing?	Yes
Paced interval	80
Identification	Ventricular-paced rhythm with pacemaker malfunction (failure to capture)

Figure answer 10-56

Ventricular rate/rhythm	34 beats/min, regular
Atrial rate/rhythm	68 beats/min, regular
PR interval	0.14 to 0.16 sec
QRS duration	0.10 sec
Identification	2:1 AV block, probably type I at 34 beats/min

Figure answer 10-57

Ventricular rate/rhythm	88 (sinus beats), regular except for the events
Atrial rate/rhythm	88 (sinus beats), regular except for the events
PR interval	0.20 sec (sinus beats)
QRS duration	0.08 sec (sinus beats)
Identification	Sinus rhythm at 88 beats/min with a PVC and run of VT, ST-segment depression, inverted T waves

Figure answer 10-58

Ventricular rate/rhythm	180 beats/min, regular
Atrial rate/rhythm	Unable to determine
PR interval	Unable to determine
QRS duration	0.04 sec
Identification	AV nodal reentrant tachycardia (AVNRT) at 180 beats/min with ST-segment elevation

Figure answer 10-59

Atrial paced activity?	Yes
Ventricular paced activity?	Yes
Paced interval rate?	Atrial = 79, ventricular = 85
Identification	AV sequential demand pacemaker

Figure answer 10-60

Ventricular rate/rhythm	300 to 375 beats/min, irregular
Atrial rate/rhythm	None
PR interval	None
QRS duration	Varies
Identification	Polymorphic ventricular tachycardia at 300 to 375 beats/min

Figure answer 10-61

Ventricular rate/rhythm	79 beats/min, regular
Atrial rate/rhythm	79 beats/min, regular
PR interval	0.18 sec
QRS duration	0.06 to 0.08 sec
Identification	Sinus rhythm at 79 beats/min

Figure 10-62 answer

Ventricular rate/rhythm	51 to 83 beats/min, irregular
Atrial rate/rhythm	88 beats/min, regular
PR interval	Lengthens
QRS duration	0.06 sec
Identification	Second-degree AV block type I at 51 to 83 beats/min

Figure answer 10-63

Ventricular rate/rhythm	None
Atrial rate/rhythm	None
PR interval	None
QRS duration	None
Identification	Coarse ventricular fibrillation

Figure answer 10-64

Ventricular rate/rhythm	64 to 83 beats/min, irregular
Atrial rate/rhythm	Unable to determine
PR interval	None
QRS duration	0.08 sec
Identification	Atrial flutter at 64 to 83 beats/min

Figure answer 10-65

Ventricular rate/rhythm	40 beats/min (sinus beats), regular except for the event
Atrial rate/rhythm	40 beats/min (sinus beats), regular except for the event
PR interval	0.36 sec (sinus beats)
QRS duration	0.06 sec (sinus beats)
Identification	Sinus bradycardia at 40 beats/min with first-degree AV block and a PJC

Figure answer 10-66

Ventricular rate/rhythm	30 beats/min, regular
Atrial rate/rhythm	68 beats/min, regular
PR interval	0.28 sec
QRS duration	0.16 sec
Identification	2:1 AV block, probably type II at 30 beats/min; ST-segment elevation, hyperacute T waves

Figure answer 10-67

Ventricular rate/rhythm	30 beats/min (sinus beats), regular except for the events
Atrial rate/rhythm	30 beats/min (sinus beats), regular except for the events
PR interval	0.12 to 0.16 sec (sinus beats)
QRS duration	0.06 sec (sinus beats)
Identification	Sinus bradycardia at 30 beats/min with ventricular bigeminy (ventricular rate approximately 60 if PVCs counted), inverted T waves, horizontal ST-segments

Figure answer 10-68

Ventricular rate/rhythm	231 beats/min, regular
Atrial rate/rhythm	Unable to determine
PR interval	Unable to determine
QRS duration	0.06 sec
Identification	AV nodal reentrant tachycardia (AVNRT) at 231 beats/min with ST-segment depression

Figure answer 10-69

Ventricular rate/rhythm	60 beats/min, regular
Atrial rate/rhythm	60 beats/min, regular
PR interval	0.20 sec
QRS duration	0.06 sec
Identification	Sinus rhythm at 60 beats/min

Figure answer 10-70

Ventricular rate/rhythm	None
Atrial rate/rhythm	40 beats/min, regular
PR interval	None
QRS duration	None
Identification	P wave asystole at 40 beats/min

Figure answer 10-71

Ventricular rate/rhythm	52 to 94 beats/min, irregular
Atrial rate/rhythm	52 to 94 beats/min, irregular
PR interval	0.12 sec
QRS duration	0.08 sec
Identification	Sinus arrhythmia at 52 to 94 beats/min

Figure answer 10-72

Ventricular rate/rhythm	215 beats/min, regular
Atrial rate/rhythm	215 beats/min, regular
PR interval	0.10 sec
QRS duration	0.08 sec
Identification	Sinus tachycardia at 215 beats/min

Figure 10-73 answer

Ventricular rate/rhythm	125 to 158 beats/min, irregular
Atrial rate/rhythm	Unable to determine
PR interval	Unable to determine
QRS duration	0.06 sec
Identification	Atrial fibrillation (uncontrolled) at 125 to 158 beats/min with ST-segment depression

Figure answer 10-74

Atrial pacing?	No
Ventricular pacing?	Yes
Paced interval	74
Identification	100% ventricular-paced rhythm; underlying rhythm is atrial flutter

Figure answer 10-75

Ventricular rate/rhythm	76 beats/min, regular
Atrial rate/rhythm	None
PR interval	None
QRS duration	0.06 sec
Identification	Accelerated junctional rhythm at 76 beats/min

Overdrive pacing: Pacing the heart at a rate faster than the rate of the tachycardia

Pacemaker: Artificial pulse generator that delivers an electrical current to the heart to stimulate depolarization

Pacemaker cells: Specialized cells of the heart's electrical conduction system, capable of spontaneously generating and conducting electrical impulses

Pacemaker generator (pulse generator): Power source that houses the battery and controls for regulating a pacemaker

Pacemaker spike: Vertical line on the ECG that indicates the pacemaker has discharged

Pacemaker syndrome: Adverse clinical signs and symptoms that limit a patient's everyday functioning, occurring in the setting of an electrically normal pacing system; pacemaker syndrome is most commonly associated with a loss of AV synchrony (e.g., VVI pacing) but may also occur because of an inappropriate AV interval or inappropriate rate modulation

Pacing interval: Period, expressed in milliseconds, between two consecutively paced events in the same cardiac chamber without an intervening sensed event (e.g., AA interval, VV interval); also known as the demand interval or basic interval

Paired beats: Two consecutive complexes

Palpitations: An unpleasant awareness of one's heartbeat

Papillary muscles: Muscles attached to the chordae tendineae of the heart valves and the ventricular muscle of the heart

Paroxysmal atrial tachycardia: AT that starts or ends suddenly

Paroxysmal supraventricular tachycardia (PSVT): A regular, narrow-QRS tachycardia that starts or ends suddenly

Pericardiocentesis: A procedure in which a needle is inserted into the pericardial space and the excess fluid is sucked out (aspirated) through the needle

Pericardium: A double-walled sac that encloses the heart and helps protect it from trauma and infection

Peripheral vascular resistance: Resistance to the flow of blood determined by blood vessel diameter and the tone of the vascular musculature

Permeability: Ability of a membrane channel to allow passage of electrolytes once it is open

Point of maximal impulse (PMI): Apical impulse; the site where the left ventricular contraction is most strongly felt

Polarized state: Period after repolarization of a myocardial cell (also called the resting state) when the outside of the cell is positive and the interior of the cell is negative

Polymorphic: Varying in shape

Potential difference: Difference in electrical charge between two points in a circuit; expressed in volts or millivolts

ppm: Abbreviation for pulses/min; ppm usually refers to a paced rate, while bpm (beats/min) refers to an intrinsic heart rate

Preexcitation: Term used to describe rhythms that originate from above the ventricles but in which the impulse travels by a pathway other than the AV node and bundle of His; thus the supraventricular impulse excites the ventricles earlier than normal.

Preload: Force exerted by the blood on the walls of the ventricles at the end of diastole

Premature complex: Early beat occurring before the next expected beat; can be atrial, junctional, or ventricular

PR interval: P wave plus the PR-segment; reflects depolarization of the right and left atria (P wave) and the spread of the impulse through the AV node, bundle of His, right and left bundle branches, and the Purkinje fibers (PR-segment)

Prophylaxis: Preventive treatment

Pulse generator: Power source that houses the battery and controls for regulating a pacemaker

Pulseless electrical activity (PEA): Organized electrical activity observed on a cardiac monitor (other than VT) without the patient having a palpable pulse

Pulmonary circulation: Flow of unoxygenated (venous) blood from the right ventricle to the lungs and oxygenated blood from the lungs to the left atrium

Purkinje fibers: Fibers found in both ventricles that conduct an electrical impulse through the heart

P wave: First wave in the cardiac cycle; represents atrial depolarization and the spread of the electrical impulse throughout the right and left atria

QRS complex: Several waveforms (Q wave, R wave, and S wave) that represent the spread of an electrical impulse through the ventricles (ventricular depolarization)

Quadrigeminy: Dysrhythmia in which every fourth beat is a premature ectopic beat

R wave: On an EGG, the first positive deflection in the QRS complex, representing ventricular depolarization; in pacing, R wave refers to the entire QRS complex, denoting an intrinsic ventricular event

Rate modulation: Ability of a pacemaker to increase the pacing rate in response to physical activity or metabolic demand; some type of physiologic sensor is used by the pacemaker to determine the need for an increased pacing rate; also known as rate adaptation or rate response

RBBB: Right bundle branch block

Reciprocal change: Mirror image ECG changes seen in the wall of the heart opposite the location of an infarction

Reentry: Spread of an impulse through tissue already stimulated by that same impulse.

Refractoriness: Period of recovery that cells need after being discharged before they are able to respond to a stimulus

Relative refractory period: Corresponds with the downslope of the T wave; cardiac cells can be stimulated to depolarize if the stimulus is strong enough.

Repolarization: Movement of ions across a cell membrane in which the inside of the cell is restored to its negative charge

Retrograde: Moving backward; moving in the opposite direction to that which is considered normal

Right axis deviation: Current flow to the right of normal (190-1180 degrees)

Run: Three or more sequential ectopic beats; also referred to as a "salvo" or "burst"

RV interval: Period from the intrinsic ventricular event and the ventricular-paced event that follows; the pacemaker's escape interval

Salvo: Three or more sequential ectopic beats; also referred to as a "run" or "burst"

Sarcolemma: Membrane that covers smooth, striated, and cardiac muscle fibers

Sarcomere: Smallest functional unit of a myofibril

Sarcoplasm: Semifluid cytoplasm of muscle cells

Sarcoplasmic reticulum: Network of tubules and sacs that plays an important role in muscle contraction and relaxation by releasing and storing calcium ions

Segment: Line between waveforms; named by the waveform that precedes and follows it

Semilunar valves: Valves shaped like half-moons that separate the ventricles from the aorta and pulmonary artery

Sensing: Ability of a pacemaker to recognize and respond to intrinsic electrical activity

Septum: An internal wall of connective tissue

Shock: Inadequate tissue perfusion that results from the failure of the cardiovascular system to deliver sufficient oxygen and nutrients to sustain vital organ function

Sick sinus syndrome: Term used to describe a sinus node dysfunction that may be manifested as severe sinus bradycardia, sinus arrest or sinus block, or bradycardia-tachycardia syndrome

Sinoatrial node: Normal pacemaker of the heart that normally discharges at a rhythmic rate of 60 to 100 beats/min

Sinus arrhythmia: Dysrhythmia originating in the sinoatrial node that occurs when the SA node discharges irregularly; sinus arrhythmia is a normal phenomenon associated with the phases of respiration and changes in intrathoracic pressure

Sinus bradycardia: Dysrhythmia originating in the sinoatrial node with a ventricular response of less than 60 beats/min

Sinus tachycardia: Dysrhythmia originating in the sinoatrial node with a ventricular response between 101 and 180 beats/min

ST segment: Portion of the ECG representing the end of ventricular depolarization (end of the R wave) and the beginning of ventricular repolarization (T wave)

Stroke volume: The amount of blood ejected from a ventricle with each heartbeat

Sulcus: Groove

Supernormal period: Period during the cardiac cycle when a weaker than normal stimulus can cause cardiac cells to depolarize; extends from the end of phase 3 to the beginning of phase 4 of the cardiac action potential

Supraventricular: Originating from a site above the bifurcation of the bundle of His, such as the SA node, atria, or AV junction

Syncytium: Unit of combined cells

Systole: Contraction of the heart (usually referring to ventricular contraction) during which blood is propelled into the pulmonary artery and aorta; when the term is used without reference to a specific chamber of the heart, the term implies ventricular systole

Tachycardia: Heart rate greater than 100 beats/min (tachy, fast)

Threshold: Membrane potential at which the cell membrane will depolarize and generate an action potential

Tone: A term that may be used when referring to the normal state of balanced tension in body tissues

Torsades de pointes (TdP): Type of polymorphic VT associated with a prolonged Q-T interval; the QRS changes in shape, amplitude, and width and appears to "twist" around the isoelectric line, resembling a spindle

T wave: Waveform that follows the QRS complex and represents ventricular repolarization

TP-segment: Interval between two successive PQRST complexes during which electrical activity of the heart is absent; begins with the end of the T wave through the onset of the following P wave and represents the period from the end of ventricular repolarization to the onset of atrial depolarization

Trifascicular block: Block in the three primary divisions of the bundle branches (i.e., right bundle branch, left anterior fascicle, and left posterior fascicle)

Trigeminy: Dysrhythmia in which every third beat is a premature ectopic beat

Triggered activity: A disorder of impulse formation that occurs when escape pacemaker and myocardial working cells fire more than once after stimulation by a single impulse resulting in atrial or ventricular beats that occur alone, in pairs, in runs, or as a sustained ectopic rhythm.

Unipolar lead: Lead that consists of a single positive electrode and a reference point; a pacing lead with a single electrical pole at the distal tip of the pacing lead (negative pole) through which the stimulating pulse is delivered. In a permanent pacemaker with a unipolar lead, the positive pole is the pulse generator case

VA interval: In dual-chamber pacing, the interval between a sensed- or ventricular-paced event and the next atrial-paced event

VV interval: Interval between two ventricular-paced events

V wave: Ventricular-paced event; the ventricular stimulus or the point in the intrinsic ventricular depolarization (R wave) during which ventricular sensing occurs

Vagal maneuver: Methods used to stimulate the vagus nerve in an attempt to slow conduction through the AV node, resulting in slowing of the heart rate

Vector: Quantity having direction and magnitude, usually depicted by a straight arrow whose length represents magnitude and whose head represents direction

Venous return: Amount of blood flowing into the right atrium each minute from the systemic circulation

Ventricle: Either of the two lower chambers of the heart

Ventricular pacing: Pacing system with a lead attached in the right ventricle

Ventricular tachycardia (VT): Dysrhythmia originating in the ventricles with a ventricular response greater than 100 beats/min

Voltage: Difference in electrical charge between two points

Wandering atrial pacemaker (multiformed atrial rhythm): Cardiac dysrhythmia that occurs because of impulses originating from various sites, including the sino-atrial node, the atria, and/or the AV junction; requires at least three different P waves, seen in the same lead, for proper diagnosis.

Waveform: Movement away from the baseline in either a positive or negative direction

Wolff-Parkinson-White syndrome: Type of preexcitation syndrome, characterized by a slurred upstroke of the QRS complex (delta wave) and wide QRS

Credits

CHAPTER 1

Figure 1-1   Herlihy B, Maebius NK: *The human body in health and illness,* ed 3, St Louis, 2007, WB Saunders.

Figure 1-2   Canobbio MM: *Cardiovascular disorders, Mosby's clinical nursing series,* vol 1, St Louis, 1990, Mosby.

Figure 1-3   Thibodeau GA, Patton KT: *Anatomy and physiology,* ed 7, St Louis, 2010, Mosby.

Figure 1-4   Drake R, Vogl W, Mitchell A: *Gray's anatomy for students,* ed 2, Philadelphia, 2010, Churchill Livingstone.

Figure 1-6   Butler HA, Caplin M, McCaully E et al (eds): *Managing major diseases, cardiac disorders,* vol 2, St Louis, 1999, Mosby.

Figures 1-7, 1-8   Thibodeau GA, Patton KT: *Anatomy and physiology,* ed 7, St Louis, 2010, Mosby.

Figures 1-9, 1-10   Canobbio MM: *Cardiovascular disorders, Mosby's clinical nursing series,* vol 1, St Louis, 1990, Mosby.

Figure 1-11   Thibodeau GA, Patton KT: *Anatomy and physiology,* ed 7, St Louis, 2010, Mosby.

Figure 1-12   Drake R, Vogl W, Mitchell A: *Gray's anatomy for students,* ed 2, Philadelphia, 2010, Churchill Livingstone.

Figure 1-13   Herlihy B, Maebius NK: *The human body in health and illness,* ed 3, St Louis, 2007, Saunders.

Figure 1-14   Canobbio MM: *Cardiovascular disorders, Mosby's clinical nursing series,* vol 1, St Louis, 1990, Mosby.

Figure 1-15   Thibodeau GA, Patton KT: *Anatomy and physiology,* ed 7, St Louis, 2010, Mosby.

Figure 1-16   Urden LD, Stacy KM, Lough ME: *Thelans's critical care nursing: diagnosis and management,* ed 5, St Louis, 2006, Mosby.

Figure 1-18   Thibodeau GA, Patton KT: *Anatomy and physiology,* ed 7, St Louis, 2010, Mosby.

CHAPTER 2

Figure 2-1   Thibodeau GA, Patton KT: *Anatomy and physiology,* ed 7, St Louis, 2010, Mosby.

Figures 2-2, 2-3, 2-4   Herlihy B, Maebius NK: *The human body in health and illness,* ed 3, St Louis, 2007, WB Saunders.

Figure 2-5   Sanders MJ: *Mosby's paramedic textbook,* ed 3, St Louis, 2005, Mosby.

Figures 2-6, 2-7, 2-8   Canobbio MM: *Cardiovascular disorders, Mosby's clinical nursing series,* vol 1, St Louis, 1990, Mosby.

Figure 2-9   Goldman L, Ausiello D: *Cecil textbook of medicine,* ed 22, Philadelphia, 2004, WB Saunders.

Figure 2-10   Urden LD, Stacy KM, Lough ME: *Thelans critical care nursing: diagnosis and management,* ed 5, St Louis, 2006, Mosby.

Figure 2-11   Crawford MV, Spence MI: *Commonsense approach to coronary care,* rev ed 6, St Louis, 1994, Mosby.

Figure 2-12   Herlihy B, Maebius NK: *The human body in health and illness,* ed 3, St Louis, 2007, WB Saunders.

Figure 2-14   Thelan L, Urden LD, Lough ME et al: *Critical care nursing,* ed 3, St Louis, 1998, Mosby.

Figure 2-15   Guyton A, Hall J: *Textbook of medical physiology,* ed 11, Philadelphia, 2006, WB Saunders.

Figure 2-16   Modified from Marriot H, Conover M: *Advanced concepts in arrhythmias,* ed 3, St Louis, 1998, Mosby.

Figure 2-17   Guyton A, Hall J: *Textbook of medical physiology,* ed 11, Philadelphia, 2006, WB Saunders.

Figure 2-18   Crawford MV, Spence MI: *Commonsense approach to coronary care,* rev ed 6, St Louis, 1994, Mosby.

Figure 2-19   Goldberger A: *Clinical electrocardiography: a simplified approach,* ed 6, St Louis, 1999, Mosby.

Figure 2-20 Methodist Hospital: *Basic electrocardiography: a modular approach*, St Louis, 1986, Mosby.

Figure 2-22 Urden LD, Stacy KM, Lough ME: *Thelan's critical care nursing: diagnosis and management*, ed 5, St Louis, 2006, Mosby.

Figure 2-23 Goldberger A: *Clinical electrocardiography: a simplified approach*, ed 6, St Louis, 1999, Mosby.

Figure 2-24 Urden LD, Stacy KM, Lough ME: *Thelan's critical care nursing: diagnosis and management*, ed 4, St Louis, 2002, Mosby.

Figure 2-25 Urden LD, Stacy KM, Lough ME: *Thelan's critical care nursing: diagnosis and management*, ed 5, St Louis, 2006, Mosby.

Figure 2-26 Phalen T, Aehlert B: *The 12-lead ECG in acute coronary syndromes*, ed 2, St Louis, 2006, Mosby.

Figure 2-28 Goldberger A: *Clinical electrocardiography: a simplified approach*, ed 6, St Louis, 1999, Mosby.

Figure 2-29 Urden LD, Stacy KM, Lough ME: *Thelan's critical care nursing: diagnosis and management*, ed 5, St Louis, 2006, Mosby.

Figures 2-30, 2-32 Modified from Noble A, Johnson R, Thomas A et al: *The cardiovascular system*, Philadelphia, 2005, Churchill Livingstone.

Figure 2-33 Phalen T, Aehlert B: *The 12-lead ECG in acute coronary syndromes*, ed 2, St Louis, 2006, Mosby.

Figure 2-34 Phillips RE, Feeney MK: *The cardiac rhythms: a systematic approach to interpretation*, ed 3, Philadelphia, 1990, WB Saunders.

Figure 2-35 Goldberger A: *Clinical electrocardiography: a simplified approach*, ed 6, St Louis, 1999, Mosby.

Figure 2-36 Modified from Noble A, Johnson R, Thomas A et al: *The cardiovascular system*, Philadelphia, 2005, Churchill Livingstone.

Figure 2-38 Goldberger A: *Clinical electrocardiography: a simplified approach*, ed 6, St Louis, 1999, Mosby.

Figure 2-39 Surawicz B, Knilans TK: *Chou's electrocardiography in clinical practice: adult and pediatric*, ed 5, Philadelphia, 2001, WB Saunders.

Figure 2-41 Modified from Noble A, Johnson R, Thomas A et al: *The cardiovascular system*, Philadelphia, 2005, Churchill Livingstone.

Figure 2-42 Urden LD, Stacy KM, Lough ME: *Thelan's critical care nursing: diagnosis and management*, ed 5, St Louis, 2006, Mosby.

Figure 2-44 Grauer K: *A practical guide to ECG interpretation*, ed 2, St Louis, 1998, Mosby.

Figure 2-45 Goldberger A: *Clinical electrocardiography: a simplified approach*, ed 6, St Louis, 1999, Mosby.

Figure 2-46 Grauer K: *A practical guide to ECG interpretation*, ed 2, St Louis, 1998, Mosby.

Figures 2-47 Modified from Noble A, Johnson R, Thomas A et al: *The cardiovascular system*, Philadelphia, 2005, Churchill Livingstone.

Figure 2-48 Grauer K: *A practical guide to ECG interpretation*, ed 2, St Louis, 1998, Mosby.

Figure 2-49, 2-50 Modified from Thibodeau GA, Patton KT: *Anatomy and physiology*, ed 7, St Louis, 2010, Mosby.

Figures 2-51, 2-52, 2-53 Sanders MJ: *Mosby's paramedic textbook*, ed 3, St Louis, 2005, Mosby.

Figure 2-54 Urden LD, Stacy KM, Lough ME: *Thelan's critical care nursing: diagnosis and management*, ed 5, St Louis, 2006, Mosby.

Figure 2-55 Crawford MV, Spence MI: *Commonsense approach to coronary care*, rev ed 6, St Louis, 1994, Mosby.

Skill 2-1, 2-2, 2-3, 2-4 Aehlert B: *Paramedic practice today*, St Louis, 2010, Mosby.

CHAPTER 4

Figure 4-1 Crawford MV, Spence MI: *Commonsense approach to coronary care*, rev ed 6, St Louis, 1994, Mosby.

Figure 4-3 Kinney MP, Packa DR: *Andreoli's comprehensive cardiac care*, ed 8, St Louis, 1996, Mosby.

Figure 4-5 Goldberger A: *Clinical electrocardiography: a simplified approach*, ed 6, St Louis, 1999, Mosby.

Figure 4-6 Zipes DP, Libby P, Bonow RO et al: *Braunwald's heart disease: a textbook of cardiovascular medicine*, ed 7, Philadelphia, 2005, WB Saunders.

Figure 4-7 Conover MB: *Understanding electrocardiography*, ed 8, St Louis, 2003, Mosby.

Figures 4-8 Goldberger A: *Clinical electrocardiography: a simplified approach*, ed 6, St Louis, 1999, Mosby.

Figure 4-9 Shade B, Rothenberg M, Wertz E et al: *Mosby's EMT-intermediate textbook*, ed 2, St Louis, 2002, Mosby.

Figure 4-10 Goldberger A: *Clinical electrocardiography: a simplified approach*, ed 6, St Louis, 1999, Mosby.

Figure 4-11 Kinney MP, Packa DR: *Andreoli's comprehensive cardiac care*, ed 8, St Louis, 1996, Mosby.

Figure 4-12 Goldman L, Braunwald E: *Primary cardiology*, Philadelphia, 1998, WB Saunders.

Figure 4-14 Urden LD, Stacy KM, Lough ME: *Thelan's critical care nursing: diagnosis and management*, ed 5, St Louis, 2006, Mosby.

Figure 4-15 Goldberger A: *Clinical electrocardiography: a simplified approach*, ed 7, St Louis, 2006, Mosby.

Figure 4-16 Surawicz B, Knilans TK: *Chou's electrocardiography in clinical practice: adult and pediatric*, ed 5, Philadelphia, 1996, WB Saunders.

Figure 4-17 Grauer K: *A practical guide to ECG interpretation*, ed 2, St Louis, 1998, Mosby.

Figure 4-18 Zipes DP, Jalife J: *Cardiac electrophysiology: from cell to bedside*, ed 4, Philadelphia, 2004, WB Saunders.

Figure 4-19 Behrman RE, Kliegman RM, Jenson HB: *Nelson textbook of pediatrics*, ed 17, Philadelphia, 2004, WB Saunders.

Figure 4-20 Shade B, Rothenberg M, Wertz E et al: *Mosby's EMT-intermediate textbook*, ed 2, St Louis, 2002, Mosby.

Figure 4-21 Grauer K: *A practical guide to ECG interpretation*, ed 2, St Louis, 1998, Mosby.

Figure 4-22 Shade B, Rothenberg M, Wertz E et al: *Mosby's EMT-intermediate textbook*, ed 2, St Louis, 2002, Mosby.

Figure 4-24 Goldberger A: *Clinical electrocardiography: a simplified approach*, ed 6, St Louis, 1999, Mosby.

Skill 4-1, 4-2 Aehlert B: *Paramedic practice today*, St Louis, 2010, Mosby.

CHAPTER 5

Figures 5-2, 5-3 Grauer K: *A practical guide to ECG interpretation,* ed 2, St Louis, 1998, Mosby.

CHAPTER 6

Figure 6-1 Grauer K: *A practical guide to ECG interpretation,* ed 2, St Louis, 1998, Mosby.

Figure 6-2 Crawford MV, Spence MI: *Commonsense approach to coronary care,* rev ed 6, St Louis, 1994, Mosby.

Figure 6-3 Kinney MP, Packa DR: *Andreoli's comprehensive cardiac care,* ed 8, St Louis, 1996, Mosby.

Figure 6-9 Surawicz B, Knilans TK: *Chou's electrocardiography in clinical practice: adult and pediatric,* ed 5, Philadelphia, 1996, WB Saunders.

Figure 6-12 Crawford MV, Spence MI: *Commonsense approach to coronary care,* rev ed 6, St Louis, 1994, Mosby.

Figure 6-18 Grauer K: *A practical guide to ECG interpretation,* ed 2, St Louis, 1998, Mosby.

Skill 6-1 Aehlert B: *Paramedic practice today,* St Louis, 2010, Mosby.

CHAPTER 7

Figure 7-7 Grauer K: *A practical guide to ECG interpretation,* ed 2, St Louis, 1998, Mosby.

CHAPTER 8

Figure 8-5 Courtesy Medtronic, Inc.

Skill 8-1 Aehlert B: *Paramedic practice today,* St Louis, 2010, Mosby.

CHAPTER 9

Figures 9-1 Urden LD, Stacy KM, Lough ME: *Thelans's critical care nursing: diagnosis and management,* ed 5, St Louis, 2006, Mosby.

Figure 9-2 Phalen T, Aehlert B: *The 12-lead ECG in acute coronary syndromes,* ed 2, St Louis, 2006, Mosby.

Figure 9-3 Aehlert B: *Paramedic practice today,* St Louis, 2010, Mosby.

Figure 9-4 Urden LD, Stacy KM, Lough ME: *Thelans's critical care nursing: diagnosis and management,* ed 4, St Louis, 2002, Mosby.

Figure 9-5 Aehlert B: *Paramedic practice today,* St Louis, 2010, Mosby.

Figure 9-6 Aehlert B: *Paramedic practice today,* St Louis, 2010, Mosby.

Figure 9-7 Aehlert B: *Paramedic practice today,* St Louis, 2010, Mosby.

Figure 9-10 Aehlert B: *Paramedic practice today,* St Louis, 2010, Mosby.

Figure 9-11 Aehlert B: *Paramedic practice today,* St Louis, 2010, Mosby.

Figure 9-12 Aehlert B: *Paramedic practice today,* St Louis, 2010, Mosby.

Figure 9-13 Aehlert B: *Paramedic practice today,* St Louis, 2010, Mosby.

Figure 9-14 Aehlert B: *Paramedic practice today,* St Louis, 2010, Mosby.

Figure 9-15 Aehlert B: *Paramedic practice today,* St Louis, 2010, Mosby.

Figure 9-16 Aehlert B: *Paramedic practice today,* St Louis, 2010, Mosby.

Figure 9-17 Aehlert B: *Paramedic practice today,* St Louis, 2010, Mosby.

Figure 9-18 Aehlert B: *Paramedic practice today,* St Louis, 2010, Mosby.

Figure 9-28 Johnson R, Schwartz M: *A simplified approach to electrocardiography,* Philadelphia, 1986, WS Saunders.

Figure 9-27 Surawicz B, Knilans TK: *Chou's electrocardiography in clinical practice: adult and pediatric,* ed 5, Philadelphia, 1996, WB Saunders.

Figure 9-28, 9-29, 9-30 Johnson R, Schwartz M: *A simplified approach to electrocardiography,* Philadelphia, 1986, WS Saunders.

Figure 9-29 Phalen T, Aehlert B: *The 12-lead ECG in acute coronary syndromes,* ed 2, St Louis, 2006, Mosby.

Figure 9-31 Kinney MP, Packa DR: *Andreoli's comprehensive cardiac care,* ed 8, St Louis, 1996, Mosby.

Index

Q